THE FIRST YEAR OF LIFE

JANET B. HARDY, M.D., C.M.
Professor of Pediatrics,
The Johns Hopkins School of Medicine;
Professor of Health Services Administration,
The Johns Hopkins School of Hygiene and Public Health

JOSEPH S. DRAGE, M.D.
Chief, Developmental Neurology Branch,
The National Institute of Neurological and Communicative
Disorders and Stroke

ESTHER C. JACKSON
Mathematical Statistician,
Office of Biometry and Epidemiology,
The National Institute of Neurological and Communicative
Disorders and Stroke

The First Year of Life

THE COLLABORATIVE PERINATAL
PROJECT OF THE NATIONAL INSTITUTE
OF NEUROLOGICAL AND COMMUNICATIVE
DISORDERS AND STROKE

JANET B. HARDY, M.D., C.M.   JOSEPH S. DRAGE, M.D.
ESTHER C. JACKSON

The Johns Hopkins University Press
Baltimore and London

Published in 1979 under the Freedom of Information Act

The Collaborative Perinatal Project of The National Institute of Neurological and Communicative Disorders and Stroke, National Institutes of Health, Public Health Service, The U.S. Department of Health, Education and Welfare

Manufactured in the United States of America

The Johns Hopkins University Press, Baltimore, Maryland 21218
The Johns Hopkins Press Ltd., London

Library of Congress Catalog Number 78–20528
ISBN 0-8018-2167-3
Library of Congress Cataloging in Publication data will be found on the last printed page of this book.

CONTENTS

TABLES

FIGURES

FOREWORD

Many of us who witnessed the early planning and organization of the NINCDS Collaborative Perinatal Project have looked forward to a definitive publication of the findings of that remarkable effort. During the years 1959 to 1966, 58,000 women were registered in the project in the twelve collaborating institutions. Although much of the factual information pertaining to immediate pregnancy outcome has been made available in the 1972 volume *The Women and Their Pregnancies*, the follow-up information for the infants is now presented in this long-awaited report.

The uniqueness of this study is in the size of the population, the prospective nature of many of the observations, and the high success in follow-up with carefully conducted developmental assessments in later childhood. We have been given previews of these observations in a number of publications concerned with the rubella epidemic that occurred during the study, reports on the relationship of hyperbilirubinemia and neurologic sequelae, and papers from some of the participating institutions focused on one or another question answerable from a smaller cohort of patients.

The excitement surrounding this publication surely is based on the extensive tabulation of observations, well organized and labeled, and a relatively brief but lucid text interpreting and highlighting well-selected findings. The authors note that many of the observations reported here have been known for a long time, but some are new, and the large number of systematic findings lends important scientific documentation to conclusions that were often based on less adequate information or only impressions. This publication should remain of historical significance as a description of the outcome of pregnancy and delivery and the relationship of events during the perinatal period on outcome of the first year of life. Extraordinary changes have taken place since this study was conducted. As a result some of the findings are recognizably dated and differ markedly from experiences in the 1970s. For example, we are told that only two of forty-five babies under 1,500 grams birthweight with a diagnosis of respiratory distress syndrome survived. We now know that approximately three-quarters of such babies survive, dramatic evidence that the interventions undertaken in the past decade have been successful. Many of them, especially artificial respiration, intravenous nutrition, attention to thermobalance, and the like, came into focus and became a part of routine care of the newborn after most of the infants had been enrolled in the study. Thus, the care of the infant now differs significantly from the 1960s and both mortality and morbidity are dramatically reduced. Indeed, it is paradoxical that perhaps the study itself induced to some extent the change that limits the generality of the conclusions or their relevance to babies born in the 1970s.

One can only reflect that perhaps the perinatal project stimulated an interest in problems of the newborn that was necessary before approaches to their solutions could be undertaken. Certainly many individuals in the collaborating institutions put more time and effort on observations pertinent to intrauterine and postnatal life than had ever been done before. Some of these individuals, first recruited into academic medicine as participants in the Collaborative Project, are now themselves either leaders of neonatal programs or of departments of pediatrics where a significant emphasis on the well being of the newborn is taken for granted.

Finally, it should be repeated that data presented in this volume should be of enduring value: as a description of events in the 1960s; as a source of information about relationships between perinatal, and particularly neonatal conditions, and outcomes during the first year; and, as an index of the frequency of specific congenital malformations and other conditions during the first year. These data should be helpful to anyone concerned with comprehensive planning for health care for mothers and infants. They can serve as a resource for the derivation of research hypotheses for further testing in the 1970s and for further analysis by examination of the information obtained from follow-up of the Collaborative Project children to age seven.

Children's Hospital Medical Center   Mary Ellen Avery, M.D.
Boston, Massachusetts 02115

ACKNOWLEDGMENTS

The Collaborative Perinatal Project of the National Institute of Neurological and Communicative Disorders and Stroke is a large, complex study, extending over a long time span and involving many thousands of people. Without the wholehearted cooperation of the mothers and their children the study could not have been carried out.

The authors wish to acknowledge the contributions of the project staffs at the fourteen collaborating institutions (listed in Table 2–1) and of the staffs of the Developmental Neurology Branch (formerly the Perinatal Research Branch) and of the Office of Biometry and Epidemiology, National Institute of Neurological and Communicative Disorders and Stroke.

Individual acknowledgments to many of these dedicated people were made in the first major monograph from the project (see *The Women and Their Pregnancies*, 1972, K. R. Niswander and M. Gordon, editors, Appendix A).

Special thanks are also expressed to the many individuals who served on the Perinatal Research Committee, ad hoc advisory committees, task forces, and as individual consultants to the project.

We wish to express our thanks to the Directors of the National Institute of Neurological and Communicative Disorders and Stroke (NINCDS), who, over the many years of the project, have supported and promoted its development: Pearce Bailey, M.D., Director, 1951 to 1959; Richard L. Masland, M.D., Director, 1959 to 1968; Edward F. MacNichol, Jr., Ph.D., Director, 1968 to 1972; and Donald B. Tower, M.D., Director, 1972 to the present.

We also wish to acknowledge the contributions of: Dr. Eldon L. Eagles, Deputy Director, NINCDS, for his consistent encouragement and backing; Dr. Heinz Berendes, Chief, Perinatal Research Branch, NINCDS, 1960 to 1971, who directed the Collaborative Perinatal Project during this period; William Weiss, Chief, Office of Biometry and Epidemiology, NINCDS, for his support in planning and carrying out the data tabulation and analysis.

The authors further wish to acknowledge the help of Dr. Lewis P. Lipsett, Brown

University, Providence, R.I., and Dr. Sarah H. Broman, Developmental Neurology Branch, NINCDS, for their contribution to the development of Chapter 13.

In addition to the above, we should like to acknowledge the assistance, in data analysis and preparation of the manuscript, of the following people at NINCDS: Frances H. Canning, Colman Fisher, James L. Hill, S. Barbara Katz (deceased), Margaret A. Meadows, Stephana P. Ney, Irene B. Ross, Dorothy N. Waters, and Catherine D. Wildman; and at the Johns Hopkins University Medical Center: Cassandra Young.

THE FIRST YEAR OF LIFE

1

INTRODUCTION

OBJECTIVES

The National Institute of Neurological and Communicative Disorders and Stroke (NINCDS) established the Collaborative Perinatal Project (NCPP) to investigate the etiology of neurological and sensory disorders of children by examining their relationship to events, conditions, and abnormalities of pregnancy, labor, and delivery. A broad prospective, multidisciplinary, epidemiological study was designed to examine the "continuum of reproductive casualty" (1). The abnormal outcomes included fetal and neonatal death, low birthweight, congenital malformations, neurological and sensory handicaps such as cerebral palsy, seizure disorders, visual and auditory impairments, and intellectual deficits ranging from severe degrees of mental retardation to the more subtle defects of learning and cognition that characterize certain communicative and learning disabilities.

The causes of these abnormal outcomes may be multidimensional and may depend, at least in part, on the complex interaction of many factors. Association between certain perinatal factors and neurological defects had been suggested by retrospective studies (2) that led to the concept of a continuum of reproductive casualty. A prospective study was deemed necessary to test this concept and possibly to extend its applicability to other and unrecognized etiological factors. As most individuals in such a study will be normal, in order to gain sufficient numbers of specific neurological defects to permit a valid statistical analysis, a large population is essential. To meet the population requirements of the project, fourteen medical centers in twelve universities joined with the Perinatal Research Branch, NINCDS, to provide information on the detailed study of over 58,000 pregnancies and the follow-up to age seven or eight years of the surviving children.

It is only within the framework of a prospective, longitudinal study, carried out over a number of years, that causal relationships between antecedent events and abnormal conditions recognized later in life can be developed and meaningfully investigated. A longitudinal follow-up of children is required, as the detection of certain neurological deficits may not be possible until the child attains a level of

1

development sufficient to permit evaluation. The characteristic evolution of neuro-logical abnormalities, with changing manifestations over time, demands repeated observations in order that the full impact of the antecedent events can be under-stood. For example, motor abnormalities present during the early weeks and months of life may be suggestive of cerebral palsy, but long-term observations ultimately allow one to observe whether the signs disappear or persist and intensify to mani-fest the characteristics of cerebral palsy. On the other hand, seizure disorders, communication deficits, and learning problems frequently are not apparent until later in childhood. It is only after the children have been followed long enough for definite and stable diagnoses to be established that meaningful etiological relation-ships can be developed.

The perinatal death rate on a national basis has declined substantially since 1959, when the project began. However, the rate remains high in some areas of the country (3,4). The related problems of perinatal mortality and the continuum of neurological handicap in survivors rank among the major health problems in the United States (Fig. 1–1). An estimated 20 million individuals suffer from some degree of neurological and/or sensory impairment that probably stemmed from factors present during the perinatal period (5). This is a problem of very large dimensions. The devastating and lifelong impact on individual children, their fami-lies, and the communities in which they live is not measurable. In addition to the tragedy of human suffering, billions of dollars are expended annually for medical and custodial care, special education, vocational rehabilitation, and the other special programs and services required for the support of the neurologically and intellec-tually handicapped. In general, these handicaps are permanent, continuing through-out the entire life span of the individual. While rehabilitation and special education may alleviate their effects, normal functioning and full participation in life is much less often attained. An estimate of the numbers of persons suffering neurological and neurosensory handicaps in the United States is provided in Table 1–1.

Prevention of perinatal problems and their potentially serious consequences is the basis upon which programs for the effective reduction of neurological handicaps must be built. The NCPP was designed to establish leads to the development of strategies for prevention and intervention by providing a frame of reference for the identification of factors associated with adverse pregnancy outcome and subsequent abnormalities of survivors.

The fact that the birth rate is declining does not lessen the need for measures to prevent neurological handicaps. The number of children born with potential handicaps may actually be increasing. Changes in the patterns of family planning can have conflicting results. On the one hand, reproduction is controlled, and the total number of babies born is reduced. On the other hand, the diagnostic and therapeutic services accorded to those parents with sterility problems may increase the likelihood of delivery of an infant at risk. This potential increase in the number of abnormal infants, coupled with the increased chances of their survival accruing from more effective neonatal care, may well be leading to an actual increase in the number of surviving individuals with neurological handicaps.

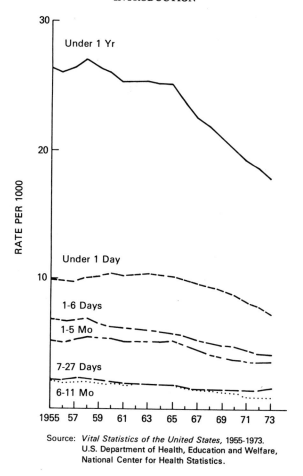

Source: *Vital Statistics of the United States*, 1955-1973.
U.S. Department of Health, Education and Welfare,
National Center for Health Statistics.

Figure 1-1. Infant Mortality by Age, U.S., 1955-1973

With the birth of fewer children, the need for optimal development of each becomes more pressing. In a highly specialized, technological and competitive society, it is essential that each child have the right to achieve his or her maximum potential for intellectual and physical development. This potential must not be reduced by preventable obstetrical or pediatric problems.

THE PURPOSE OF THIS VOLUME

This report describes the abnormalities, conditions, and events reported, during the nursery stay and the remainder of the first year of life, for 18,481 white and 19,504 black infants, single liveborn, with known birthweight, of women registered, for the first time, in the NCPP. It is intended that the information presented here stand alone, and the report deals with a specific segment of the longitudinal data in the NCPP; it covers that period extending from the moment of birth through

Table 1-1. Disability from Various Neurologic Entities Which May Represent in Part a Continuum of Reproductive Wastage

Disability Category	Total Estimated Number of Disabled Persons in U.S.
Cerebral palsy	555,000
Mental retardation	5,000,000*
Epilepsy	1,500,000
Visual handicap (legally blind)	345,000
Auditory handicap (legally deaf)	760,000
Disorder of speech	†

Source: Material prepared by the National Institute of Neurological Diseases and Blindness from morbidity estimates, received from the relevant voluntary agencies, Feb. 5, 1960; reproduced from *The Women and Their Pregnancies*, p. 2.

*Three percent of population; 126,000 mentally retarded born annually.
†Two to five percent of all children.

the first year of life. It follows the volume, *The Women and Their Pregnancies*, published in 1972, which is briefly described in the following section.

The present report provides a global description of the broad spectrum of specific abnormalities encountered during the first year of life and the frequency of their occurrence within these large and varied groups of children. This description of the characteristics of the infants during the first year represents another step in attaining the basic objectives of the NCPP. An objective here is to provide a frame of reference for the continuing longitudinal study of the data through the seven and eight-year levels and a related purpose is to provide leads for the development of new research hypotheses in the perinatal field.

The descriptive data presented, particularly those concerned with the prevalence of certain diagnoses during the newborn period, should prove useful in the planning of efficient and optimal care for high-risk infants. For example, the infrequent occurrence of most conditions requiring special diagnostic facilities and surgical intervention has possible implications regarding the development of regional centers for the special care of "high-risk" newborns (see Chapter 12).

THE WOMEN AND THEIR PREGNANCIES

As indicated, the first comprehensive report from the NCPP, *The Women and Their Pregnancies* (6) was published in 1972. That volume provides a basic description of the NCPP and its objectives. The selection of subjects, the protocol, and the measures taken to assure the quality of the data collected over time are described in some detail. An important section deals with the evaluation of the quality of the data and their comparability over time and across the collaborating institutions.

A substantial part of the first monograph is devoted to a description of the large samples of white and black women enrolled. The characteristics of the women are described in terms of their relationship to the pregnancy outcome observed, measured by rates of fetal loss (stillbirth, and neonatal death), low birthweight (i.e., below 2501 gms.), and definite neurological abnormality at one year, and by the mean, or average, birthweight observed for babies of groups of women with various conditions. The pregnancy outcome for women with specific characteristics or conditions is compared with that for women without these conditions. A brief summary of some of the more important relationships observed between maternal characteristics and pregnancy outcome follows in Chapter 5.

REFERENCES

(1) A. M. Lilienfeld and E. Parkhurst. 1951. A study of the association of the factors of pregnancy and parturition with the development of cerebral palsy. *American Journal of Hygiene* 53: 262–82.

(2) W. J. Little. 1862. On the influence of abnormal parturition, difficult labours, premature birth, and asphyxia neonatorum, on the mental and physical condition of the child, especially in relation to deformities. *Transactions of the Obstetrical Society of London* 3: 293–344.

(3) S. Shapiro, E. R. Schlesinger, and R. E. L. Nesbitt, Jr. 1968. *Infant, Perinatal, Maternal and Childhood Mortality in the United States*. Cambridge, Mass.: Harvard University Press.

(4) National Center for Health Statistics. *Vital Statistics of the United States, 1955–1973*. U.S. Department of Health, Education, and Welfare, Public Health Service, Health Resources Administration. Washington, D.C.: U.S. Government Printing Office.

(5) *Human Communication and Its Disorders: An Overview*. 1970. A report prepared and published by the Subcommittee on Human Communication and Its Disorders, R. Carhart, chairman. National Advisory Neurological Diseases and Stroke Council. NINCDS, Monograph No. 10, U.S. Department of Health, Education, and Welfare, Public Health Service. Washington, D.C. U.S. Government Printing Office.

(6) K. R. Niswander and M. Gordon (eds.). 1972. *The Women and Their Pregnancies*. Philadelphia: W. B. Saunders Co.

2

THE STUDY POPULATION

SELECTION OF THE COLLABORATING CENTERS AND THE STUDY POPULATION

Initially, fifteen university-affiliated medical centers participated in the study. One participant withdrew within the first year after registering a small number of pregnancies that have been excluded because of lack of follow-up. The remaining fourteen hospitals are affiliated with twelve universities. At two universities the obstetric and pediatric hospitals were separate. The collaborating institutions and the abbreviations used to designate them in the tables and charts, contained in this volume, are listed in Table 2–1.

The Perinatal Research Branch (PRB) was organized within the NINCDS to provide the coordination and supporting services essential to the operation of so large a study.

Gravidas were selected for the study during the seven-year period extending from January 2, 1959 through December 31, 1965. The processes by which random selection from each hospital population was accomplished are described elsewhere (1). The most important criterion was registration in the hospital clinic for prenatal care. An exception was Buffalo, where the study gravidas were the private patients of participating obstetricians. Exclusions from the sample were based on factors that precluded long-term follow-up, such as unwed gravidas who planned to place their babies for adoption, transients (i.e., women who lived beyond a defined geographic area). "Walk-ins" (i.e., women who give birth within twenty-four hours of registration in the study) were also excluded. While there were differences observed, with respect to marital status, maternal age and duration of pregnancy at registration, between the various study populations and the hospital populations from which they were selected, the differences are negligible.

Table 2-1. The Collaborating Institutions

Abbreviation	Collaborating Institution
BO	Boston Hospital for Women (Lying-in Division) and Children's Hospital Medical Center Harvard Medical School Boston, Massachusetts
BU	Children's Hospital State University of New York at Buffalo Buffalo, New York
CH	Charity Hospital Tulane University School of Medicine and Medical Center, Louisiana State University New Orleans, Louisiana
CO	Columbia-Presbyterian Medical Center Columbia University College of Physicians and Surgeons New York, New York
JH	The Johns Hopkins Hospital The Johns Hopkins University School of Medicine Baltimore, Maryland
VA	Medical College of Virginia Virginia Commonwealth University Richmond, Virginia
MN	University of Minnesota Hospitals Health Sciences Center Minneapolis, Minnesota
NY	Metropolitan Hospital New York Medical College New York, New York
OR	University of Oregon Medical School Portland, Oregon
PA	Pennsylvania Hospital and the Children's Hospital of Philadelphia University of Pennsylvania Philadelphia, Pennsylvania
PR	Child Study Center Brown University Providence, Rhode Island
TN	Gailor Hospital University of Tennessee College of Medicine Memphis, Tennessee

COMPOSITION OF THE STUDY POPULATION

A total of 58,828 pregnancies was enrolled in the study; of these, 298 "walk-ins" and 2622 "noncore" cases (i.e., women selected outside the usual sampling procedure because of special interest of the hospital) have been excluded, leaving a total of 55,908 records available for study. The 3795 pregnancies of Puerto Rican women, the 256 Oriental, and the 317 of other races were also excluded from this report, as were the 1420 white and the 686 black gravidas for whom neither labor and delivery data nor pediatric data could be obtained. These exclusions reduced the number of "core" white and black pregnancies to 49,434 cases that conformed to the hospitals' sampling procedures.

Preliminary investigation of the data demonstrated the necessity for analysis and presentation for each race separately. The data from Puerto Rican subjects were sufficiently different from that of both whites and blacks to preclude their combination with either one. As the sample size for Puerto Ricans (3795) was not sufficient for comparable analysis, the data are not presented.

Some women were included in the study for more than one pregnancy. If a woman registered more than once for prenatal care at a participating center during the period of the study and she met the criteria for the random sampling procedure at each registration, she was included again in the study. These pregnancies are termed "repeat" pregnancies; they too have been excluded from this report. It should be emphasized that the term "first study pregnancy" is not necessarily synonymous with the woman's first pregnancy (primigravidity); it merely represents her first registered pregnancy in the NCPP, and may have been, for example, her first or her sixth. It is the purpose of this report to describe the study infants, and in so doing to avoid the possible biases that inclusion of the "repeat" pregnancies of the same women might introduce.

The cases included in this volume, for the most part, are the 18,481 white and 19,504 black, single, liveborn, core, first-study pregnancies of twenty weeks or more gestation with known birthweight. The small number (152 white and 206 black) infants with unknown birthweight have been excluded because of the importance of the relationship between birthweight and outcome (see Table 2–6).

SAMPLE MAINTENANCE THROUGH THE FIRST YEAR

A considerable effort was expended to obtain follow-up examinations on all children. Reasonable success has been achieved, in spite of the difficulties inherent in a longitudinal study of large dimensions within a highly mobile, free society.

Tables 2–2 and 2–3 show the rate of successful follow-up of infants from the study, by race, during the period from birth to one year. It will be noted that almost 97 percent of the white and 98 percent of the black babies were examined in the nursery. As the first detailed pediatric examination for the study (PED–2, *Neonatal Examination*) was scheduled at twelve to twenty-four hours of age, infants who died during the first few hours did not receive this evaluation.

Overall, more than 85 percent of all children were examined at four months and about 85 percent received the one-year neurological evaluation. Children who missed one examination did not necessarily miss subsequent ones. In fact, the missing of an evaluation led to intensified efforts to have the child return for the next one. While the combined rates of successful follow-up were high, it should be pointed out that rates were higher for some institutions than for others. However, examination of rates of major abnormalities by institution shows reasonable consistency, indicating that the case loss was random. In one institution (Johns Hopkins), in 1962, a study of fifty consecutive infants missing the one-year examination

Table 2-2. Infants Examined, Deaths and Attrition, Through One Year — White

Description	BO	BU	CH	CO	JH	VA	MN	NY	OR	PA	PR	TN	Total
Total births	7823	1926	0	603	667	741	2623	253	1894	728	1769	21	19048
Stillbirths	194	57	0	13	9	10	53	4	30	14	31	0	415
Livebirths	7629	1869	0	590	658	731	2570	249	1864	714	1738	21	18633
No. with nursery exam.	7420	1839	0	582	643	705	2439	237	1742	686	1708	20	18021
% with nursery exam.	97.3	98.4	-	98.6	97.7	96.4	94.9	95.2	93.5	96.1	98.3	95.2	96.7
Neonatal deaths	93	26	0	10	7	8	28	5	33	16	27	0	253
Deaths at 1 thru 3 mo.	17	2	0	1	0	4	9	1	12	3	6	0	55
Alive at 4 mo.	7519	1841	0	579	651	719	2533	243	1819	695	1705	21	18325
No. with 4 mo. exam.	6743	1770	0	545	522	440	2153	197	1384	458	1239	16	15467
% with 4 mo. exam.	89.7	96.1	-	94.1	80.2	61.2	85.0	81.1	76.1	65.9	72.7	76.2	84.4
Deaths at 4 thru 7 mo.	16	1	0	0	1	0	7	0	4	1	8	0	38
Alive at 8 mo.	7503	1840	0	579	650	719	2526	243	1815	694	1697	21	18287
No. with 8 mo. exam.	6243	1729	0	492	507	384	2040	178	1260	407	1166	12	14418
% with 8 mo. exam.	83.2	94.0	-	85.0	78.0	53.4	80.8	73.3	69.4	58.6	68.7	57.1	78.8
Deaths at 8 thru 11 mo.	2	2	0	0	1	0	4	0	2	0	0	0	11
Alive at 1 yr.	7501	1838	0	579	649	719	2522	243	1813	694	1697	21	18276
No. with 1 yr. exam.	6084	1720	0	530	502	474	2060	178	1471	455	1173	15	14662
% with 1 yr. exam.	81.1	93.6	-	91.5	77.3	65.9	81.7	73.3	81.1	65.6	69.1	71.4	80.2

Source: *The Women and Their Pregnancies,* p. 16.

Table 2-3. Infants Examined, Deaths and Attrition, Through One Year — Black

Description	BO	BU	CH	CO	JH	VA	MN	NY	OR	PA	PR	TN	Total
Total births	913	52	2380	842	2210	1840	17	1455	603	6158	501	3196	20167
Stillbirths	26	4	51	19	60	46	1	26	14	147	14	49	457
Livebirths	887	48	2329	823	2150	1794	16	1429	589	6011	487	3147	19710
No. with nursery exam.	867	48	2320	805	2088	1747	14	1374	559	5881	478	3114	19295
% with nursery exam.	97.7	100.0	99.6	97.8	97.1	97.4	87.5	96.2	94.9	97.8	98.2	99.0	97.9
Neonatal deaths	15	0	39	13	56	21	0	28	9	147	10	50	388
Deaths at 1 thru 3 mo.	0	0	14	3	8	7	0	8	2	33	5	11	91
Alive at 4 mo.	872	48	2276	807	2086	1766	16	1393	578	5831	472	3086	19231
No. with 4 mo. exam.	816	47	2195	748	1918	1528	14	1155	523	5064	399	2949	17356
% with 4 mo. exam.	93.6	97.9	96.4	92.7	91.9	86.5	87.5	82.9	90.5	86.8	84.5	95.6	90.3
Deaths at 4 thru 7 mo.	2	0	4	2	2	9	0	3	2	18	3	7	55
Alive at 8 mo.	870	48	2272	805	2081	1757	16	1390	576	5813	469	3079	19176
No. with 8 mo. exam.	767	46	2110	686	1915	1443	14	1061	488	4413	379	2626	15948
% with 8 mo. exam.	88.2	95.8	92.9	85.2	92.0	82.1	87.5	76.3	84.7	75.9	80.8	85.3	83.2
Deaths at 8 thru 11 mo.	0	0	1	1	5	1	0	3	0	3	1	6	21
Alive at 1 yr.	870	48	2271	804	2076	1756	16	1387	576	5810	468	3073	19155
No. with 1 yr. exam.	766	48	2110	732	1928	1613	13	1137	533	4984	384	2875	17123
% with 1 yr. exam.	88.0	100.0	92.9	91.0	92.9	91.9	81.3	82.0	92.5	85.8	82.1	93.6	89.4

Source: *The Women and Their Pregnancies,* p.16 .

was made. A home visit was made by a pediatric-neurologist and a nurse to examine each infant. Only one of the fifty children was in any way abnormal, and most of the children had failed to return because their mothers were burdened with other young children, family illness, or other problems, rather than for reasons related to the presence or absence of abnormalities of the study child. Thus, no bias was detected.

Table 2-4. Comparison of Characteristics of Gravidas Whose Infants Missed the One-Year Neurological Examination with Those Examined

	WHITE				BLACK			
	Number		Percent		Number		Percent	
	Missed Exam	With Exam	Missed Exam	With Exam	Missed Exam	With Exam	Missed Exam	With Exam
Age of gravida (yr)								
Under 20	794	2883	22.0	19.7	610	5406	30.0	31.6
20–29	2289	8882	63.3	60.6	1141	8613	56.2	50.3
30+	531	2897	14.7	19.8	281	3103	13.8	18.1
Total	3614	14662	100.0	100.0	2032	17122	100.0	100.0
Parity								
0	1323	5847	38.5	40.0	583	5877	29.5	34.4
1	833	3272	24.3	22.4	485	3331	24.5	19.5
2	522	2087	15.2	14.3	289	2449	14.6	14.3
3–4	509	2324	14.8	15.9	367	3095	18.6	18.1
5+	248	1101	7.2	7.5	252	2348	12.8	13.7
Total	3435	14631	100.0	100.0	1976	17100	100.0	100.0
Schooling of gravida (yr)								
Under 9	507	1810	15.5	12.6	331	3249	16.8	19.2
9–12	1999	9575	61.2	66.6	1527	12810	77.7	75.7
13+	761	2993	23.3	20.8	108	857	5.5	5.1
Total	3267	14378	100.0	100.0	1966	16916	100.0	100.0

Source: *The Women and Their Pregnancies,* p.35.

Table 2-5. Comparison of Characteristics of Infants Who Missed the One-Year Neurological Examination with Those Examined

	WHITE				BLACK			
	Number		Percent		Number		Percent	
	Missed Exam	With Exam	Missed Exam	With Exam	Missed Exam	With Exam	Missed Exam	With Exam
Sex								
Male	1829	7610	51.0	52.0	1026	8518	50.7	49.8
Female	1755	7037	49.0	48.0	997	8597	49.3	50.2
Total	3584	14647	100.0	100.0	2023	17115	100.0	100.0
Birthweight (gm)								
Under 1501	10	42	0.3	0.3	15	122	0.8	0.7
1501–2000	40	144	1.1	1.0	46	356	2.3	2.1
2001–2500	185	735	5.2	5.0	190	1614	9.6	9.5
2501–3000	714	2877	20.2	19.7	619	5115	31.3	30.0
3001+	2593	10819	73.2	74.0	1107	9846	56.0	57.7
Total	3542	14617	100.0	100.0	1977	17053	100.0	100.0
One-minute APGAR Score								
0–1	41	197	1.4	1.4	28	180	1.6	1.2
2	62	249	2.1	1.8	31	267	1.8	1.7
3	53	294	1.8	2.1	41	297	2.4	1.9
4	74	402	2.5	2.9	53	380	3.1	2.5
5	131	685	4.4	4.9	56	605	3.3	3.9
6	223	1042	7.5	7.5	127	1029	7.4	6.6
7	300	1450	10.1	10.5	148	1324	8.7	8.5
8	674	3517	22.6	25.4	294	2750	17.2	17.7
9	1306	5641	43.8	40.8	754	6825	44.1	44.0
10	115	364	3.9	2.6	177	1839	10.4	11.9
Total	2979	13841	100.0	100.0	1709	15496	100.0	100.0

Table 2-6. Case Counts for Various Tables

		WHITE	BLACK
A.	All births		
	1. Total	19048	20167
	2. With known birthweight	18779	19877
	3. With known birthweight and gestation	18668	19717
B.	Livebirths		
	1. Total	18633	19710
	2. With known birthweight	18481	19504
	3. With known gestation	18473	19527
	4. With known birthweight and gestation	18373	19346
	5. With known birthweight, gestation, and 1-min. APGAR score	16992	17471
	6. With known birthweight, gestation, and 5-min. APGAR score	17156	17916
	7. With known birthweight, gestation, and bilirubin	17195	17880
	8. With known birthweight and gestation and with Coombs' test	17497	18351
C.	Livebirths with newborn exam		
	1. With known birthweight	18029	19259
	2. With known birthweight and gestation	17939	19149
	3. With known birthweight, gestation, and type of delivery	17919	19107
D.	Number seen after nursery period		
	1. With known birthweight	16521	18121
E.	Number having 8-month exam at 7.5 to 8.5 months of age		
	1. With known birthweight	11534	13516
	2. With known birthweight and parity	11511	13501
	3. With known birthweight, gestation, and motor score	11468	13398
	4. With known birthweight, gestation, and mental score	11471	13399
	5. With known birthweight, age of gravida, and motor score	11525	13507
	6. With known birthweight, age of gravida, and mental score	11528	13508
	7. With known birthweight, education of gravida, and motor score	11323	13360
	8. With known birthweight, education of gravida, and mental score	11326	13361
F.	Number with 1-year exam		
	1. Total	14662	17123
	2. With known birthweight	14617	17053
	3. With known birthweight and gestation	14540	16939
G.	Number having 1-year exam at 48 to 56 weeks of age		
	1. With known birthweight	12703	15142
	2. With known birthweight and locomotor development	11001	13320

An evaluation of the introduction of possible bias, as the result of loss to follow-up, was carried out for the NCPP as a whole. The question was addressed by the comparisons of those infants receiving the twelve-month neurological examination with those who failed to receive it, with respect to certain variables collected earlier and known to relate to abnormal pregnancy outcome, for example, selected maternal characteristics and low birthweight (Tables 2–4 and 2–5). If the frequency of these predictive variables is randomly distributed between the two groups then, by inference, little bias was present. For the study as a whole, relatively small differences along a number of important parameters existed between those infants examined at twelve months and those who were not. With respect to the three maternal characteristics of age, parity, and education, differences were slight and inconsistent; with respect to sex of child, birthweight, and Apgar score, essentially no difference existed between the groups.

NUMBERS OF CASES IN VARIOUS CATEGORIES

One of the problems in the study of large bodies of longitudinally collected data is that occasioned by the fluctuation in numbers of cases available at successive points in time. This problem results from death, cases that were missed at one or more examinations, and the unavoidable or inadvertent failure to collect desired observations. The largest number of missing examinations was the Eight-Month Developmental Evaluation and is largely due to the delays of protocol development. Thus, standardized observations at eight months were not available for several thousand infants born during the early years of the study, as the observations made were used for pretesting purposes.

Table 2–6 provides a numerical frame of reference by listing the number of white and black infants included in each of the major categories presented in this volume.

REFERENCE

(1) K. R. Niswander and M. Gordon (eds.). 1972. *The Women and Their Pregnancies*, p. 7. Philadelphia: W. B. Saunders Co.

3

THE DATA: COLLECTION
AND PROCESSING

Special challenges were inherent in data collection in the NCPP. The complexities involved: (1) data collection over a sixteen-year time span; (2) the requirement for large amounts of reliable, standardized, highly specific and detailed information on each mother-child pair; (3) the very large number of women and children enrolled; (4) the geographic distribution of the twelve university medical centers that necessitated special attention to communication; (5) the study personnel, which changed over time and varied in professional orientation. Figure 3–1 provides a visual summary of the types of information and the time intervals over which various data were collected. While this volume is concerned primarily with the first year of life, the figure provides a perspective of the pediatric and developmental follow-up through age eight.

FORMS AND MANUALS

Specific forms and manuals were developed collaboratively by staff members from PRB, the participating institutions, and consultants, because hospital records, which are maintained primarily for patient care, were judged to be inadequate for this type of research.

These detailed forms provided for the direct recording of the observations collected for collaborative study purposes. In many instances the new forms prepared for the study were adopted by the hospital and became the official hospital record. Procedure manuals were developed to promote uniformity of data collection. Important considerations in the development of the forms were: (1) inclusion of the detailed and comprehensive information necessary for thorough studies of etiology; (2) reduction to a minimum of ambiguity of meaning, assuring reproducibility and comparability of information collected over time by different examiners and institutions; (3) simplification and standardization of the processing of the information

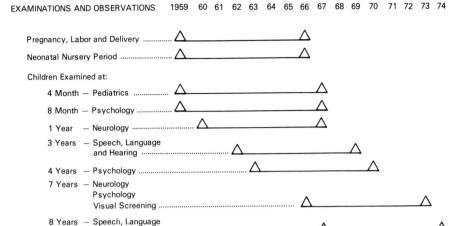

Figure 3-1. Collaborative Perinatal Project Data Collection Time Span — 16 Years (1959-1974).

at all stages of data collection and handling. Wherever possible the items on the forms were structured to facilitate completeness of history taking and examination. Separate precoded check boxes for both positive and negative information permitted direct key punching and minimized coding errors. Ample space was provided on each page for unstructured narrative information to supplement the precoded material.

Throughout the period of the study, continuing efforts were made to ensure the consistency and accuracy of the data collected. Staff members from the participating medical centers met in workshops; films describing the neonatal and one-year neurological examinations were produced and used in training pediatricians and neurologists. There was an interchange of visits among personnel of the centers and the PRB to exchange views and to standardize examining techniques and recording of data.

At each hospital the study records of the patient were reviewed by a trained editor for consistency and completeness. In addition, before the record forms were sent to the PRB for processing to the data file, they were reviewed in detail by senior medical personnel for consistency and accuracy. Further editing and review were carried out at PRB and efforts were made to retrieve missing data and to resolve inconsistencies.

A list of record forms pertaining to the study of the infants from birth through the first year of life appears in Table 3–1. Several of these forms are presented in the Appendix. Copies of all forms and their accompanying manuals are available upon request from the Developmental Neurology Branch, Neurological Disorders Program, NINCDS, National Institutes of Health, Bethesda, Maryland 20205.

A flow chart, Figure 3–2, shows the sequence of data collection from the time of delivery through the first year of life.

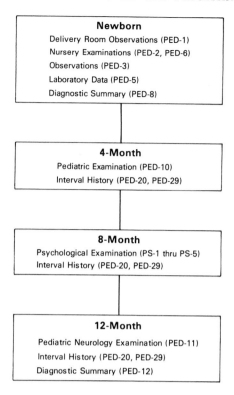

Figure 3-2. Flow Chart of Examinations and Observations
at Specified Ages.

DATA PROCESSING

As has been described elsewhere (1), an effective system was developed that included comprehensive reviews and tests at each step of data processing in the PRB. Some six million punch cards have been generated and converted to computer tape for storage and analysis.

THE EVALUATION OF THE INFANTS

The collection and recording of clinical research information by those responsible for the care of the patient may lead to unavoidable biases and inaccuracies. The study protocol was designed to minimize these problems. While the NCPP required the collection of detailed observations from each patient, wherever possible those administratively responsible to the study had no decision-making responsibilities for patient care. They were specially trained and supervised to make the required objective observations that were recorded on study forms.

As this was *not* an intervention study, standard hospital routines and staff practices, which differed somewhat among the participating institutions, were used in caring for the babies. However, the presence of the senior study pediatricians served

Table 3-1. Collaborative Perinatal Study Forms for the First Year of Life

PED-1	Delivery Room Observation of the Neonate
PED-2	Neonatal Examination
PED-3	Nursery History
PED-4	Report of Fetal or Infant Death
PED-5	Results of Tests and Procedures Done on the Neonate
PED-6	Neonatal Neurological Examination
PED-8	Newborn Diagnostic Summary
PED-10	Four-Month Pediatric Examination
PED-11	One-Year Neurological Examination
PED-12	Summary of the First Year of Life
PED-14	Physical Growth Measurements
PED-20	Interval Medical History
PED-29	Summary of Medical Records of Illness or Hospitalization
SE-1	Socio-Economic Interview
PATH-3	Autopsy Protocol
PS-1	COLR Research Form of Bayley Scales of Mental Development
PS-2	COLR Research Form of Bayley Scales of Motor Development
PS-3	Infant Behavior Profile
PS-4	Additional Observations
PS-5	Maternal Behavior in Testing Situation

as a stimulus to the more detailed observation of the newborn, enhancing both the quality of neonatal care and the completeness of hospital record keeping. Project directors reported that the routine hospital examination of babies improved in quality, diagnostic evaluations became more complete, and the teaching improved. Particular importance was placed on routine use of neonatal neurological evaluations. "Feedback" to nursery staffs from the follow-up of study infants at later ages reinforced interest in the early detection of abnormalities. The presence of the study encouraged and promoted communication and closer cooperation between obstetric and pediatric personnel at all levels.

The Neonatal Period

The collection of data from the newborn infants began in the delivery room at birth. The observations were made by the study observer who was present at the delivery and who had responsibility for collecting the labor and delivery data. At first these observers were physicians, but reliability studies in several institutions indicated that specially trained nurse-midwives, nurses, and senior medical students employed by the study were equally satisfactory. The delivery room information included the exact time of delivery, breathing and crying times, Apgar scores, and any procedures carried out (e.g., resuscitation) and therapy administered. A brief physical evaluation of the baby was made to document any externally manifest abnormalities and to provide a baseline for later, more detailed observations. These findings were recorded on PED-1, *Delivery Room Observation of the Neonate* (see Appendix).

The collection of information continued during the hospital stay of the neonate. The number of days spent in the nursery varied among institutions and depended upon the routine hospital practice, on the one hand, and the condition of the infant, on the other; small or sick infants staying longer than babies considered normal.

Table 3–2. Usual Length of Nursery Stay* by Institution by Race

Institution	Length (days)	
	WHITE	BLACK
BO	5–6	5–6
BU	5	†
CH	–	3
CO	5	5
JH	3	2
VA	2–3	2
MN	5–6	†
NY	3	3
OR	3–4	3–4
PA	5	5
PR	4–5	4–5
TN	†	3

*Modal stay for babies, with birthweight over 2500 gm, discharged alive. Where a second
period has almost as many releases as the modal period, both periods are shown.
† Less than 100 cases.

Table 3–2 shows the usual duration of hospital stay for those infants weighing more than 2500 grams at birth and discharged alive from the nursery. There was considerable variation by institution.

Various study evaluations were scheduled at specific times during the nursery stay. The nature of each and the age at which each set of observations was made are listed in Table 3–1 and are described below. The PED–2, *Neonatal Examination*, a general pediatric examination, was carried out by a pediatrician at approximately twelve hours of age and repeated at forty-eight hours. Careful measurements, following manual instructions, were made of body length and of the maximum suboccipital-bregmatic head circumference. If the baby remained more than twenty-four hours in the nursery after the second examination, a third was performed by study personnel at discharge. In the event that the infant's stay was prolonged, he was examined at weekly intervals until discharge. These evaluations identified evidence of congenital malformations, birth injury, and other abnormal conditions.

The PED–6, *Neonatal Neurological Examination*, was completed at forty-eight hours. This examination was designed by pediatric neurologists specially proficient in neonatal neurology. By the use of films, workshops, and training sessions, pediatricians also became proficient in this examination. The study neurologist was available for consultation and to reexamine infants thought to be suspect or abnormal. The neurological examination was repeated on a weekly basis when the infant remained more than one week in the hospital. The purpose of the neonatal neurological examination was assessment of central nervous system function and identification of suspected or definite neurological abnormality.

The PED–3, *Nursery History*, summarizing the infant's nursery course, including information on feeding, body temperature and weight, environmental conditions (oxygen, incubator, etc.), medications, procedures, and other pertinent factors, was usually completed on a daily basis by a study nurse, from hospital records and queries of housestaff and nursery nurses. As a minimum, this information was recorded on each occasion when a neonatal examination was done.

The PED–4, *Report of Fetal or Infant Death*, was completed by the study pediatrician. This form was used to record the provisional cause of death and whether or not an autopsy was obtained. Every effort was made to obtain detailed pathological studies; autopsies were carried out on over 90 percent of the infants dying during the neonatal period and 72 percent of infants dying later in the first year.

Certain laboratory data were routinely obtained at specified times on the babies and recorded on PED–5, *Results of Tests and Procedures Done on the Neonate*. These included, among others, determination of ABO and Rh blood types and a Coombs' test. These determinations were usually made using a sample of cord blood or, if this was not available, on capillary or venous blood drawn shortly after birth. Additionally, cord blood serum was frozen and shipped to the Perinatal Research Laboratory for storage and use with the mother's serum in later studies of perinatal infection.

Serum bilirubin and *microhematocrit* determinations were carried out on a routine basis on capillary blood drawn at approximately forty-eight hours. If the bilirubin level was 10 mg% or above, the determination was repeated at least once every twenty-four hours until the level fell below 10 mg%. If the baby weighed less than 2250 grams (5 lbs.) at birth, the determination was repeated at four to five days of age. Additional determinations were made as clinically indicated to monitor bilirubin levels. All results were recorded on PED–5. In order to assure comparability in laboratory results, a committee developed a quality control program. Unknown samples were sent periodically to each bilirubin laboratory to check on the comparability of results over time and between institutions. A description of these procedures has been published (2). While serious discrepancies were found initially in a few institutions, the techniques were quickly improved.

The results of all other laboratory determinations, radiological examinations, and diagnostic procedures carried out in the course of patient care were also recorded on PED–5.

The PED–8, *Newborn Diagnostic Summary*, was completed, by or under the supervision of a senior pediatrician on the study staff, when the baby was discharged from the nursery. Both hospital nursery and study records were reviewed in order to make a judgment regarding the presence, suspected presence, or absence of certain specific abnormalities. Thus, the diagnostic summary permitted the separation of the children into three mutually exclusive groups with respect to certain abnormalities: those who appeared, on the basis of specifically defined criteria, to have the abnormality in question, i.e., the diagnosis was definite; those who were suspected of having it; and those who did not have it and were therefore judged to be "normal" in that respect. For the purposes of the descriptive analyses to be included in this report, only definite abnormalities are considered; the infants with "suspect" abnormalities are grouped with the very large number of those without the particular abnormality.

The *Newborn Diagnostic Summary* (PED–8) also provided for the recording of major procedures: (a) diagnostic, such as lumbar punctures, X-ray examinations, bacterial and serological tests, etc.; and (b) therapeutic, such as surgery, with anesthesia, and the administration of therapeutic agents such as antibiotics.

As this study has been concerned primarily with neurologic outcomes, emphasis was placed on documentation of these outcomes. If a neurologic abnormality was detected, the reviewing pediatrician was requested to decide whether this represented malfunction of the brain, as opposed to the peripheral nervous system, and to check those manifestations which, in his judgment, reflected the infant's brain abnormality.

Information about various pediatric and neurologic conditions drawn from the *Newborn Diagnostic Summary* (PED–8) forms the basis for much of the information presented in the part of this report concerned with the neonate. Each definite diagnosis is evaluated by race in terms of its association with low birthweight, mean birthweight, risk of neonatal death, and of neurologic abnormality at one year of age. It should be noted that the comparisons are between babies with a given condition, for example, congenital hydrocephalus, and for that large group with no abnormalities of the central nervous system, though they may have abnormalities in some other system.

At Four Months

The infant was brought back to the study center at four months of age, when a thorough pediatric evaluation was carried out. The primary purposes of this examination were the search for congenital malformations not recognized in the newborn period and the evaluation of changes in neurological status since the neonatal period. The data collected on a routine basis at four months of age are included in the PED–12, *Summary of the First Year of Life*, but are not otherwise considered in this volume.

Physical Growth

Body length, weight, and the maximum suboccipital bregmatic head circumference were measured in the newborn period and at each follow-up visit. These measurements were made with calibrated scales and measuring devices, according to a standard protocol, which yielded reproducible results between observers measuring the same child. The techniques used and the results obtained form the subject of a monograph describing the physical growth characteristics of the study children that is nearing completion.

Interval Medical History

Each time an infant was returned to the study center, PED–20, *Interval Medical History* was completed to document routine health care and to elicit information about illness or accident and certain diagnostic and/or therapeutic procedures, such as X-rays, examination of cerebro-spinal fluid or the administration of blood or parenteral fluids. This historical information was systematically verified by means of review of hospital records, letters to physicians, and the like. The findings were recorded on the PED–29, *Summary of Medical Records of Illness or Hospitalization*. The information thus collected provides the basis for much of the information about intercurrent events included in the PED–12, *Summary of the First Year of Life*.

At Eight Months

At eight months of age (plus or minus two weeks), the child was brought back to the study center for a developmental evaluation by a trained psychologist, using the *Bayley Scales of Mental and Motor Development* (3) (as modified in 1958 for use in the NCPP). These tests, which will be described in more detail in Chapter 13, were standardized and provided scaled numerical scores.

At One Year

An extensive *pediatric neurological examination* was carried out on each child at twelve months (50 to 56 weeks). This evaluation was made by a neurologist, or by a pediatrician trained under his supervision to carry out the examination. To assure comparability of information, between many physicians in the various centers over the entire period of the study, workshops were held, a movie demonstrating the standardized examination technique was produced, and a special form (PED–11, *One-Year Neurological Examination*) and accompanying manual were provided. While the standard age requirements for this examination were 50 to 56 weeks of age, and most infants were processed within these limits, a small proportion was not. The observations obtained between 50 and 56 weeks have been compared for a number of items with those obtained by including all children examined between 48 and 60 weeks. Except for developmental items, the differences were minimal; the results described here, unless otherwise indicated, are based on the broader time interval. For developmental observations the age range has been restricted to 48 to 56 weeks.

After the completion of the one-year evaluation and any diagnostic or referral examinations indicated by its findings or history, the study neurologist or pediatrician reviewed the child's record since nursery discharge and completed the PED–12, *Summary of the First Year of Life*.

PED–12 has provided a major information source for this monograph. It should be noted that PED–12 includes diagnostic information, by source, on events occurring from the time of discharge from the hospital nursery through the time of the twelve-month examination, including diagnostic studies that may have been initiated at that examination. Information about nursery events was not included on this form. If the baby died after leaving the nursery, or was not followed until one year for some other reason, the form was completed insofar as possible, and the information available has been used in this report. A copy of PED–12 is included in the Appendix.

REFERENCES

(1) K. R. Niswander and M. Gordon (eds.). 1972. *The Women and Their Pregnancies,* p. 18. Philadelphia: W. B. Saunders Co.

(2) M. Westphal, E. Viergiver, and R. Roth. 1962. Analysis of a bilirubin survey. *Pediatrics* 30: 12–16.

(3) N. Bayley. 1933. Mental growth during the first three years: A developmental study of sixty-one children by repeated tests. *Genetic Psychology Monographs* 14:1–92.

4

DATA ASSESSMENT AND
INTERPRETATION

GENERAL ASSESSMENT OF THE DATA

The Perinatal Research Committee, an official advisory committee to the Director, NINCDS, on the NCPP and a number of special ad hoc committees devoted much time and attention to all aspects of data collection and production. Many prominent obstetricians, pediatricians, neurologists, epidemiologists, biostatisticians, pathologists, and behavioral scientists participated in the design and evaluation of the program. Various committees have devoted attention to all aspects of data production, including assessment of the quality of data and appropriateness of statistical methodology. More recently, the overall plans for analysis and presentation were the responsibility of the Coordinating Committee for Data Analysis. Some methodological considerations are discussed in *The Women and Their Pregnancies*, pages 20–35 (1). In general, the data were found to be satisfactory to meet the objectives of the study, and combination, or pooling, of the data from the individual collaborating institutions was appropriate for analytical purposes.

The data base providing the information presented here has been reviewed in detail by the authors and is generally consistent by institution. Inconsistencies were identified in a small number of instances, but they were of little consequence to the issues of interest and the reasons for their presence could usually be identified. For example, the data may have been too sparse by institution (i.e., too few cases) to provide precise information concerning the likelihood that an association observed might be spurious. In rare instances, the quality control procedures indicated individual-observer bias in the recording of clinical observations. Such bias, when it occurred, appeared in relation to isolated, relatively unimportant physical findings that represented a particular interest of one examiner.

While, for the most part, the observations presented in this report reflect examination of the pooled data, the information from each institution was prepared and studied individually in the same manner as the combined data. The pooled data rather consistently reflected the associations noted by institutions.

There was general agreement that the data for white and black gravidas and their offspring should be considered and reported separately as their demographic characteristics were very different. In addition, there were differences between white and black babies, in rates of mortality, in average birthweight (about 200 grams), and in gestational age (nine days). Nonetheless, there was rather striking similarity between white and black infants with respect to the frequency distributions of many pediatric, neurological, and development observations during the first year. These similarities are of considerable biological interest and lend support to the validity of the observations from the various institutions.

STATISTICAL INTERPRETATION

The data presented in this report, like those in *The Women and Their Pregnancies*, are largely descriptive. The methodology, therefore, is simple and straightforward and is that required for the development of distributions, rates, mean values, and cross tabulations of one variable by another. Comparisons have been made by race, sex, birthweight, and other variables thought to be relevant. Sometimes the differences observed have been substantial; at other times, there has been no difference, or it has been quite small. How should observed differences be interpreted? Among those advising on statistical methodology, there has been considerable discussion about the issue of the significance of such differences, both in a practical, clinical sense, and in a statistical sense. The resolution is not a simple matter. On the practical level, clinical experience and common sense indicate the importance of substantial differences between comparable groups, regardless of whether the sample sizes are very large or include only a relatively few cases in the comparison. For example, if there were ten persons with condition X in one group and five of them died, and an otherwise comparable group of 2010 without condition X with a mortality experience of five cases, no statistical test of significance is required to indicate the clinical importance of condition X.

A problem exists in the NCPP as the result of the large sample size; almost 59,000 pregnancies were enrolled. When sample size is very large the standard tests for statistical significance frequently indicate high levels of significance, even in the presence of very small differences between groups. Care must then be exercised in the interpretation of the biological (or practical) significance involved. For example, in very large samples, small differences, such as 0.3 cm. in average height at age seven years, may have statistical significance but little practical meaning.

Another consideration in the interpretation of the data concerns the relative importance of differing rates between comparison groups. The practical significance of a given finding is determined not only by the rates but also by the size of the populations to which the rates are applied. For example, the neonatal mortality rate for white infants weighing between 1501 and 2000 grams at birth was 121 per 1000 livebirths, almost four times that (31.5) of the next higher birthweight group of

2001 to 2500 grams. However, only 223 babies, of whom 27 died, were included in the smaller group, as compared with 954 of whom 30 died in the larger group. Thus the larger babies actually made a slightly greater contribution to the overall number of deaths. Among blacks, 98 of the 336 neonatal deaths occurred among babies weighing over 2500 grams at birth. Thus, even though the rates for babies of 2501 grams and above were in themselves relatively quite low, this group contributed 29.2 percent of the total neonatal deaths, a point that is easily overlooked when one is preoccupied solely with the magnitude of rates experienced by the very small infants.

Other difficulties or pitfalls in proper interpretation result because the associations that appear to exist among two, three, or more variables may not always precisely reflect the complexity of their interrelationships. Furthermore, the demonstration of an association in the data does not necessarily imply a causal relationship, nor does it preclude the possibility that the association may be an indirect one, or fortuitous.

REFERENCE

(1) K. R. Niswander and M. Gordon (eds.). 1972. *The Women and Their Pregnancies,* pp. 20–35. Philadelphia: W. B. Saunders Co.

5

MATERNAL CHARACTERISTICS AND PERINATAL OUTCOME

The first comprehensive report from the NCPP addressed pregnancy outcome in relation to many antecedent factors. A wide range of maternal characteristics, conditions, and abnormalities were considered in relation to perinatal mortality, birthweight, and neurological abnormality at one year; an elaboration of these outcomes represents a major aspect of this volume. For the convenience of the reader and to provide certain background information, pertinent material has been abstracted from the more detailed discussions, tables, and graphs presented in *The Women and Their Pregnancies* (1).

DEMOGRAPHIC CHARACTERISTICS

Race

The race of the mother was that reported by the mother herself at the time of her enrollment in the study. While the father's race was also reported by the mother, the mother's race was assigned to the child. The data presented here are concerned with the single-born infants resulting from the white and black gravidas' first entry into the study. The racial components of the study reflect the urban location of the collaborating centers and the enrollment of clinic patients, excepting for the center in Buffalo, where only private patients were enrolled. Of the 39,215 such registrants in the study, 19,048 were white and 20,167 were black. The registration of black women ranged from 0.6 percent at the University of Minnesota to 100 percent at Charity Hospital in New Orleans.

Maternal Education

In both white and black infants, a relationship was observed between the years of schooling completed by the mother and the outcome. As the educational level of the mother increased there was a progressive decrease in the rates of birthweight below 2501 grams and of neurological abnormalities at one year. A similar, though less clear-cut, relationship with perinatal mortality and its components (stillbirths and neonatal deaths) was observed, but there was an increase in neonatal deaths for white women with sixteen or more years of schooling, which may perhaps reflect advanced maternal age and primigravidity in this group of women.

Maternal Age

In general, the perinatal death rates become progressively greater with increasing maternal age above 18 years. The optimal age for childbearing on the basis of the risk of perinatal death was 18 to 19 years.

The rate of low birthweight was highest for the infants of women of both races who were below 16 years of age. For the white infants the rate was lowest where maternal age was between 18 and 29 years, for black infants where it was 25 to 29 years. Mean birthweight for infants of both races was progressively higher with increasing maternal age. There are interactions between maternal age and other variables affecting birthweight; in particular, the prepregnant weight and weight gain during pregnancy, socioeconomic status, parity, and cigarette smoking, all of which tend to increase somewhat with increasing age.

Parity

Perinatal death rates for white and black infants for each parity category of the mother tend to increase with increasing maternal age. The babies of primigravidas over thirty years of age have far higher rates of perinatal death and low birthweight than those of younger women. The interrelationships between age and parity make for difficulty in assessing the effect of either variable alone.

Socioeconomic Status

As mentioned in *The Women and Their Pregnancies*, and previously reported by Myrianthopoulos and French (2), the socioeconomic characteristics of the study families were, in general, somewhat different from those prevailing nationally for similar ethnic groups. The whites, in terms of income and socioeconomic index, based on family income and education and occupation of head of household, were generally somewhat below the whites, nationally; whereas the black families in the study were somewhat above the national average for blacks. Similarly, the white gravidas in the study had fewer years of schooling, were younger, and included a higher proportion of primigravidas as compared with their racial counterparts on a national basis. The black women had relatively more education, but tended to be younger than their racial counterparts.

Not unexpected was the consistent relationship observed between race and adverse fetal outcome, with black infants generally having higher rates than whites with respect to perinatal death and low birthweight. The average birthweight for black infants was also lower.

Cigarette Smoking

Smoking was more frequent among white gravidas; 50.4 percent smoked two cigarettes or more per day, as compared with 36.2 percent of the blacks. Among blacks, the perinatal death rates were progressively higher as the number of cigarettes smoked per day increased; in whites the relationship was less clear. However, heavy smoking (i.e., thirty or more cigarettes per day) was clearly associated with increased perinatal mortality in both ethnic groups.

A clear relationship between birthweight and maternal smoking was observed. The rate of low birthweight progressively increased and the mean birthweight decreased with the number of cigarettes smoked per day. The mean birthweight was over 400 grams less in whites and 250 grams less in blacks in women who smoked more than forty cigarettes per day, and the rate of low birthweight more than doubled for the infants of women smoking more than twenty cigarettes per day, as compared with the infants of nonsmokers.

The long-range effect of maternal smoking during pregnancy on infants surviving the neonatal period is less clear. Data from the British Perinatal Study (3) suggest that the seven-year-old children of women who smoked after the first four months of pregnancy are slightly shorter and have some delay (about three months) in the acquisition of reading skills than the seven-year-olds of women who did not smoke. Conversely, in a matched pair study of infants in the Johns Hopkins sample (4), no significant differences at age seven years, in either physical or intellectual growth and academic achievement, were noted between the offspring of women who smoked ten cigarettes or more per day throughout pregnancy and those of women who did not smoke. The women who smoked were matched, on a number of parameters known to affect birthweight, with comparable nonsmokers in an effort to isolate the effect of smoking. A 250-gram difference in birthweight was observed, and the infants of smokers were still significantly smaller in both weight and length at one year, but by age four and seven years the differences were not significant.

Comment

Of all the demographic characteristics, race and socioeconomic parameters probably bear the strongest overall relationship to fetal outcome, both immediate and long-range. In this study, the analyses were made separately for whites, and blacks. The interactions between socioeconomic variables and other factors that affect fetal outcome, such as parity, maternal age, marital status, timing and quality of medical care, and the opportunity for infection, among others, make for problems in the analysis of data. The complexity of these interactions is beyond the scope of this descriptive volume, but these relationships will be addressed in a subsequent monograph focusing on birthweight and gestational age.

An earlier report of an analysis of 142,017 livebirths and 3115 infant deaths (death during the first year), in New York City in 1973, by Kessner et al. (5), is of interest in this context. That study focused on the relationships among variables concerned with the obstetrical risk of the mother, the maternal health services she received, and the survival of her infant through the first year of life. Fifty-five percent of the mothers were considered to have one or more demographic, social, medical and/or obstetrical handicaps that could exert an adverse influence on the pregnancy outcome. The distribution of risks varied by race; black women were at risk three times as frequently as white. More than three-fifths of the whites were at no risk at all, whereas only one-fourth of the blacks were at no risk. Pregnancy outcome was clearly related to the degree of risk, and those women at no risk had a superior pregnancy outcome, as compared with those at risk.

PHYSICAL CHARACTERISTICS OF THE MOTHER

Relationships between the mother's height, prepregnant weight and weight gain during pregnancy, and fetal outcome were extensively investigated and the results published in *The Women and Their Pregnancies* (pp. 80–153), and other publications of NCPP data. Each of the three variables mentioned, when examined singly, was strongly related to birthweight and risks of mortality.

When appropriately controlled on gestational age, weight gain in pregnancy and prepregnant weight were found to be strongly related to birthweight and fetal outcome; a weight gain during pregnancy of 25 to 30 lbs. being optimal in relation to highest average birthweight and lowest rates of perinatal mortality. Maternal height appeared to be of importance only insofar as it related to the weight of the mother (6).

The interrelationships between the variables make assessment of their individual effect difficult. Furthermore, the effect of other characteristics, such as socioeconomic status, age, parity, and smoking must be considered, as they also have important relationships with outcome.

HISTORY OF LAST PRIOR PREGNANCY

The risks of fetal or neonatal death and low birthweight for infants in this study were greatly increased if the mother's last prior pregnancy had terminated in a stillbirth or neonatal death. For whites, if the birthweight of the last prior child was below 2501 grams, the chances were one in four that the study infant would also weigh under 2501 grams; for blacks, the risks were one in three.

HISTORY OF INFERTILITY

Infertility, based on a history of a sterility investigation, has an association with low birthweight and an increase in the perinatal mortality rate. Among those gravida who reported that they had been trying to become pregnant for at least one year, an association was observed between increasing time to become pregnant and risk of perinatal mortality. While numbers of cases were small, the trend was stronger for stillbirths than for neonatal deaths. The relationship with birthweight was equiv-

Table 5-1. Characteristics and Conditions of Pregnancy

Condition	WHITE with Condition			BLACK with Condition		
	Percent	Perinatal Death Rate*	Birthweight Rate Below 2501 gm	Percent	Perinatal Death Rate*	Birthweight Rate Below 2501 gm
Organic heart disease	1.44	55.2	176.5	1.76	71.4	189.0
Pneumonia during pregnancy	.57	27.8	103.8	.44	56.8	139.5
Bronchial asthma	.93	28.4	105.3	1.42	70.4	159.3
Diabetes	.66	144.0	95.7	.65	139.5	149.1
Convulsions, not eclamptic	.35	30.3	46.9	.21	119.1	194.4
Psychosis or neurosis	4.71	36.0	89.7	1.69	29.6	186.8
Hyperemesis gravidarum	1.64	35.7	66.7	.71	35.5	117.7
Incompetent cervix	.34	323.1	614.0	.36	478.9	679.3
Hydramnios	1.54	137.9	86.5	1.26	99.2	87.9
Placenta previa	.77	176.1	328.2	.56	190.9	529.4
Abruptio placentae	2.39	195.5	263.0	1.90	360.7	476.9
Prolapse of cord	1.10	168.3	118.6	.78	298.0	235.3
All cases	–	35.1	71.4	–	41.9	134.2

Source: *The Women and Their Pregnancies,* inside front cover.
*Perinatal deaths include stillbirths and neonatal deaths.

ocal; while the relationship with rate of neurological abnormality at one year was reversed, the risk of abnormality decreased as the time of becoming pregnant increased.

DISEASE STATES AND CONDITIONS OF PREGNANCY, LABOR, AND DELIVERY

Maternal Diseases and Conditions

The relationships observed between fetal outcome and a number of disease states and conditions affecting the mother are listed in Table 5–1. The frequency with which these maternal abnormalities was observed is also given. Some, such as organic heart disease and abruptio placentae, were quite frequent in women of both racial groups and were accompanied by increased risk to the fetus; others, such as psychiatric disturbances and hyperemesis, were also relatively frequent, but without any apparent increase in fetal risk.

Adverse fetal outcomes associated with pregnancy hypertension are the subject of a special detailed study based on NCPP data that have been reported by Friedman and Neff (7).

Vaginal Bleeding

The occurrence of vaginal bleeding during pregnancy has long been suspected to have an association with abnormal fetal outcome, and such was found to be the case in the NCPP. The perinatal death rates for both white and black infants were higher when vaginal bleeding occurred, particularly for those infants whose mothers reported vaginal bleeding during the second trimester.

Premature Rupture of Membranes

The membranes ruptured prematurely (i.e., before the onset of labor) in 45 percent of the white and 44 percent of black women in whom there was spontaneous onset of labor and spontaneous rupture of membranes. Among those with premature rupture of membranes, 78 percent of the whites and 65 percent of the blacks experienced the onset of labor within twelve hours of the rupture of their membranes. A delay in the onset of labor beyond forty-eight hours was noted in 5 percent of white and 10 percent of black women; a marked increase in both stillbirths and neonatal deaths (approximately tenfold in whites and fourfold in blacks) was observed in these patients, as compared to those whose onset of labor was less than eight hours after rupture. Both the birthweight and the maturity of the infant was related to prolongation of the time elapsed from membrane rupture to the onset of labor. The rate of low birthweight was about three times higher, the mean birthweight decreased, and the rate of neurological abnormality at one year increased for infants of both races delivered after having had forty-eight hours of ruptured membranes before labor as compared with those who delivered within twenty-four hours. An additional factor contributing to the high risk of adverse outcome following prolonged rupture of membranes was the increasing likelihood of intrauterine and fetal infection with the increasing elapsed time from the rupture. The relationship between low birthweight, short gestation, and premature rupture of the membranes should be borne in mind when interpreting the degrees of adverse outcome associated with premature rupture of membranes.

Duration of Labor

The duration of both first and second stages of labor was very similar for women of both racial groups having spontaneous vertex deliveries. In primiparas, 47 percent of the whites and 49 percent of the blacks had a first stage of labor of more than eight hours, and 7 percent of the former and 10 percent of the latter were in the first stage for more than eighteen hours. In women of both ethnic groups, a short first stage (i.e., under two hours), and a first stage prolonged over ten hours were associated with increased perinatal mortality.

The second stage of labor lasted more than two hours in 13 percent of white primiparas and 0.6 percent of white multiparas, as compared with 6 percent of primiparas and 0.3 percent multiparas in blacks. A short second stage of less than thirty minutes was noted in 29 percent of primiparas and 84 percent of multiparas among whites, and 51 percent of primiparas and 91 percent of multiparas in blacks. The rates of adverse fetal outcome were increased with both short (i.e., less than thirty minutes) and prolonged second stage of labor (more than two hours).

Type of Delivery

Approximately 92 percent of study babies were delivered vaginally following vertex presentation. In 5 percent, Cesarean section was used to effect delivery, and the remaining 3 percent were delivered by breech. Breech delivery was associated

Table 5-2. Fetal Outcome by Type of Delivery

Type of Delivery	Number	Percent	Rates* — Adverse Outcome		
			Perinatal Deaths	Low Birthweight	Neurological Abnormality†
WHITE					
Vaginal					
Vertex	17176	91.7	19.2	62.6	16.4
Breech	626	3.3	207.7	230.2	30.5
Cesarean section	921	4.9	66.2	144.3	27.3
BLACK					
Vaginal					
Vertex	18406	92.4	26.4	125.5	15.1
Breech	519	2.6	314.1	385.2	41.7
Cesarean section	992	5.0	62.5	185.5	23.1

Source: *The Women and Their Pregnancies,* pp. 381–2.
*Perinatal deaths per 1000 births, low birthweight per 1000 livebirths, neurological abnormality per 1000 examinations.
†Definite neurological abnormality at one year.

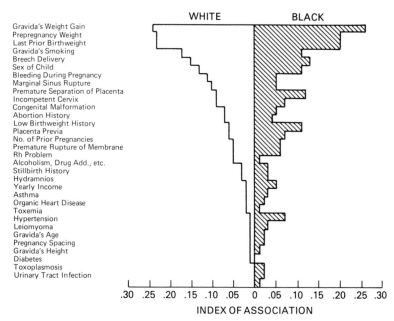

Based on data from the Collaborative Perinatal Project, NINCDS, NIH.
Weiss, W., and Jackson, E.: Maternal Factors Affecting Birth Weight.
PAHO: Scientific Pub. 185: 54-59, 1969.

Figure 5-1. Factors Associated with Birthweight-Multiparas

with the highest mortality rates and lowest mean birthweights, and vertex delivery with the lowest mortality and highest average birthweight. A major factor in the high mortality associated with breech delivery was the marked association with low birthweight (Table 5–2).

Summary

Many factors, biological and environmental, affect the gravida, her pregnancy, and her infant. Their effects may be apparent through associations with perinatal outcome, birthweight, and long-range physical and intellectual development. The precise effects and their relative importance may be difficult to ascertain because of interactions and interrelationships between the factors, for example, those between age and parity. In an attempt to rank the order of their importance, thirty-two factors thought to be associated with birthweight were assessed by Weiss and his co-workers (8). A multiple regression analysis was utilized to examine the factors simultaneously and to rank them on the basis of the strength of their association with birthweight (Fig. 5–1). Maternal weight gain in pregnancy and pre-pregnant weight showed the strongest correlations with the weight of the infant at birth. It should be noted that this analysis was limited to multiparous women, so that the effect of variables related to prior pregnancies could be included.

REFERENCES

(1) K. R. Niswander and M. Gordon (eds.). 1972. *The Women and Their Pregnancies.* Philadelphia: W. B. Saunders Co.

(2) N. C. Myrianthopoulos and K. S. French. 1968. An application of the U.S. Bureau of the Census socioeconomic index to a large, diversified patient population. *Social Science and Medicine* 2: 283–99.

(3) H. Goldstein. 1971. Factors influencing the height of seven-year-old children. Results from the National Child Development Study. *Human Biology* 43: 92–111.

(4) J. B. Hardy and E. D. Mellits. 1972. Does maternal smoking during pregnancy have a long-term effect on the child? *Lancet* 2: 1332–36.

(5) D. M. Kessner, J. Singer, C. E. Kalk, and E. R. Schlesinger. 1973. *Infant Death: An Analysis by Maternal Risk and Health Care.* Washington, D.C.: National Academy of Sciences, Vol. 1.

(6) K. R. Niswander, J. Singer, M. Westphal, Jr., and W. Weiss. 1969. Weight gain during pregnancy and prepregnancy weight. *Obstetrics and Gynecology* 33: 482–91.

(7) E. A. Friedman and R. K. Neff. 1977. *Pregnancy Hypertension.* Littleton, Mass.: Publishing Sciences Group, Inc.

(8) W. Weiss and E. C. Jackson. 1969. Maternal factors affecting birthweight. In *Perinatal Factors Affecting Human Development.* Washington, D.C.: Pan American Health Organization, Scientific Publication No. 185, pp. 54–59.

6

MAJOR PREGNANCY OUTCOME
CATEGORIES

OBSERVATIONS DURING THE FIRST YEAR OF LIFE

This chapter presents a brief summary of pregnancy outcome in terms of perinatal mortality (stillbirths and neonatal death rates), infant mortality rates, mean birthweight and rates of low birthweight and definite neurological abnormality at one year. Differences in the population characteristics, particularly race of mother and socioeconomic status and differences between institutions were reported in *The Women and Their Pregnancies*. Outcomes by institution are shown in Tables 6–1 and 6–2.

It is interesting to consider the mortality experience observed in this study in the context of the larger experience described by Shapiro, Schlesinger, and Nesbitt (1968) (1) for the United States. Their extensive study describes the trends in infant and perinatal mortality observed over the fifty years ending with 1965, and some of the variables relating to those trends. Because its later years almost coincide with the period during which infants in the NCPP were being delivered, it provides background description of the national United States experience as a whole against which the more detailed and specific experiences of the NCPP may be viewed.

Shapiro described the substantial decline in perinatal and first-year deaths that occurred during the five-year period from 1945 to 1950, followed by a leveling off of the mortality experience in the ten-year period between 1956 and 1965. When the data were examined in greater detail, it was found that immediate perinatal deaths (under one day) actually showed a minimal increase during the period (1956–65) and those deaths under six months showed little change. Shapiro's publication reports mortality trends in relation to race, sex of infant, certain specific causes of death, and for certain geographic regions in the country. The data from the NCPP reflect trends for the period of the study that are consistent with those of Shapiro.

Table 6-1. Stillbirths by Institution by Race

| | WHITE | | | | | BLACK | | | | |
| | | Total Stillbirths | | Fresh Stillbirths | | | Total Stillbirths | | Fresh Stillbirths | |
	Births	No.	Rate	No.	Rate	Births	No.	Rate	No.	Rate
Total	19048	415	21.79	200	10.50	20167	457	22.66	246	12.20
BO	7823	194	24.80	89	11.38	913	26	28.48	14	15.33
BU	1926	57	29.60	21	10.90	52	4	76.92	0	0
CH	0	0	—	0	—	2380	51	21.43	27	11.34
CO	603	13	21.56	5	8.29	842	19	22.57	10	11.88
JH	667	9	13.49	5	7.50	2210	60	27.15	28	12.67
VA	741	10	13.50	8	10.80	1840	46	25.00	32	17.39
MN	2623	53	20.21	29	11.06	17	1	58.82*	1	58.82*
NY	253	4	15.81	2	7.91	1455	26	17.87	15	10.31
OR	1894	30	15.84	18	9.50	603	14	23.22	9	14.93
PA	728	14	19.23	8	10.99	6158	147	23.87	77	12.50
PR	1769	31	17.52	15	8.48	501	14	27.94	4	7.98
TN	21	0	0	0	0	3196	49	15.33	29	9.07

Source: *The Women and Their Pregnancies,* p. 43.
*Based on less than 20 cases.

Table 6-2. Neonatal Deaths by Institution by Race

| | WHITE | | | BLACK | | |
	Livebirths	Neonatal Deaths	Rate	Livebirths	Neonatal Deaths	Rate
Total	18633	253	13.58	19710	388	19.69
BO	7629	93	12.19	887	15	16.91
BU	1869	26	13.91	48	0	0
CH	0	0	—	2329	39	16.75
CO	590	10	16.95	823	13	15.80
JH	658	7	10.64	2150	56	26.05
VA	731	8	10.94	1794	21	11.71
MN	2570	28	10.89	16	0	0 *
NY	249	5	20.08	1429	28	19.59
OR	1864	33	17.70	589	9	15.28
PA	714	16	22.41	6011	147	24.46
PR	1738	27	15.54	487	10	20.53
TN	21	0	0	3147	50	15.89

Source: *The Women and Their Pregnancies,* p. 44.
*Based on less than 20 cases.

Between January 2, 1959 and December 31, 1965, 19,048 white and 20,167 black singleborn infants were delivered to the women enrolled for the first time in the NCPP. Of these, 18,481 whites and 19,504 blacks were liveborn, with known birthweight of 400 grams or more. Data on abortions are not presented, because the selection procedure with varying gestations at the time of prenatal registration precluded the collection of adequate data. In general, the data in this report are restricted to first study infants with known birthweight, in contrast to *The Women and Their Pregnancies*, where the birthweight restriction was not applied. There were 152 white and 206 black infants with unknown birthweight (a very small fraction of the total births), whose exclusion accounts for minor differences in numbers and rates.

STILLBIRTHS

Stillbirths are deaths of fetuses of twenty weeks or more gestation prior to delivery. The stillbirth rate, per 1000 single births, was 21.79 for the 19,048 white, and 22.66 for the 20,167 black infants. The rates by race and birthweight are summarized in the accompanying tables and graphs. There were 200 classified as "fresh" among the 415 white stillbirths and among the black, 246 of the 457 were classified as "fresh," indicating death during or shortly before labor and delivery.

LIVEBIRTHS

The first study pregnancy terminated in a single, liveborn infant, of twenty weeks or longer gestation, for 18,633 white and 19,710 black women. Of these 18,481 whites and 19,504 blacks had known birthweights. The observations on these liveborn infants with known birthweights provided data for most of this report.

NEONATAL DEATHS

The neonatal death rate per 1000 single, liveborn infants was 13.58 for the whites and 19.69 for the blacks. There were 253 white and 388 black infants dying during the first twenty-eight days after birth.

The pathological conditions underlying the perinatal and later infant deaths in the NCPP are the subject of an intensive investigation to be reported separately.

GESTATION

A difference between black and white gravidas was observed in the average duration of gestation. The mean gestational age at delivery of white infants was 40.1 weeks, approximately nine days longer than that of 38.8 weeks of black infants. Only minimal (one-day) sex differences in gestational age were observed. Birthweight-gestational age relationships are discussed in greater detail in Chapter 7.

BIRTHWEIGHT

The *mean birthweight* for single, liveborn infants was 3272 grams for the white and 3039 grams for the black infants, a difference of 233 grams. Because considerable variation existed in mean birthweight among the collaborating institutions, the data are presented in the next chapter (Tables 7–7 and 7–8) for each participating center. An average difference by institution of 60 to 120 grams between male and female infants of each race was noted. In general, the larger difference was noted in those institutions where the mean birthweight was highest. Also, in general, the risks of perinatal mortality were lowest in those institutions with the highest average birthweight. The percentage distribution of infants by birthweight is presented in Chapter 7.

Extremes of Birthweight

The three smallest babies surviving to at least one year were all black females. They weighed 737, 822, and 879 grams, respectively. They were reported to be 35.4, 40, and 36 centimeters in length and 34, 27, and 27 weeks in gestational age.

The three largest survivors to one year weighed 6237, 5556, and 5550 grams and were 55, 59, and 57 centimeters in length. The largest was a white female, the second a black male and the third a white male.

Low birthweight (i.e., 2500 grams or below) was observed, with a rate of 71.37 in white and 134.18 in black infants. The rates tended to be higher in those institutions where the mean birthweight was low.

The dimensions of the problem of low birthweight are illustrated by examination of the distributions of the various birthweight subgroups. Among the 18,481 white infants with known birthweight, 1319 (7.14 percent) weighed 2500 grams or less. Two-thirds, 954 of these low-weight infants, weighed between 2001 and 2500 grams and 365 (less than 2 percent of all white infants) weighed 2000 grams or less. Among the 19,504 black infants, the frequency of low birthweight observed was approximately twice that of the whites, 2617 (13.42 percent). Among the low-weight black infants, 1855 (9.51 percent of total births) weighed between 2001 and 2500 grams, and 762 (3.91 percent) were 2000 grams and below. The risks of mortality and later abnormality in surviving infants were much higher for those under 2000 grams than for those weighing between 2000 and 2500 grams, but the relatively greater numbers in the heavier birthweight category tended to outweigh in importance the greater risks of smaller babies by contributing substantially larger numbers of children at risk.

The frequency of low birthweight observed in the NCPP is similar to that reported by Shapiro et al. (1968) (1) for the nation as a whole. They also reported a considerable variation in the proportion of low-birthweight infants (2500 grams and below) by geographic region that is consistent with the variation in mean birthweight by institution noted in this study.

INFANT DEATHS

Among white infants 104, and among blacks 167, died between twenty-eight days of age and their first birthday. More than half of these deaths occurred before four months of age. Some of the conditions relating to specific causes of infant death are listed in the One-Year Diagnostic Summary (tables presented in Chapter 15). Detailed information is being developed as part of an intensive investigation of all deaths in the NCPP, and pathological findings will be reported in a subsequent monograph.

NEUROLOGICAL ABNORMALITIES AT ONE YEAR

Neurological evaluations carried out between forty-eight and sixty weeks of age are considered in this report. Of the white infants, 14,662, and among blacks, 17,123 were examined within this time span, and 253 whites and 274 blacks were considered to be abnormal. Neurological abnormality was designated definite when in the examiner's opinion strong evidence of organic deficit was present. Children with "soft" signs were diagnosed as neurologically suspect, and for the purposes of this report are included with those who were thought to be neurologically normal. The rates of neurological abnormality per 1000 examinations, of 17.26 for the whites and 16.00 for the blacks are not essentially different. The general category of "neurological abnormality" was developed to provide a gross measure of outcome at one year of age, and it has proven useful in that context. However, for more detailed analytical studies the use of specific diagnostic categories may be necessary.

REFERENCE

(1) S. Shapiro, E. R. Schlesinger, and R. E. L. Nesbitt, Jr. 1968. *Infant, Perinatal, Maternal, and Childhood Mortality in the United States*. Cambridge, Mass.: Harvard University Press.

7

INTRAUTERINE GROWTH

INTRODUCTION

Both the risk of neonatal death and the long-range outcome of survivors are strongly influenced by weight at birth, which in turn is intimately related to the gestational age of the fetus at delivery. Therefore, a description of these characteristics as they pertain to the study population is basic to the evaluation of all other clinical observations. The weight of the infant at birth in conjunction with the duration of gestation at the time of delivery provides an assessment of intrauterine growth. However, estimations of fetal growth obtained in this fashion must be interpreted with caution, as the weights of infants delivered at a given time in gestation are not necessarily representative of the fetuses remaining in utero at that same gestational age (1,2).

COLLECTION OF DATA

For this study, gestational age was the elapsed time between the first day of the last menstrual period (LMP) reported by the woman and the date of delivery. Information pertaining to gestational age has well-recognized shortcomings, the most notable being the difficulty in establishing an exact date for the onset of the LMP. This date depends upon the gravida's recollection of the date of onset of the LMP prior to the onset of pregnancy; this date may not be accurately remembered or, in fact, may not be clearly known or discernible. For example, postconceptual bleeding during the early months of pregnancy may be mistaken for a menstrual period. Pregnancy may sometimes recur without intervening menstruation. From the LMP and the date of birth, the gestation was calculated knowing full well that variations in the length of the menstrual cycle, time of ovulation, and conception further complicate the matter.

In the NCPP, the date of the LMP was ascertained at the time of prenatal registration by a specially trained interviewer (without administrative responsibility for patient care), who recorded not only the date of the LMP but also the date of onset of the period preceding the LMP. A systematic inquiry was made about the nature of the LMP. Information pertaining to the LMP was also independently collected by the hospital staff and by the obstetrician, who in addition was required to provide an estimate, based on physical findings and history, of the duration of pregnancy, this estimate being reevaluated at each prenatal visit. Furthermore, after the termination of pregnancy, the study obstetrician, reviewing the hospital and study records, made note of any inconsistencies in the data, though previously recorded dates were maintained.

The results of a careful attempt to assess the reliability of the gestational age data gathered from the black sample (which is lower and lower-middle class) in the Johns Hopkins Collaborative Study have been reported by Cushner and Mellits (3). They concluded that, in spite of the problems mentioned above, when carefully collected, the LMP data in this study are reliable and useful.

The *birthweight* was obtained within one hour of delivery by the NCPP observer of labor and delivery, using calibrated scales.

The sources of the data presented here was the date of onset of the LMP as recorded at the *initial* study interview (Form OB–4) and the date of birth (Form PED–1). The duration of gestation was computed in days from the onset of the LMP to delivery, then transposed to weeks, rounded to the nearest week. No attempt was made to correct or adjust gestational age, even in the rare instance where the data seemed incompatible, for example, when an infant of twenty-five weeks reported gestation weighed 4000 grams. However, in this report those gestations of less than twenty or more than fifty weeks were included with unknown gestations.

DISTRIBUTIONS OF GESTATIONAL AGE

The data presented in this section display the percent distribution of duration of gestation, by week, and the mean gestation for each race, for each institution, separately. Tables 7–1 through 7–3 and Figure 7–1 show the data, in addition, by sex, for each race and institution.

It is of considerable interest and importance to note that the gestational age distributions for white and black liveborn infants were quite dissimilar. The curve for black infants indicated generally shorter periods of gestation for blacks. The validity of this observation was substantiated by the finding that the average period of gestation for black infants was 38.8 weeks, as compared with 40.1 weeks for white infants; a difference of 1.3 weeks (approximately 9 days). When examined by institution, the difference in mean gestational age was consistently longer for whites than for blacks in those institutions with a sufficient sample size to permit a comparison. The substantial difference in average length of gestation between the two races has important implications and, as was demonstrated by an analysis of data from the Johns Hopkins Collaborative Study (4), undoubtedly contributes in a major way to the observed difference between the two races in average birthweight.

Table 7-1. Gestation at Delivery by Race

Gestation (wk)	WHITE Livebirths with Known Birthweight	Percent	Cumulative Percent	BLACK Livebirths with Known Birthweight	Percent	Cumulative Percent
Under 25	35	0.2	0.2	81	0.4	0.4
25	11	0.1	0.3	50	0.3	0.7
26	25	0.1	0.4	77	0.4	1.1
27	31	0.2	0.6	59	0.3	1.4
28	26	0.1	0.7	90	0.5	1.9
29	36	0.2	0.9	105	0.5	2.4
30	41	0.2	1.1	136	0.7	3.1
31	51	0.3	1.4	198	1.0	4.1
32	79	0.4	1.8	287	1.5	5.6
33	113	0.6	2.4	291	1.5	7.1
34	175	1.0	3.4	506	2.6	9.7
35	254	1.4	4.8	710	3.7	13.4
36	424	2.3	7.1	850	4.4	17.8
37	711	3.8	10.9	1210	6.3	24.1
38	1292	7.0	17.9	2000	10.3	34.4
39	2662	14.5	32.4	3180	16.4	50.8
40	4074	22.2	54.6	3602	18.6	69.4
41	3835	20.9	75.5	2671	13.8	83.2
42	2300	12.5	88.0	1446	7.5	90.7
43	1043	5.7	93.7	667	3.4	94.1
44	474	2.6	96.3	473	2.4	96.5
45	283	1.5	97.8	264	1.4	97.9
46	171	0.9	98.7	169	0.9	98.8
47	102	0.6	99.3	90	0.5	99.3
48	58	0.3	99.6	54	0.3	99.6
49	36	0.2	99.8	41	0.2	99.8
50	31	0.2	100.0	39	0.2	100.0
Total	18373	100.0		19346	100.0	
Unknown	108	0.6		158	0.8	
Grand total	18481	100.0		19504	100.0	

Updated from: *The Women and Their Pregnancies,* p. 50.

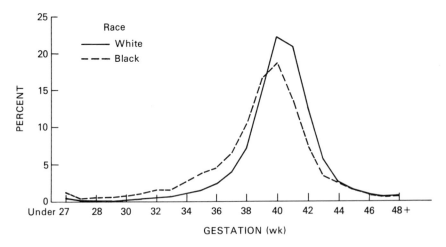

Updated from: *The Women and Their Pregnancies,* p. 50.

Figure 7-1. Gestation at Delivery by Race

Table 7-2. Mean Gestation at Delivery by Institution by Sex — White

| Institution | Male | | Female | | Unknown Sex | Total | |
	Livebirths with Known Gestation	Mean Gestation	Livebirths with Known Gestation	Mean Gestation	Livebirths with Known Gestation	Livebirths with Known Gestation	Mean Gestation
BO	3967	39.9	3582	40.0	18	7567	40.0
BU	953	40.0	909	40.1	0	1862	40.1
CH	0	-	0	-	0	0	-
CO	318	39.7	270	40.1	0	588	39.9
JH	337	39.7	314	39.7	2	653	39.7
VA	359	39.9	355	40.4	1	715	40.2
MN	1351	40.1	1199	40.3	1	2551	40.3
NY	128	39.6	121	39.4	0	249	39.5
OR	919	40.4	901	40.4	25	1845	40.4
PA	352	39.8	347	39.3	5	704	39.5
PR	863	39.8	855	40.3	0	1718	40.0
TN	11	37.1	10	40.1	0	21	38.5
Total	9558	40.0	8863	40.1	52	18473	40.1

Table 7-3. Mean Gestation at Delivery by Institution by Sex — Black

| Institution | Male | | Female | | Unknown Sex | Total | |
	Livebirths with Known Gestation	Mean Gestation	Livebirths with Known Gestation	Mean Gestation	Livebirths with Known Gestation	Livebirths with Known Gestation	Mean Gestation
BO	434	39.0	448	39.4	1	883	39.3
BU	24	39.2	23	39.1	0	47	39.2
CH	1151	38.8	1162	39.0	0	2313	38.9
CO	424	38.9	393	39.0	1	818	39.0
JH	1045	38.5	1077	39.0	2	2124	38.8
VA	909	38.9	857	39.1	1	1767	38.9
MN	6	38.1	9	39.8	0	15	39.2
NY	710	38.8	706	39.0	4	1420	38.9
OR	296	39.2	282	39.7	4	582	39.4
PA	2964	38.6	2968	38.6	15	5947	38.6
PR	232	39.2	246	39.4	1	479	39.3
TN	1559	38.9	1573	38.8	0	3132	38.9
Total	9754	38.8	9744	38.9	29	19527	38.8

As little difference between males and females was noted in gestational age, only 0.1 weeks, or less than one day on the average, gestational age cannot be a major factor in the average birthweight difference between the two sexes.

BIRTHWEIGHT

The *percentage distribution of birthweight* in 500-gram increments and the cumulative percentages are shown for each race and sex. The percentage distributions of birthweight observed by race were unimodal and, as expected, the curve for black infants indicates generally lower birthweights for black babies. The average birthweight for the two races differed by 233 grams. (Fig. 7–2 and Tables 7–4 and 7–5.)

Table 7-4. Birthweight by Sex — White

Birthweight (gm)	Male			Female			Total*		
	Livebirths with Known Birthweight	Percent	Cumulative Percent	Livebirths with Known Birthweight	Percent	Cumulative Percent	Livebirths with Known Birthweight	Percent	Cumulative Percent
Under 501	2	0.02	0.02	0	0	0	2	0.01	0.01
501–1000	29	0.30	0.32	30	0.34	0.34	59	0.32	0.33
1001–1500	58	0.61	0.93	23	0.26	0.60	81	0.44	0.77
1501–2000	106	1.11	2.04	112	1.26	1.86	223	1.21	1.98
2001–2500	397	4.14	6.18	557	6.27	8.13	954	5.16	7.14
2501–3000	1613	16.84	23.02	2039	22.96	31.09	3653	19.77	26.90
3001–3500	3758	39.24	62.26	3655	41.16	72.25	7424	40.17	67.07
3501–4000	2755	28.76	91.02	1980	22.30	94.55	4738	25.64	92.71
4001–4500	720	7.52	98.54	433	4.88	99.43	1155	6.25	98.96
4501+	140	1.46	100.00	51	0.57	100.00	192	1.04	100.00
Total	9578	100.00		8880	100.00		18481	100.00	

*Includes unknown sex.

Table 7-5. Birthweight by Sex — Black

Birthweight (gm)	Male			Female			Total*		
	Livebirths with Known Birthweight	Percent	Cumulative Percent	Livebirths with Known Birthweight	Percent	Cumulative Percent	Livebirths with Known Birthweight	Percent	Cumulative Percent
Under 501	6	0.06	0.06	7	0.07	0.07	14	0.07	0.07
501–1000	45	0.46	0.52	60	0.62	0.69	105	0.54	0.61
1001–1500	110	1.13	1.65	93	0.96	1.64	203	1.04	1.65
1501–2000	203	2.08	3.73	237	2.43	4.08	440	2.26	3.91
2001–2500	811	8.31	12.04	1044	10.72	14.80	1855	9.51	13.42
2501–3000	2566	26.29	38.33	3248	33.35	48.15	5817	29.82	43.24
3001–3500	3958	40.55	78.88	3671	37.70	85.85	7629	39.12	82.36
3501–4000	1708	17.50	96.37	1177	12.09	97.94	2886	14.80	97.15
4001–4500	299	3.06	99.44	168	1.73	99.66	467	2.39	99.55
4501+	55	0.56	100.00	33	0.34	100.00	88	0.45	100.00
Total	9761	100.00		9738	100.00		19504	100.00	

*Includes unknown sex.

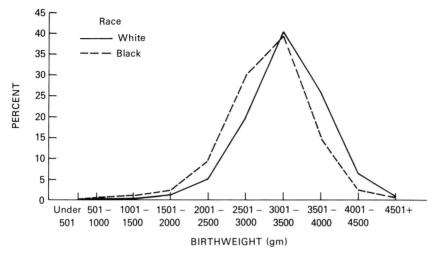

Figure 7-2. Birthweight by Race

Table 7-6. Birthweights Under 2501 gm by Institution by Race

	WHITE			BLACK		
	Livebirths with Known Birthweight	Birthweights Under 2501 gm	Rate	Livebirths with Known Birthweight	Birthweights Under 2501 gm	Rate
Total	18481	1319	71.37	19504	2617	134.18
BO	7588	544	71.69	882	100	114.38
BU	1862	89	47.80	48	2	41.67
CH	0	0	—	2320	292	125.86
CO	588	40	68.03	820	100	121.95
JH	654	76	116.21	2126	327	153.81
VA	716	50	69.83	1780	225	126.40
MN	2548	151	59.26	16	2	125.00*
NY	245	27	110.20	1392	188	135.05
OR	1832	131	71.51	576	50	86.81
PA	695	57	82.01	5934	830	139.87
PR	1732	150	86.61	485	74	152.58
TN	21	4	190.48	3125	427	136.64

Source: *The Women and Their Pregnancies,* p. 46.
*Based on less than 20 cases.

The term "low birthweight" designates those infants weighing less than 2501 grams or 5.5 pounds at birth. The rate of "low birthweight" per 1000 livebirths, observed in this study, was 71.37 for the white and 134.18 for the black babies. Where the number of cases permitted evaluation, the rates for whites varied considerably by institution, from a low of 47.80 at the University of Buffalo to a high of 116.21 at Johns Hopkins. The rate of 71.37 (7.1 percent) of low birthweight for whites compares quite closely with that of 6.7 percent observed in the British Perinatal Study (5) and in the study of Shapiro et al. (6). The rates for blacks ranged from a low of 86.81 to a high of 153.81. The variations in the distributions

Table 7-7. Mean Birthweight by Institution by Sex — White

Institution	Male		Female		Unknown Sex	Total	
	Livebirths with Known Birthweight	Mean Birthweight	Livebirths with Known Birthweight	Mean Birthweight	Livebirths with Known Birthweight	Livebirths with Known Birthweight	Mean Birthweight
BO	3986	3333	3594	3212	8	7588	3277
BU	958	3347	904	3240	0	1862	3300
CH	0	–	0	–	0	0	–
CO	318	3321	270	3224	0	588	3276
JH	339	3174	315	3112	0	654	3144
VA	361	3334	354	3233	1	716	3285
MN	1346	3364	1202	3254	0	2548	3312
NY	125	3312	120	3092	0	245	3204
OR	916	3330	902	3221	14	1832	3278
PA	352	3319	343	3127	0	695	3232
PR	866	3283	866	3164	0	1732	3224
TN	11	2773	10	3042	0	21	2901
Total	9578	3327	8880	3209	23	18481	3272

of maternal characteristics with recognized effect on birthweight, such as socio-economic status, maternal age and parity, prepregnant weight and weight gained during pregnancy, and complications of pregnancy and delivery, probably account for much of the institutional variability in birthweight. (Table 7–6.)

The *mean birthweight* for the 18,481 white infants was 3272 grams, 233 grams greater than the average of 3039 grams observed for the 19,504 black infants. Within each racial group, the male babies weighed more than the female; white males 3327 grams compared to 3209 grams for the white females, a difference of 118 grams. The black males weighed, on the average, 3093 grams and the black females 2980 grams, a difference of 113 grams. These race and sex relationships were consistent by institution, but the magnitude of the difference between males and females, within race, differed from 220 grams between white males and females at the New York Medical College to a low of 62 grams at Johns Hopkins. (Tables 7–7 and 7–8.)

BIRTHWEIGHT-GESTATIONAL AGE RELATIONSHIPS

The graphs and tables display the gestational age-birthweight relationships observed, for male and female, white and black infants. The information presented is reported as collected, no adjustments or exclusions have been made. The means, where shown, were computed from the individual observations, not grouped data.

Birthweight at Each Week of Gestation

The distributions of white and black infants by weight and gestational age at delivery are shown in Figure 7–3 and Table 7–9.

The graph showing the mean birthweight, of whites and blacks, observed at each week of gestation is of particular interest. Only 102 liveborn white infants were

Table 7-8. Mean Birthweight by Institution by Sex — Black

Institution	Male Livebirths with Known Birthweight	Male Mean Birthweight	Female Livebirths with Known Birthweight	Female Mean Birthweight	Unknown Sex Livebirths with Known Birthweight	Total Livebirths with Known Birthweight	Total Mean Birthweight
BO	434	3165	448	3097	0	882	3131
BU	25	3252	23	3149	0	48	3203
CH	1158	3125	1162	3035	0	2320	3080
CO	427	3114	393	3056	0	820	3090
JH	1050	3010	1076	2951	0	2126	2982
VA	916	3120	863	2983	1	1780	3054
MN	6	2816	10	3283	0	16	3108
NY	696	3073	695	2982	1	1392	3027
OR	297	3218	278	3087	1	576	3159
PA	2965	3103	2967	2949	2	5934	3034
PR	235	3121	250	2947	0	485	3031
TN	1552	3043	1573	2943	0	3125	2994
Total	9761	3093	9738	2980	5	19504	3039

Table 7-9. Mean Birthweight by Gestation at Delivery by Race

Gestation (wk)	WHITE Livebirths with Known Birthweight	WHITE Mean Birthweight	BLACK Livebirths with Known Birthweight	BLACK Mean Birthweight
Under 25	35	1856	81	1739
25	11	1598	50	2026
26	25	1508	77	2058
27	31	1546	59	2206
28	26	1713	90	2117
29	36	2314	105	2337
30	41	2100	136	2252
31	51	2256	198	2616
32	79	2285	287	2533
33	113	2492	291	2572
34	175	2534	506	2671
35	254	2760	710	2773
36	424	2892	850	2847
37	711	2943	1210	2897
38	1292	3040	2000	2959
39	2662	3195	3180	3072
40	4074	3315	3602	3163
41	3835	3420	2671	3261
42	2300	3481	1446	3269
43	1043	3486	667	3230
44	474	3445	473	3215
45	283	3450	264	3239
46	171	3441	169	3183
47	102	3391	90	3210
48	58	3409	54	3130
49	36	3442	41	3258
50	31	3291	39	3076
Total	18373	3271	19346	3038
Unknown	108	3442	158	3180
Grand total	18481	3272	19504	3039

Updated from: *The Women and Their Pregnancies*, p. 50.

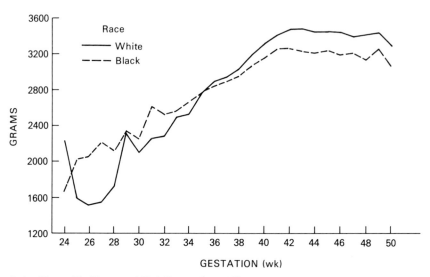

Updated from: *The Women and Their Pregnancies*, p. 50.

Figure 7-3. Mean Birthweight by Gestation at Delivery by Race

reported to be of 20 to 27 weeks gestation and only 35 of these were of 24 weeks or less. Below 30 weeks, the mean birthweight fluctuates considerably for each gestational age, probably reflecting, in large part, the small number of cases at each week and misreporting of gestational age. Above 29 weeks there was a steady increase in birthweight with increasing gestational age until the 42nd week, when the curves level off. It is of interest that the birthweight of white infants, on the average, was less than black infants at each week of gestation until the 35th. However, from the 36th week until the 42nd week, the mean for the white infants increased at a more rapid rate than that for blacks, so that at 42 weeks the white infants weighed in excess of 200 grams more than the blacks. This apparent acceleration in weight gain helped to accentuate the birthweight difference, as did the generally longer gestations observed in white infants. Similar differences, between white and black children, in weight at different gestational ages, were also observed in the Johns Hopkins cases (4).

Percentiles of Birthweight by Gestational Age

The data presented in Figures 7–4 through 7–7 and Tables 7–10 through 7–13 display the percentile distributions of birthweight for males and females, by race, by week of gestation between 30 and 45 weeks and above. Because of relatively small sample size for the early weeks of gestation, the data are not shown below 30 weeks.

There is a broad spread between the 10th and 90th percentiles of weight at 30 weeks, from 1890 grams for white females (1540–3430) to 2240 for white males (1080–3320). The spread at 42-weeks gestation is less, 1223 grams for white males (2966–4189) and 1178 grams for black males (2743–3921). The wide

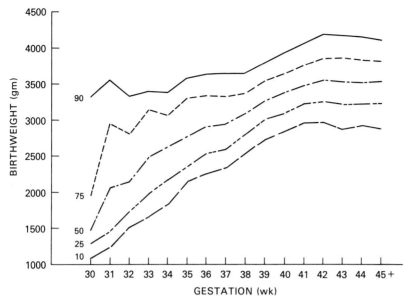

Figure 7-4. Percentiles of Birthweight by Gestation — White Male

Table 7-10. Selected Percentiles of Birthweight
by Gestation at Delivery — White Male

Gestation at Delivery (wk)	Livebirths with Known Birthweight	Percentile				
		10	25	50	75	90
30	24	1080	1286	1480	1950	3320
31	27	1235	1450	2050	2950	3553
32	43	1510	1725	2140	2813	3335
33	60	1650	1971	2480	3143	3400
34	86	1820	2166	2623	3063	3385
35	142	2138	2348	2771	3300	3586
36	245	2250	2529	2906	3340	3642
37	399	2329	2591	2945	3330	3651
38	681	2526	2791	3086	3374	3652
39	1430	2722	3009	3269	3546	3789
40	2162	2840	3096	3386	3647	3933
41	1889	2957	3225	3481	3767	4060
42	1134	2966	3260	3554	3860	4189
43	524	2867	3215	3530	3867	4170
44	259	2916	3224	3519	3832	4153
45+	339	2869	3230	3535	3816	4106

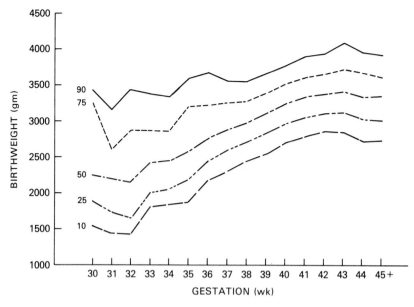

Figure 7-5. Percentiles of Birthweight by Gestation — White Female

Table 7-11. Selected Percentiles of Birthweight
by Gestation at Delivery — White Female

Gestation at Delivery (wk)	Livebirths with Known Birthweight	Percentile				
		10	25	50	75	90
30	17	1540	1883	2250	3250	3430
31	24	1440	1733	2200	2600	3160
32	36	1424	1650	2150	2867	3440
33	53	1808	2006	2415	2870	3380
34	89	1845	2050	2442	2861	3340
35	112	1871	2183	2585	3200	3595
36	179	2180	2441	2773	3221	3675
37	312	2302	2600	2889	3260	3561
38	610	2448	2707	2984	3278	3554
39	1229	2544	2838	3121	3395	3672
40	1909	2710	2971	3250	3532	3780
41	1943	2795	3056	3352	3623	3908
42	1164	2861	3109	3384	3663	3947
43	519	2846	3122	3417	3729	4097
44	215	2731	3023	3336	3679	3959
45+	340	2745	3014	3353	3611	3925

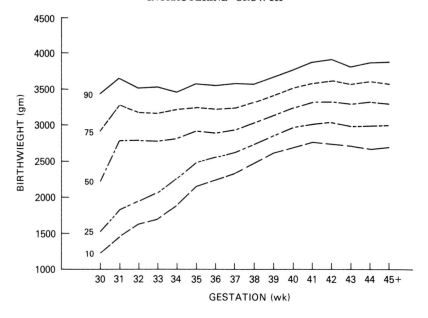

Figure 7-6. Percentiles of Birthweight by Gestation — Black Male

Table 7-12. Selected Percentiles of Birthweight by Gestation at Delivery — Black Male

Gestation at Delivery (wk)	Livebirths with Known Birthweight	Percentile				
		10	25	50	75	90
30	65	1225	1525	2220	2917	3434
31	107	1449	1819	2783	3277	3652
32	147	1629	1944	2787	3173	3515
33	152	1693	2057	2777	3160	3526
34	289	1882	2259	2814	3218	3457
35	340	2150	2483	2918	3246	3568
36	432	2237	2560	2895	3222	3551
37	615	2325	2625	2934	3237	3583
38	1018	2471	2733	3031	3317	3572
39	1632	2614	2854	3137	3415	3672
40	1735	2692	2963	3243	3525	3773
41	1315	2760	3013	3325	3592	3885
42	711	2743	3035	3330	3621	3921
43	331	2712	2984	3296	3569	3817
44	236	2670	2984	3328	3614	3878
45+	322	2698	3006	3296	3581	3885

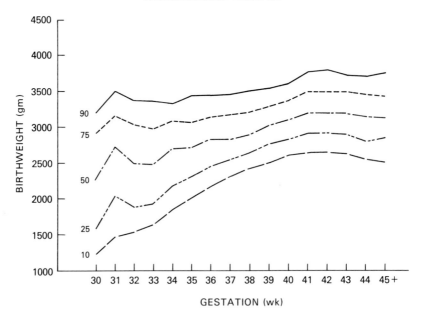

Figure 7-7. Percentiles of Birthweight by Gestation — Black Female

Table 7-13. Selected Percentiles of Birthweight
by Gestation at Delivery — Black Female

Gestation at Delivery (wk)	Livebirths with Known Birthweight	Percentile				
		10	25	50	75	90
30	71	1225	1583	2272	2912	3197
31	91	1469	2038	2722	3154	3498
32	140	1533	1892	2495	3031	3366
33	139	1635	1930	2475	2967	3362
34	217	1844	2175	2700	3080	3325
35	370	2000	2302	2712	3061	3440
36	417	2164	2452	2827	3135	3439
37	594	2307	2543	2825	3168	3451
38	982	2422	2635	2895	3203	3502
39	1548	2492	2760	3017	3285	3534
40	1867	2604	2826	3099	3370	3601
41	1355	2642	2912	3197	3495	3759
42	734	2646	2914	3194	3485	3787
43	336	2624	2894	3190	3487	3714
44	237	2547	2795	3142	3447	3698
45+	335	2508	2843	3119	3420	3744

spread at the lower gestations reflects the inclusion of the babies who are large for their stated gestational age. While some of these represent larger than expected infants, who have had true acceleration of growth, others were undoubtedly misclassified as the result of inaccurate gestational age. However, data from The Johns Hopkins Collaborative Study suggested that the group of babies large for gestational age included some who were of short gestations, and that as a group the "large for dates" babies had a less favorable outcome than babies of similar weight born at 38-weeks gestation (4).

Birthweight-gestational age relationships, the prenatal factors that influence them, their concomitants in terms of placental weight, body length, and other findings during the neonatal period, and their relationship to the subsequent outcome for the child are the subject of a detailed investigation of the data, the results of which will be published in monograph form.

GESTATION, BIRTHWEIGHT, AND MORTALITY

Stillbirths

Among the 18,779 singleborn white infants with known birthweight there were 298 stillbirths, for an overall rate of 15.87 per 1000 births; among the 19,877 blacks there were 373 stillbirths, a rate of 18.77. In whites, the rate of 15.74 for females was slightly greater than that of 14.81 for males. In blacks, the relationship was reversed with a rate of 16.07 for the females and 19.29 for males. These rates are not essentially different by sex. The stillbirth rates observed for whites in the gestational age groups below 39 weeks were appreciably higher than those for blacks; however, the rates for blacks at gestations of 40 to 42 weeks and 43 weeks and above were higher as compared with the whites.

The curves showing the relationship between stillbirth rates and birthweight are similar in shape to those showing the relationship between stillbirth rates and gestational age at delivery. For infants of both races, the risk of stillbirth is greatest at low birthweights and progressively decreases with increasing weight to about 3500 grams. The rates for white infants are higher than those for blacks up to 3000 grams. Above this point, the rates for black infants are higher than those for whites. While the stillbirth rate for infants weighing over 3000 grams was lower than the rates for smaller babies, the deaths among the large number of infants weighing over 3000 grams accounts for the larger overall number of stillbirths among blacks as compared with whites. (Figs. 7–8 and 7–9 and Tables 7–14 through 7–19.)

Neonatal Deaths

There were 223 neonatal deaths recorded among the 18,481 white, singleborn infants, giving a rate of 12.07 per 1000 liveborn. There were 336 neonatal deaths among the 19,504 blacks, a rate of 17.23. The neonatal death rate among males was higher than that for females of the same race; for white males it was 13.78; white females 10.25; black males 18.75, and black females 15.61.

Table 7-14. Stillbirths by Gestation at Delivery by Race

	WHITE			BLACK		
Gestation (wk)	Births with Known Birthweight	Stillbirths	Rate	Births with Known Birthweight	Stillbirths	Rate
Under 34	576	128	222.22	1555	181	116.40
34–36	895	42	46.93	2113	47	22.24
37–39	4723	58	12.28	6453	63	9.76
40–42	10253	44	4.29	7769	50	6.44
43+	2221	23	10.36	1827	30	16.42
Total	18668	295	15.80	19717	371	18.82
Unknown	111	3	27.03	160	2	12.50
Grand total	18779	298	15.87	19877	373	18.77

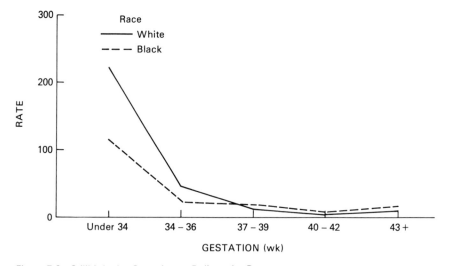

Figure 7-8. Stillbirths by Gestation at Delivery by Race

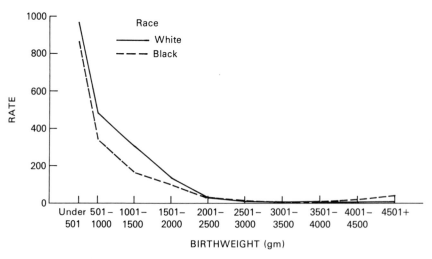

Figure 7-9. Stillbirths by Birthweight by Race

Table 7-15. Stillbirths by Gestation at Delivery by Sex — White

Gestation (wk)	Male			Female		
	Births with Known Birthweight	Stillbirths	Rate	Births with Known Birthweight	Stillbirths	Rate
Under 34	301	64	212.62	255	52	203.92
34–36	487	14	28.75	408	28	68.63
37–39	2544	34	13.36	2175	24	11.03
40–42	5206	21	4.03	5039	23	4.56
43+	1132	10	8.83	1087	13	11.96
Total	9670	143	14.79	8964	140	15.62
Unknown	52	1	19.23	58	2	34.48
Grand total	9722	144	14.81	9022	142	15.74

Table 7-16. Stillbirths by Gestation at Delivery by Sex — Black

Gestation (wk)	Male			Female		
	Births with Known Birthweight	Stillbirths	Rate	Births with Known Birthweight	Stillbirths	Rate
Under 34	802	92	114.71	733	69	94.13
34–36	1082	21	19.41	1029	25	24.30
37–39	3294	29	8.80	3158	34	10.77
40–42	3787	26	6.87	3980	24	6.03
43+	912	23	25.22	914	6	6.56
Total	9877	191	19.34	9814	158	16.10
Unknown	76	1	13.16	83	1	12.05
Grand total	9953	192	19.29	9897	159	16.07

Table 7-17. Stillbirths by Birthweight by Race

Birthweight (gm)	WHITE			BLACK		
	Births with Known Birthweight	Stillbirths	Rate	Births with Known Birthweight	Stillbirths	Rate
Under 501	65	63	969.23	103	89	864.08
501–1000	114	55	482.46	160	55	343.75
1001–1500	116	35	301.72	243	40	164.61
1501–2000	258	35	135.66	488	48	98.36
2001–2500	983	29	29.50	1896	41	21.62
2501–3000	3688	35	9.49	5860	43	7.34
3001–3500	7448	24	3.22	7658	29	3.79
3501–4000	4758	20	4.20	2902	16	5.51
4001–4500	1157	2	1.73	475	8	16.84
4501+	192	0	0	92	4	43.48
Total	18779	298	15.87	19877	373	18.77

Table 7-18. Stillbirths by Birthweight by Sex — White

Birthweight (gm)	Male			Female		
	Births with Known Birthweight	Stillbirths	Rate	Births with Known Birthweight	Stillbirths	Rate
Under 501	26	24	923.08	28	28	1000.00
501–1000	60	31	516.67	54	24	444.44
1001–1500	75	17	226.67	40	17	425.00
1501–2000	118	12	101.69	135	23	170.37
2001–2500	411	14	34.06	572	15	26.22
2501–3000	1632	19	11.64	2055	16	7.79
3001–3500	3774	16	4.24	3663	8	2.18
3501–4000	2765	10	3.62	1990	10	5.03
4001–4500	721	1	1.39	434	1	2.30
4501+	140	0	0	51	0	0
Total	9722	144	14.81	9022	142	15.74

Table 7-19. Stillbirths by Birthweight by Sex — Black

Birthweight (gm)	Male			Female		
	Births with Known Birthweight	Stillbirths	Rate	Births with Known Birthweight	Stillbirths	Rate
Under 501	49	43	877.55	33	26	787.88
501–1000	68	23	338.24	91	31	340.66
1001–1500	133	23	172.93	110	17	154.55
1501–2000	227	24	105.73	260	23	88.46
2001–2500	831	20	24.07	1065	21	19.72
2501–3000	2592	26	10.03	3265	17	5.21
3001–3500	3977	19	4.78	3681	10	2.72
3501–4000	1715	7	4.08	1186	9	7.59
4001–4500	303	4	13.20	172	4	23.26
4501+	58	3	51.72	34	1	29.41
Total	9953	192	19.29	9897	159	16.07

As expected, when examined by *gestational age* at delivery, the risk of neonatal death was highest for the infants of shortest gestational age. The rate decreased progressively until 40 to 42 weeks for babies of both races and then increased slightly with longer gestations. At the early gestations, the rate for white babies was higher than for blacks, but at 40 weeks and longer the rate for blacks was higher. As large numbers of babies were delivered at 40 weeks and beyond, the net result was a higher overall rate of neonatal deaths observed in the black babies. For babies of both races, the males showed somewhat higher rates than the females, particularly at the shorter gestational ages.

Similar relationships were found between *birthweight* and risk of neonatal death, with highest rates for the smallest babies. Below 3000 grams the black babies had slightly lower rates than whites. (Figs. 7–10 and 7–11 and Tables 7–20 through 7–25.)

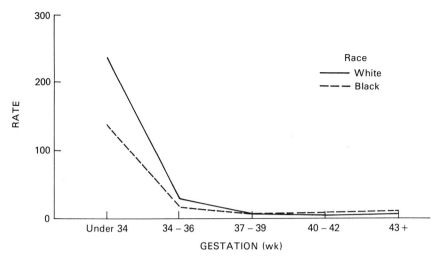

Figure 7-10. Neonatal Deaths by Gestation at Delivery by Race

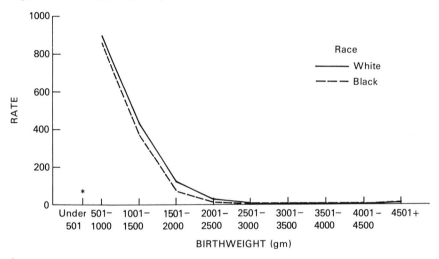

*Based on less than 20 cases.

Figure 7-11. Neonatal Deaths by Birthweight by Race

Table 7-20. Neonatal Deaths by Gestation at Delivery by Race

Gestation (wk)	WHITE			BLACK		
	Livebirths with Known Birthweight	Neonatal Deaths	Rate	Livebirths with Known Birthweight	Neonatal Deaths	Rate
Under 34	448	107	238.84	1374	189	137.55
34–36	853	26	30.48	2066	34	16.46
37–39	4665	32	6.86	6390	40	6.26
40–42	10209	38	3.72	7719	40	5.18
43+	2198	16	7.28	1797	18	10.02
Total	18373	219	11.92	19346	321	16.59
Unknown	108	4	37.04	158	15	94.94
Grand total	18481	223	12.07	19504	336	17.23

Table 7-21. Neonatal Deaths by Gestation at Delivery by Sex — White

Gestation (wk)	Male			Female		
	Livebirths with Known Birthweight	Neonatal Deaths	Rate	Livebirths with Known Birthweight	Neonatal Deaths	Rate
Under 34	237	66	278.48	203	41	201.97
34–36	473	13	27.48	380	13	34.21
37–39	2510	21	8.37	2151	11	5.11
40–42	5185	19	3.66	5016	19	3.79
43+	1122	10	8.91	1074	6	5.59
Total	9527	129	13.54	8824	90	10.20
Unknown	51	3	58.82	56	1	17.86
Grand total	9578	132	13.78	8880	91	10.25

Table 7-22. Neonatal Deaths by Gestation at Delivery by Sex — Black

Gestation (wk)	Male			Female		
	Livebirths with Known Birthweight	Neonatal Deaths	Rate	Livebirths with Known Birthweight	Neonatal Deaths	Rate
Under 34	710	101	142.25	664	88	132.53
34–36	1061	21	19.79	1004	13	12.95
37–39	3265	26	7.96	3124	14	4.48
40–42	3761	19	5.05	3956	21	5.31
43+	889	9	10.12	908	9	9.91
Total	9686	176	18.17	9656	145	15.02
Unknown	75	7	93.33	82	7	85.37
Grand total	9761	183	18.75	9738	152	15.61

Table 7-23. Neonatal Deaths by Birthweight by Race

Birthweight (gm)	WHITE			BLACK		
	Livebirths with Known Birthweight	Neonatal Deaths	Rate	Livebirths with Known Birthweight	Neonatal Deaths	Rate
Under 501	2	2	1000.00*	14	14	1000.00*
501–1000	59	53	898.31	105	90	857.14
1001–1500	81	35	432.10	203	76	374.38
1501–2000	223	27	121.08	440	32	72.73
2001–2500	954	30	31.45	1855	26	14.02
2501–3000	3653	31	8.49	5817	41	7.05
3001–3500	7424	27	3.64	7629	41	5.37
3501–4000	4738	11	2.32	2886	13	4.50
4001–4500	1155	6	5.19	467	2	4.28
4501+	192	1	5.21	88	1	11.36
Total	18481	223	12.07	19504	336	17.23

*Based on less than 20 cases.

Table 7-24. Neonatal Deaths by Birthweight by Sex — White

Birthweight (gm)	Male			Female		
	Livebirths with Known Birthweight	Neonatal Deaths	Rate	Livebirths with Known Birthweight	Neonatal Deaths	Rate
Under 501	2	2	1000.00*	0	0	–
501–1000	29	25	862.07	30	28	933.33
1001–1500	58	28	482.76	23	7	304.35
1501–2000	106	20	188.68	112	7	62.50
2001–2500	397	11	27.71	557	19	34.11
2501–3000	1613	15	9.30	2039	16	7.85
3001–3500	3758	18	4.79	3655	9	2.46
3501–4000	2755	7	2.54	1980	4	2.02
4001–4500	720	5	6.94	433	1	2.31
4501+	140	1	7.14	51	0	0
Total	9578	132	13.78	8880	91	10.25

*Based on less than 20 cases.

Table 7-25. Neonatal Deaths by Birthweight by Sex — Black

Birthweight (gm)	Male			Female		
	Livebirths with Known Birthweight	Neonatal Deaths	Rate	Livebirths with Known Birthweight	Neonatal Deaths	Rate
Under 501	6	6	1000.00*	7	7	1000.00*
501–1000	45	41	911.11	60	49	816.67
1001–1500	110	45	409.09	93	31	333.33
1501–2000	203	19	93.60	237	13	54.85
2001–2500	811	19	23.43	1044	7	6.70
2501–3000	2566	20	7.79	3248	21	6.47
3001–3500	3958	23	5.81	3671	18	4.90
3501–4000	1708	9	5.27	1177	4	3.40
4001–4500	299	1	3.34	168	1	5.95
4501+	55	0	0	33	1	30.30
Total	9761	183	18.75	9738	152	15.61

*Based on less than 20 cases.

Perinatal Death and Birthweight-Gestational Age Interactions

The data available from the large numbers of pregnancies in the study made possible the assessment of birthweight-gestational age interactions and their relationship to outcome. The use of birthweight alone (2500 grams and below) as the single criterion of prematurity has been traditional: however, greater accuracy in predicting various outcomes can be achieved by the addition of gestational age. Classification by both gestational age and birthweight can lead to better understanding of underlying physiological problems and thus to more appropriate clinical management.

Extensive studies of birthweight-gestational age relationships have emphasized the increased risks of mortality of the growth-retarded fetus ("small for dates")

Table 7-26. Perinatal Deaths by Birthweight
by Gestation at Delivery — White Male

| | Births with Known Birthweight | | | | | | | |
| | Gestation (wk) | | | | | | | |
Birthweight (gm)	Under 34	34–36	37–39	40–42	43+	Total	Unknown	Grand Total
Under 1001	80	4	1	0	0	85	1	86
1001–1500	53	10	6	3	1	73	2	75
1501–2000	44	29	35	6	4	118	0	118
2001–2500	37	115	158	83	18	411	0	411
2501–3000	31	142	666	645	142	1626	6	1632
3001–3500	37	124	1104	2121	370	3756	18	3774
3501–4000	13	51	489	1772	420	2745	20	2765
4001–4500	4	10	73	485	145	717	4	721
4501+	2	2	12	91	32	139	1	140
Total	301	487	2544	5206	1132	9670	52	9722
	Perinatal Deaths							
Under 1001	76	4	1	0	0	81	1	82
1001–1500	32	2	6	3	0	43	2	45
1501–2000	12	6	12	1	1	32	0	32
2001–2500	6	7	6	3	3	25	0	25
2501–3000	2	5	13	9	5	34	0	34
3001–3500	0	1	13	15	5	34	0	34
3501–4000	1	1	3	7	4	16	1	17
4001–4500	1	1	0	2	2	6	0	6
4501+	0	0	1	0	0	1	0	1
Total	130	27	55	40	20	272	4	276
	Rate							
Under 1001	950.00	1000.00*	1000.00	–	–	952.94	1000.00*	953.49
1001–1500	603.77	200.00*	1000.00	1000.00*	0 *	589.04	1000.00*	600.00
1501–2000	272.73	206.90	342.86	166.67*	250.00*	271.19	–	271.19
2001–2500	162.16	60.87	37.97	36.14	166.67*	60.83	–	60.83
2501–3000	64.52	35.21	19.52	13.95	35.21	20.91	0 *	20.83
3001–3500	0	8.06	11.78	7.07	13.51	9.05	0 *	9.01
3501–4000	76.92*	19.61	6.13	3.95	9.52	5.83	50.00	6.15
4001–4500	250.00*	100.00*	0	4.12	13.79	8.37	0 *	8.32
4501+	0 *	0 *	83.33*	0	0	7.19	0 *	7.14
Total	431.89	55.44	21.62	7.68	17.67	28.13	72.92	28.39

*Based on less than 20 cases.

(1,2,7). Data in the British Perinatal Study (8) showed that growth-retarded infants of between thirty-five and forty-one weeks gestation have a risk of mortality about six times greater than infants of appropriate weight for their gestational age.

Data pertaining to the possible effect of intrauterine growth on outcome are presented in this section in terms of rates of perinatal and neonatal death and neurological abnormality at one year. Perinatal deaths include both stillbirths and neonatal deaths. This grouping provides a larger base number and permits evaluation, for infants of each sex and race, of a larger number of birthweight-gestational age combinations than would be possible for either stillbirths or neonatal deaths separately. The results are presented in detail in Tables 7–26 through 7–29 and sum-

Table 7-27. Perinatal Deaths by Birthweight by Gestation at Delivery — White Female

Births with Known Birthweight

Birthweight (gm)	Gestation (wk)					Total	Unknown	Grand Total
	Under 34	34–36	37–39	40–42	43+			
Under 1001	70	8	2	0	1	81	1	82
1001–1500	25	12	1	1	0	39	1	40
1501–2000	37	48	30	17	3	135	0	135
2001–2500	39	112	223	156	42	572	0	572
2501–3000	41	114	741	959	185	2040	15	2055
3001–3500	31	63	840	2265	441	3640	23	3663
3501–4000	8	38	270	1351	306	1973	17	1990
4001–4500	4	13	65	260	91	433	1	434
4501+	0	0	3	30	18	51	0	51
Total	255	408	2175	5039	1087	8964	58	9022

Perinatal Deaths

Birthweight (gm)	Under 34	34–36	37–39	40–42	43+	Total	Unknown	Grand Total
Under 1001	69	8	1	0	1	79	1	80
1001–1500	11	11	1	0	0	23	1	24
1501–2000	6	8	9	7	0	30	0	30
2001–2500	5	7	8	8	6	34	0	34
2501–3000	2	4	10	14	2	32	0	32
3001–3500	0	3	0	7	6	16	1	17
3501–4000	0	0	4	6	4	14	0	14
4001–4500	0	0	2	0	0	2	0	2
4501+	0	0	0	0	0	0	0	0
Total	93	41	35	42	19	230	3	233

Rate

Birthweight (gm)	Under 34	34–36	37–39	40–42	43+	Total	Unknown	Grand Total
Under 1001	985.71	1000.00*	500.00*	–	1000.00*	975.31	1000.00*	975.61
1001–1500	440.00	916.67*	1000.00*	0 *	– *	589.74	1000.00*	600.00
1501–2000	162.16	166.67	300.00	411.76*	0 *	222.22	–	222.22
2001–2500	128.21	62.50	35.87	51.28	51.28	59.44	–	59.44
2501–3000	48.78	35.09	13.50	14.60	10.81	15.69	0 *	15.57
3001–3500	0	47.62	0	3.09	13.61	4.40	43.48	4.64
3501–4000	0 *	0	14.81	4.44	13.07	7.10	0 *	7.04
4001–4500	0 *	0 *	30.77	0	0	4.62	0 *	4.61
4501+	–	–	0 *	0	0 *	0	–	0
Total	364.71	100.49	16.09	8.33	17.48	25.66	51.72	25.83

*Based on less than 20 cases.

marized in three-dimensional graphs (Figs. 7–12 through 7–15). Small numbers of cases in the low gestations dictated combination of groups, and it should be noted that the data presented in the tables is in greater detail than that summarized in the graphs. The graphs for white and black infants of like sex resemble each other more closely than the graphs for boys and girls within each race. All four graphs for perinatal death show clearly that the smallest infants of lowest gestational ages (i.e., those of less than 2000 grams and 34-weeks gestation) have substantially greater risks of mortality than infants in any other group. It is also clear that, as expected, infants who are "small for dates" or growth-retarded (i.e., low birthweight for gestational age) have a greater risk of mortality than that ob-

Table 7-28. Perinatal Deaths by Birthweight by Gestation at Delivery — Black Male

Births with Known Birthweight

Birthweight (gm)	Gestation (wk)					Total	Unknown	Grand Total
	Under 34	34–36	37–39	40–42	43+			
Under 1001	106	4	1	0	0	111	6	117
1001–1500	102	22	6	1	1	132	1	133
1501–2000	116	60	30	11	6	223	4	227
2001–2500	113	226	312	134	38	823	8	831
2501–3000	129	333	1108	816	192	2578	14	2592
3001–3500	170	324	1337	1727	390	3948	29	3977
3501–4000	51	96	427	888	243	1705	10	1715
4001–4500	14	15	65	170	35	299	4	303
4501+	1	2	8	40	7	58	0	58
Total	802	1082	3294	3787	912	9877	76	9953

Perinatal Deaths

Birthweight (gm)	Under 34	34–36	37–39	40–42	43+	Total	Unknown	Grand Total
Under 1001	103	3	1	0	0	107	6	113
1001–1500	55	7	4	0	1	67	1	68
1501–2000	20	10	7	3	2	42	1	43
2001–2500	12	14	5	4	4	39	0	39
2501–3000	3	6	22	9	6	46	0	46
3001–3500	0	2	13	17	10	42	0	42
3501–4000	0	0	2	8	6	16	0	16
4001–4500	0	0	0	3	2	5	0	5
4501+	0	0	1	1	1	3	0	3
Total	193	42	55	45	32	367	8	375

Rate

Birthweight (gm)	Under 34	34–36	37–39	40–42	43+	Total	Unknown	Grand Total
Under 1001	971.70	750.00*	1000.00*	–	–	963.96	1000.00*	965.81
1001–1500	539.22	318.18	666.67*	0 *	1000.00*	507.58	1000.00*	511.28
1501–2000	172.41	166.67	233.33	272.73*	333.33*	188.34	250.00*	189.43
2001–2500	106.19	61.95	16.03	29.85	105.26	47.39	0 *	46.93
2501–3000	23.26	18.02	19.86	11.03	31.25	17.84	0 *	17.75
3001–3500	0	6.17	9.72	9.84	25.64	10.64	0	10.56
3501–4000	0	0	4.68	9.01	24.69	9.38	0 *	9.33
4001–4500	0 *	0 *	0	17.65	57.14	16.72	0 *	16.50
4501+	0 *	0 *	125.00*	25.00	142.86*	51.72	–	51.72
Total	240.65	38.82	16.70	11.88	35.09	37.16	105.26	37.68

*Based on less than 20 cases.

served for infants of the same gestational age but higher birthweight. The greater rate of mortality for the "large" infants of short gestational age is also evident, even though the degree of risk is considerably less than that for the small infant of comparably low gestational age.

The graphs demonstrating the risks of neonatal death observed in the white and black infants (sexes combined) show the stepwise progression in risks a little more emphatically than those, by sex, above. (Figs. 7–16 and 7–17 and Tables 7–30 and 7–31.)

Table 7-29. Perinatal Deaths by Birthweight
by Gestation at Delivery — Black Female

Births with Known Birthweight

Birthweight (gm)	Gestation (wk) Under 34	34–36	37–39	40–42	43+	Total	Unknown	Grand Total
Under 1001	106	8	4	2	0	120	4	124
1001–1500	77	17	7	6	2	109	1	110
1501–2000	107	79	42	23	8	259	1	260
2001–2500	120	259	399	211	66	1055	10	1065
2501–3000	155	351	1290	1172	260	3228	37	3265
3001–3500	131	248	1106	1788	388	3661	20	3681
3501–4000	32	59	272	656	157	1176	10	1186
4001–4500	3	7	33	103	26	172	0	172
4501+	2	1	5	19	7	34	0	34
Total	733	1029	3158	3980	914	9814	83	9897

Perinatal Deaths

Birthweight (gm)	Under 34	34–36	37–39	40–42	43+	Total	Unknown	Grand Total
Under 1001	97	8	3	1	0	109	4	113
1001–1500	37	6	2	1	1	47	1	48
1501–2000	15	10	6	3	2	36	0	36
2001–2500	2	8	8	7	2	27	1	28
2501–3000	3	5	12	13	4	37	1	38
3001–3500	3	1	8	12	4	28	0	28
3501–4000	0	0	4	6	2	12	1	13
4001–4500	0	0	3	2	0	5	0	5
4501+	0	0	2	0	0	2	0	2
Total	157	38	48	45	15	303	8	311

Rate

Birthweight (gm)	Under 34	34–36	37–39	40–42	43+	Total	Unknown	Grand Total
Under 1001	915.09	100.00*	750.00*	500.00*	–	908.33	1000.00*	911.29
1001–1500	480.52	352.94*	285.71*	166.67*	500.00*	431.19	1000.00*	436.36
1501–2000	140.19	126.58	142.88	130.43	250.00*	139.00	0 *	138.46
2001–2500	16.67	30.89	20.05	33.18	30.30	25.59	100.00*	26.29
2501–3000	19.35	14.25	9.30	11.09	15.38	11.46	27.03	11.64
3001–3500	22.90	4.03	7.23	6.71	10.31	7.65	0	7.61
3501–4000	0	0	14.71	9.15	12.74	10.20	100.00*	10.96
4001–4500	0 *	0 *	90.91	19.42	0 *	29.07	–	29.07
4501+	0 *	0 *	400.00*	0 *	0 *	58.82	–	58.82
Total	214.19	36.93	15.20	11.31	16.41	30.87	96.39	31.42

*Based on less than 20 cases.

BIRTHWEIGHT-GESTATIONAL AGE CATEGORY IN RELATION TO
ABNORMAL NEUROLOGICAL STATUS

The longer-range effects of patterns of intrauterine growth are presented in Tables 7–32 and 7–33 and in three-dimensional graphs (Figs. 7–18 and 7–19) relating the birthweight-gestational age category to the presence of definite neurological abnormalities at one year (see Chapter 14 for discussion of the one-year neurological examination). Again, similarity in the distribution of neurological abnormalities was observed in infants of both races, with the smallest infants displaying the highest rates of abnormalities per 1000 examinations. Among the white infants,

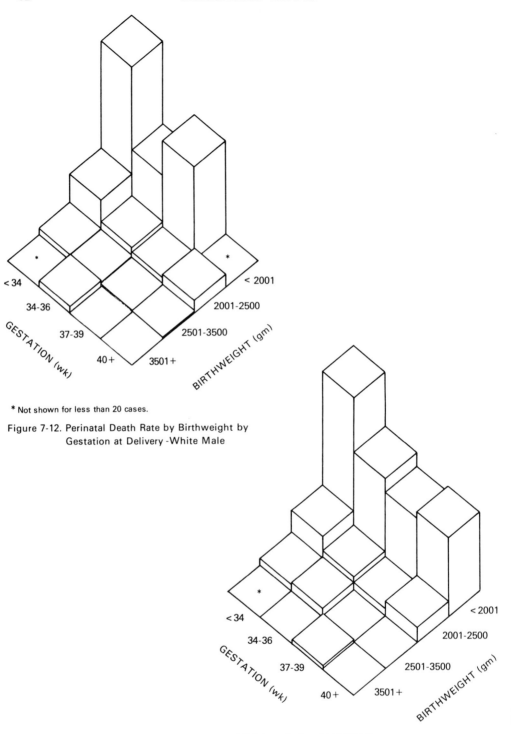

* Not shown for less than 20 cases.

Figure 7-12. Perinatal Death Rate by Birthweight by
        Gestation at Delivery -White Male

* Not shown for less than 20 cases.

Figure 7-13. Perinatal Death Rate by Birthweight by
        Gestation at Delivery-White Female

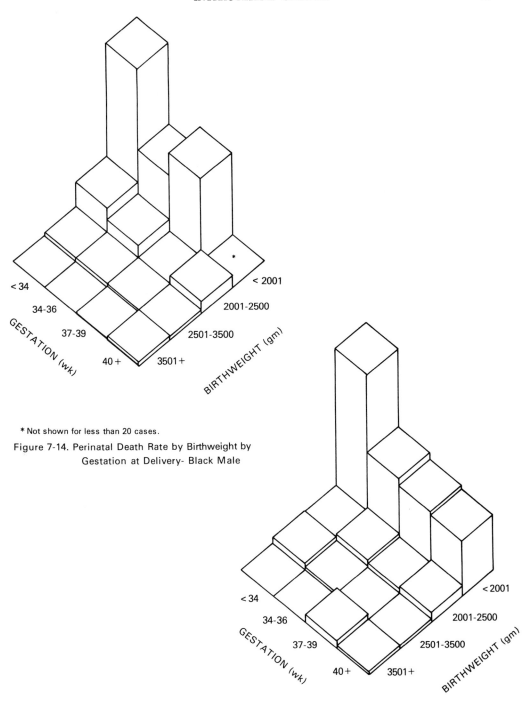

* Not shown for less than 20 cases.

Figure 7-14. Perinatal Death Rate by Birthweight by
Gestation at Delivery- Black Male

Figure 7-15. Perinatal Death Rate by Birthweight by
Gestation at Delivery-Black Female

Table 7-30. Neonatal Deaths by Birthweight by Gestation at Delivery — White

Livebirths with Known Birthweight

Birthweight (gm)	Gestation (wk)							
	Under 34	34–36	37–39	40–42	43+	Total	Unknown	Grand Total
Under 1001	59	1	1	0	0	61	0	61
1001–1500	63	11	2	1	1	78	3	81
1501–2000	82	66	50	18	7	223	0	223
2001–2500	74	224	374	230	52	954	0	954
2501–3000	69	252	1395	1593	323	3632	21	3653
3001–3500	71	186	1939	4380	807	7383	41	7424
3501–4000	20	88	752	3119	722	4701	37	4738
4001–4500	8	23	137	747	235	1150	5	1155
4501+	2	2	15	121	51	191	1	192
Total	448	853	4665	10209	2198	18373	108	18481

Neonatal Deaths

Birthweight (gm)	Under 34	34–36	37–39	40–42	43+	Total	Unknown	Grand Total
Under 1001	54	1	0	0	0	55	0	55
1001–1500	28	2	2	0	0	32	3	35
1501–2000	14	3	6	3	1	27	0	27
2001–2500	9	11	7	2	1	30	0	30
2501–3000	1	5	10	12	3	31	0	31
3001–3500	0	3	5	12	7	27	0	27
3501–4000	0	0	0	7	3	10	1	11
4001–4500	1	1	1	2	1	6	0	6
4501+	0	0	1	0	0	1	0	1
Total	107	26	32	38	16	219	4	223

Rate

Birthweight (gm)	Under 34	34–36	37–39	40–42	43+	Total	Unknown	Grand Total
Under 1001	915.25	1000.00*	0 *	–	–	901.64	–	901.64
1001–1500	444.44	181.82*	1000.00*	0 *	0 *	410.26	1000.00*	432.10
1501–2000	170.73	45.45	120.00	166.67*	142.86*	121.08	–	121.08
2001–2500	121.62	49.11	18.72	8.70	19.23	31.45	–	31.45
2501–3000	14.49	19.84	7.17	7.53	9.29	8.54	0	8.49
3001–3500	0	16.13	2.58	2.74	8.67	3.66	0	3.64
3501–4000	0	0	0	2.24	4.16	2.13	27.03	2.32
4001–4500	125.00*	43.48	7.30	2.68	4.26	5.22	0 *	5.19
4501+	0 *	0 *	66.67*	0	0	5.24	0 *	5.21
Total	238.84	30.48	6.86	3.72	7.28	11.92	37.04	12.07

*Based on less than 20 cases.

the growth-retarded infants (i.e., those below 2001 grams at 40+ weeks gestation) showed the highest rate of abnormality, while in the blacks, the smallest immature infants were at greatest risk. The "large" infants at low gestations showed only a minimally increased risk of abnormalities.

For each gestational age category, the highest risk of neurological abnormality was for those infants with the lowest birthweight. This relationship was similar to the relationship with perinatal mortality. However, when the data were examined by birthweight category, the babies over 2500 grams birthweight behaved as one might expect, with the lowest gestational age group having the highest neurological abnormality rate. Inversely, in the intermediate birthweight (2001–2500 grams)

Table 7-31. Neonatal Deaths by Birthweight
by Gestation at Delivery — Black

Livebirths with Known Birthweight

Birthweight (gm)	Gestation (wk)							
	Under 34	34–36	37–39	40–42	43+	Total	Unknown	Grand Total
Under 1001	100	6	1	1	0	108	11	119
1001–1500	152	32	10	6	1	201	2	203
1501–2000	208	127	62	28	11	436	4	440
2001–2500	230	472	699	338	98	1837	18	1855
2501–3000	281	678	2381	1979	447	5766	51	5817
3001–3500	300	571	2436	3501	772	7580	49	7629
3501–4000	83	155	695	1538	396	2867	19	2886
4001–4500	17	22	95	270	59	463	4	467
4501+	3	3	11	58	13	88	0	88
Total	1374	2066	6390	7719	1797	19346	158	19504

Neonatal Deaths

Birthweight (gm)	Under 34	34–36	37–39	40–42	43+	Total	Unknown	Grand Total
Under 1001	88	5	0	0	0	93	11	104
1001–1500	65	6	3	0	0	74	2	76
1501–2000	20	8	3	0	1	32	0	32
2001–2500	11	9	1	4	0	25	1	26
2501–3000	3	4	16	12	5	40	1	41
3001–3500	2	2	14	15	8	41	0	41
3501–4000	0	0	2	7	4	13	0	13
4001–4500	0	0	0	2	0	2	0	2
4501+	0	0	1	0	0	1	0	1
Total	189	34	40	40	18	321	15	336

Rate

Birthweight (gm)	Under 34	34–36	37–39	40–42	43+	Total	Unknown	Grand Total
Under 1001	880.00	833.33*	0 *	0 *	—	861.11	1000.00*	873.95
1001–1500	427.63	187.50	300.00*	0 *	0 *	368.16	1000.00*	374.38
1501–2000	96.15	62.99	48.39	0	90.91*	73.39	—	72.73
2001–2500	47.83	19.07	1.43	11.83	0	13.61	55.55	14.02
2501–3000	10.68	5.90	6.72	6.06	11.19	6.94	19.61	7.05
3001–3500	6.67	3.50	5.75	4.28	10.36	5.41	0	5.37
3501–4000	0	0	2.88	4.55	10.10	4.53	0 *	4.50
4001–4500	0	0	0	7.41	0	4.32	0 *	4.28
4501+	0 *	0 *	90.91*	0	0 *	11.36	—	11.36
Total	137.55	16.46	6.26	5.18	10.02	16.59	94.94	17.23

*Based on less than 20 cases.

the lowest rate of abnormality was in the lowest gestational age group, the highest in the 40-week and above group. For those two birthweight groups the findings are similar for both whites and blacks. However, the smallest babies (i.e., those under 2001 grams) were not consistent by race. In the babies of less than 2001 grams, for both races, the lowest rate of neurological abnormality was for those of 37- to 39-weeks gestation. In white infants, the highest rate of neurological abnormality was in those of 40-weeks or more gestation (i.e., the small for dates). In blacks, this group of babies was also at increased risk, but for those infants weighing less than 2001 the highest rates of abnormality was for babies of less than 37-weeks gestation. Increased risks of abnormality were experienced by babies of both races with gestational age longer or shorter than 37 to 39 weeks.

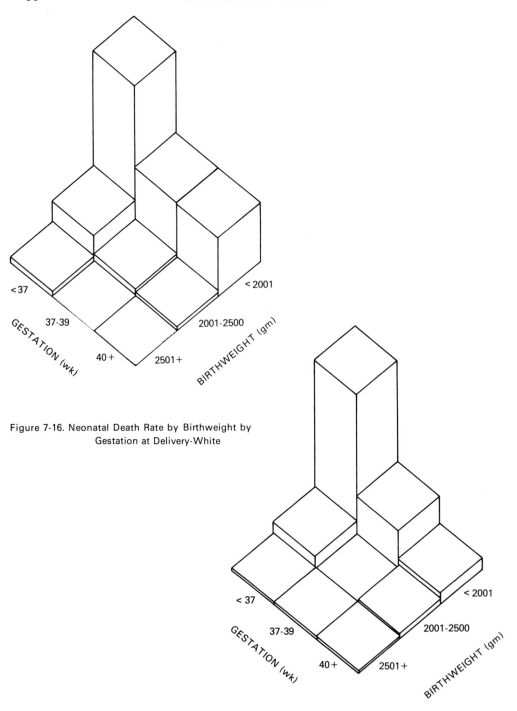

Figure 7-16. Neonatal Death Rate by Birthweight by
Gestation at Delivery-White

Figure 7-17. Neonatal Death Rate by Birthweight by
Gestation at Delivery-Black

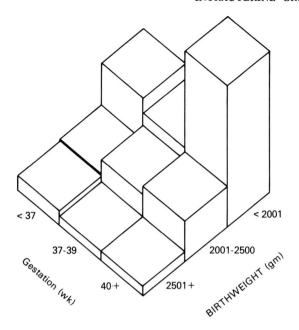

Figure 7-18. Neurological Abnormality Rate at One Year by
Birthweight by Gestation at Delivery-White

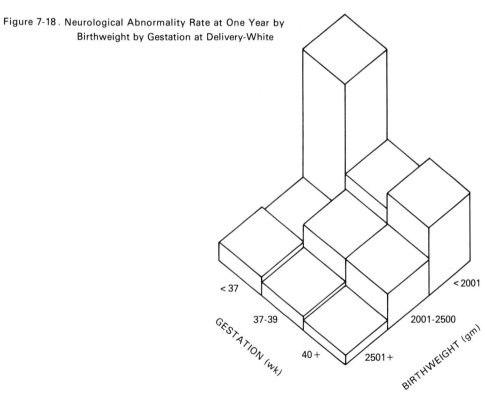

Figure 7-19. Neurological Abnormality Rate at One Year by
Birthweight by Gestation at Delivery-Black

Table 7–32. Children Neurologically Abnormal at One Year
by Birthweight, by Gestation at Delivery — White

	One Year Exam with Known Birthweight							
	Gestational Age (wk)							
Birthweight (gm)	Under 34	34–36	37–39	40–42	43+	Total	Unknown	Grand Total
Under 1501	31	8	1	1	1	42	0	42
1501–2000	43	52	32	13	5	145	0	145
2001–2500	43	172	291	188	40	734	0	734
2501–3000	45	199	1126	1254	242	2866	11	2877
3001–3500	49	147	1568	3487	619	5870	31	5901
3501–4000	20	73	605	2546	563	3807	31	3838
4001–4500	7	17	106	593	190	913	4	917
4501+	2	0	11	106	44	163	0	163
Total	240	668	3740	8188	1704	14540	77	14617
Abnormals								
Under 1501	4	0	1	1	0	6	0	6
1501–2000	5	2	1	3	0	11	0	11
2001–2500	2	3	13	12	1	31	0	31
2501–3000	3	5	19	23	4	54	0	54
3001–3500	3	1	18	49	7	78	1	79
3501–4000	0	0	9	36	10	55	0	55
4001–4500	0	0	1	7	2	10	0	10
4501+	0	0	0	1	1	2	0	2
Total	17	11	62	132	25	247	1	248
Rate								
Under 1501	129.03	0 *	1000.00*	1000.00*	0 *	142.86	–	142.86
1501–2000	116.28	38.46	31.25	230.77*	0 *	75.86	–	75.86
2001–2500	46.51	17.44	44.67	63.83	25.00	42.23	–	42.23
2501–3000	66.67	25.13	16.87	18.34	16.53	18.84	0 *	18.77
3001–3500	61.22	6.80	11.48	14.05	11.31	13.29	32.26	13.39
3501–4000	0	0	14.88	14.14	17.76	14.45	0	14.33
4001–4500	0 *	0 *	9.43	11.80	10.53	10.95	0 *	10.91
4501+	0 *	–	0 *	9.43	22.73	12.27	–	12.27
Total	70.83	16.47	16.58	16.12	14.67	16.99	12.99	16.97

*Based on less than 20 cases.

SUMMARY

Fetal outcome, as measured by neonatal death or survival to one year, with or without neurological abnormality, showed strong relationships with body weight at birth for both white and black children. Gestational age at delivery was also a factor of importance in determining outcome. There was a decreasing risk of adverse outcome with increasing birthweight and gestational age through the normal ranges of these parameters. Gestational age and birthweight considered together provided an index of intrauterine growth. Outcome was influenced by patterns of intrauterine growth. The risks of mortality and neurological abnormality were greatest for the small infants, particularly those of short gestations, but infants who were of low weight for gestational age experienced considerably greater risk than

Table 7-33. Children Neurologically Abnormal at One Year by Birthweight, by Gestation at Delivery — Black

One Year Exam with Known Birthweight

Birthweight (gm)	Under 34	34–36	37–39	40–42	43+	Total	Unknown	Grand Total
				Gestational Age (wk)				
Under 1501	87	21	7	7	1	123	0	123
1501–2000	157	112	51	28	8	356	0	356
2001–2500	181	420	627	297	88	1613	0	1613
2501–3000	238	586	2098	1744	402	5068	47	5115
3001–3500	262	501	2210	3131	673	6777	44	6821
3501–4000	76	131	612	1365	344	2528	19	2547
4001–4500	14	17	89	226	55	401	4	405
4501+	2	3	7	50	11	73	0	73
Total	1017	1791	5701	6848	1582	16939	114	17053

Abnormals

Birthweight (gm)	Under 34	34–36	37–39	40–42	43+	Total	Unknown	Grand Total
Under 1501	11	1	0	2	0	14	0	14
1501–2000	15	8	3	1	0	27	0	27
2001–2500	2	6	23	10	4	45	0	45
2501–3000	6	12	19	23	4	64	1	65
3001–3500	5	8	38	23	9	83	1	84
3501–4000	1	3	10	14	3	31	0	31
4001–4500	0	0	2	3	0	5	0	5
4501+	0	0	0	1	0	1	0	1
Total	40	38	95	77	20	270	2	272

Rate

Birthweight (gm)	Under 34	34–36	37–39	40–42	43+	Total	Unknown	Grand Total
Under 1501	126.44	47.62	0 *	285.71*	0 *	113.82	–	113.82
1501–2000	95.54	71.43	58.82	35.71	0 *	75.84	–	75.84
2001–2500	11.05	14.29	36.68	33.67	45.45*	27.90	–	27.90
2501–3000	25.21	20.48	9.06	13.19	9.95	12.63	21.28	12.71
3001–3500	19.08	15.97	17.19	7.35	13.37	12.25	22.73	12.31
3501–4000	13.16	22.90	16.34	10.26	8.72	12.26	0 *	12.17
4001–4500	0 *	0 *	22.47	13.27	0	12.47	0 *	12.35
4501+	0 *	0 *	0 *	20.00	0 *	13.70	–	13.70
Total	39.33	21.22	16.66	11.24	12.64	15.94	17.54	15.95

*Based on less than 20 cases.

babies whose weight was within the normal range for gestation. There was a suggestion in the data that the "large for dates" baby might also be at increased risk.

The relationships presented here are not new; they have been reported previously. However, this study was based on a very large number of infants from diverse backgrounds, each prospectively followed over a considerable time span. The findings lend importance to the original observations by providing a wealth of detailed data not previously available.

There have been earlier investigations in the NCPP data, relating to birthweight and to factors that influence it and to its effect on outcome. Birthweight was one of the five major outcome variables considered in the first major publication from this study (*The Women and Their Pregnancies*). Other publications from the

NCPP (9,10,11) have made major contributions to our understanding of the important role of birthweight. This presentation includes, in addition, a consideration of gestational age and investigates some aspects of birthweight-gestational age relationships. A more definitive study of the large and complex subject of interrelationships between a number of physical parameters at birth and their effect on outcome is under way and will be reported separately.

REFERENCES

(1) L. O. Lubchenco, C. Hansman, M. Dressler, and E. Boyd. 1963. Intrauterine growth as estimated from liveborn birth weight data at 24 to 42 weeks of gestation. *Pediatrics* 32: 793–800.

(2) P. Gruenwald. 1966. Growth of the human fetus: I. Normal growth and its variation. *American Journal of Obstetrics and Gynecology* 94: 1112–32.

(3) I. M. Cushner and E. D. Mellits. 1971. The relationship between fetal outcome and the gestational age and birthweight of the fetus. *Johns Hopkins Medical Journal* 128: 252–60.

(4) V. B. Penchaszadeh, J. B. Hardy, E. D. Mellits, B. H. Cohen, and V. A. McKusick. 1972. Growth and development in an "inner city" population: An assessment of possible biological and environmental influences. I. Intra-uterine growth. *Johns Hopkins Medical Journal* 130: 384–97.

(5) N. R. Butler and E. D. Alberman (eds.). 1969. *Perinatal Problems. The Second Report of the 1958 British Perinatal Mortality Survey*. Edinburgh and London: Livingstone.

(6) S. Shapiro, E. R. Schlesinger, and R. E. L. Nesbitt, Jr. 1968. *Infant, Perinatal, Maternal and Childhood Mortality in the United States*. Cambridge, Mass.: Harvard University Press.

(7) J. Yerushalmy. 1967. The classification of newborn infants by birthweight and gestational age. *Journal of Pediatrics* 71: 164–72.

(8) P. Gruenwald. 1969. Growth and maturation of the foetus and its relationship to perinatal mortality. In N. R. Butler and E. D. Alberman (eds.), *Perinatal Problems. The Second Report of the 1958 British Perinatal Mortality Survey*, pp. 141–62. Edinburgh and London: Livingstone.

(9) N. J. Eastman and E. Jackson. 1968. Weight relationships in pregnancy. I. The bearing of maternal weight gain and pre-pregnancy weight on birth weight in full term pregnancies. *Obstetrical and Gynecological Survey* 23: 1003–25.

(10) W. Weiss, E. C. Jackson, K. Niswander, and N. J. Eastman. 1969. The influence on birthweight of change in maternal weight gain in successive pregnancies of the same woman. *International Journal of Gynaecology and Obstetrics* 7: 210–33.

(11) K. Niswander and E. C. Jackson. 1974. Physical characteristics of the gravida and their association with birth weight and perinatal death. *American Journal of Obstetics and Gynecology* 119: 306–13.

8

NEONATAL BODY LENGTH AND HEAD CIRCUMFERENCE

BODY LENGTH OF NEONATE

The graphs and tables presented in this section display the distribution of body length, for white and black neonates. The length for each baby was obtained using a standardized procedure within twenty-four hours of birth (at approximately twelve hours). The black infants had, on the average, somewhat shorter lengths than white infants; this is consistent with lower average birthweight and gestational age. (Fig. 8–1 and Table 8–1.)

The mean birthweight observed by various groupings of body length for white and black infants is presented (Fig. 8–2). For each length examined, the whites have a consistently larger average birthweight than the black infants; this was in excess of 600 grams for the babies of less than 35 cm. and approximately 100 grams for the longest babies (i.e., those of 55 cm. or greater length). (Table 8–2.)

Table 8-1. Body Length of Newborn by Race

Body Length (cm)	WHITE				BLACK		
	Livebirths with Known Birthweight	Percent	Cumulative Percent		Livebirths with Known Birthweight	Percent	Cumulative Percent
Under 35	26	0.15	0.15		36	0.19	0.19
35–39	50	0.28	0.43		103	0.55	0.74
40–44	288	1.63	2.06		730	3.87	4.60
45–49	5559	31.53	33.59		8239	43.64	48.24
50–54	10929	61.99	95.58		9437	49.98	98.22
55+	779	4.42	100.00		336	1.78	100.00
Total	17631	100.00			18881	100.00	
Unknown	850	4.60			623	3.19	
Grand total	18481	100.00			19504	100.00	

71

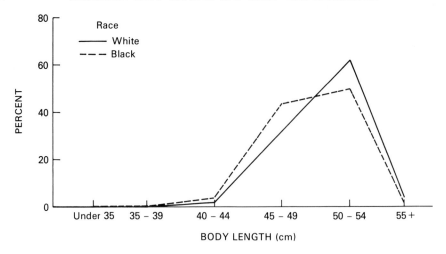

Figure 8-1. Body Length of Newborn by Race

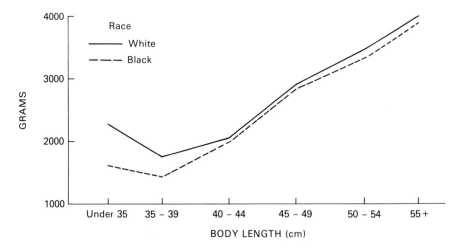

Figure 8-2. Mean Birthweight by Body Length of Newborn by Race

Table 8–2. Mean Birthweight by Body Length of Newborn by Race

Body Length (cm)	WHITE		BLACK	
	Livebirths with Known Birthweight	Mean Birthweight	Livebirths with Known Birthweight	Mean Birthweight
Under 35	26	2276	36	1614
35–39	50	1750	103	1436
40–44	288	2058	730	1987
45–49	5559	2914	8239	2836
50–54	10929	3464	9437	3322
55+	779	3998	336	3894
Total	17631	3285	18881	3055
Unknown	850	3002	623	2566
Grand total	18481	3272	19504	3039

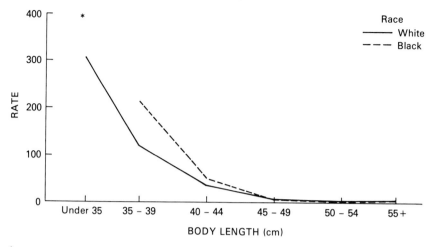

* Unplotted Rate is 527.78.

Figure 8-3. Neonatal Deaths by Body Length of Newborn by Race

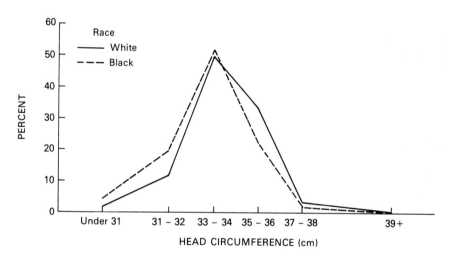

Figure 8-4. Head Circumference of Newborn by Race

As might be anticipated, the curves demonstrating the neonatal death rates by body length (Fig. 8–3) are very similar to those for birthweight and gestational age, excepting that at the shorter lengths white infants have somewhat lower rates than blacks, in contrast to the lower rates experienced by blacks at the lower birthweights and shorter gestations. (Table 8–3.)

HEAD CIRCUMFERENCE OF NEONATE

The distribution of maximum suboccipital-bregmatic head circumference (meas-ured with a narrow, flexible nonstretch tape), at approximately twelve hours of

Table 8-3. Neonatal Deaths by Body Length of Newborn by Race

Body Length (cm)	WHITE			BLACK		
	Livebirths with Known Birthweight	Neonatal Deaths	Rate	Livebirths with Known Birthweight	Neonatal Deaths	Rate
Under 35	26	8	307.67	36	19	527.78
35–39	50	6	120.00	103	22	213.59
40–44	288	10	34.72	730	36	49.32
45–49	5559	28	5.04	8239	46	5.58
50–54	10929	26	2.38	9437	22	2.33
55+	779	3	3.85	336	1	2.98
Total	17631	81	4.59	18881	146	7.73
Unknown	850	142	167.06	623	190	304.98
Grand total	18481	223	12.07	19504	336	17.23

Table 8-4. Head Circumference of Newborn by Race

Head Circumference (cm)	WHITE			BLACK		
	Livebirths with Known Birthweight	Percent	Cumulative Percent	Livebirths with Known Birthweight	Percent	Cumulative Percent
Under 31	330	1.86	1.86	829	4.38	4.38
31–32	2108	11.91	13.77	3741	19.76	24.13
33–34	8752	49.43	63.20	9827	51.90	76.03
35–36	5922	33.45	96.65	4192	22.14	98.17
37–38	582	3.29	99.93	334	1.76	99.93
39+	12	0.07	100.00	13	0.07	100.00
Total	17706	100.00		18936	100.00	
Unknown	775	4.19		568	2.91	
Grand total	18481	100.00		19504	100.00	

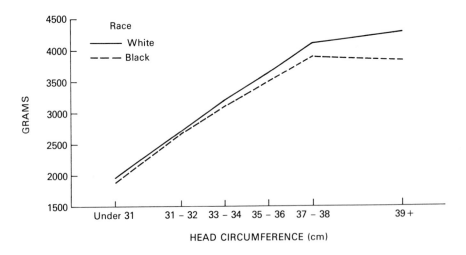

Figure 8-5. Mean Birthweight by Head Circumference of Newborn by Race

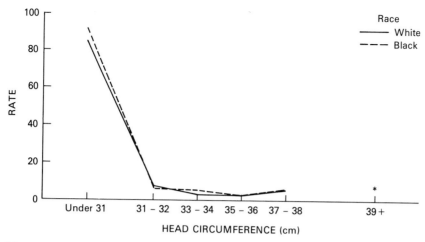

*Based on less than 20 cases

Figure 8-6. Neonatal Deaths by Head Circumference of Newborn by Race

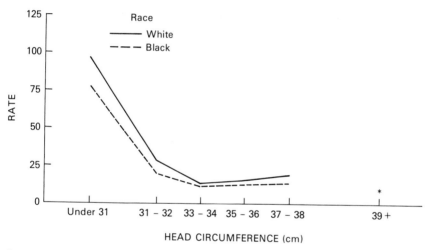

*Based on less than 20 cases.

Figure 8-7. Children Neurologically Abnormal at One Year by Head Circumference by Race

age, is displayed in this section (Fig. 8–4). Again, as with other neonatal measurements, black infants had, on the average, a somewhat smaller head circumference than whites. (Table 8–4.)

The relationship observed between head circumference and average birthweight was similar to that with length; white infants had slightly higher birthweight in each head circumference category than blacks (Fig. 8–5). However, in this instance, the difference was least where the head circumference was smallest and greatest where the head was largest. (Table 8–5.)

The neonatal death rates observed in each head circumference category are dis-

Table 8-5. Mean Birthweight by Head Circumference of Newborn by Race

Head Circumference (cm)	WHITE		BLACK	
	Livebirths with Known Birthweight	Mean Birthweight	Livebirths with Known Birthweight	Mean Birthweight
Under 31	330	1954	829	1874
31–32	2108	2706	3741	2659
33–34	8752	3191	9827	3090
35–36	5922	3620	4192	3487
37–38	582	4106	334	3885
39+	12	4276	13	3823
Total	17706	3284	18936	3054
Unknown	775	2987	568	2546
Grand total	18481	3272	19504	3039

Table 8-6. Neonatal Deaths by Head Circumference of Newborn by Race

Head Circumference (cm)	WHITE			BLACK		
	Livebirths with Known Birthweight	Neonatal Deaths	Rate	Livebirths with Known Birthweight	Neonatal Deaths	Rate
Under 31	330	28	84.85	829	76	91.68
31–32	2108	16	7.59	3741	22	5.88
33–34	8752	23	2.63	9827	48	4.88
35–36	5922	15	2.53	4192	9	2.15
37–38	582	3	5.15	334	2	5.99
39+	12	0	0*	13	1	76.92*
Total	17706	85	4.80	18936	158	8.34
Unknown	775	138	178.06	568	178	313.38
Grand total	18481	223	12.07	19504	336	17.23

*Based on less than 20 cases.

Table 8-7. Children Neurologically Abnormal at One Year by Head Circumference of Newborn by Race

Head Circumference (cm)	WHITE			BLACK		
	One Year Exam*	Abnormals	Rate	One Year Exam*	Abnormals	Rate
Under 31	237	23	97.05	653	51	78.10
31–32	1663	47	28.26	3318	65	19.59
33–34	7158	92	12.85	8729	95	10.88
35–36	4823	72	14.93	3794	48	12.65
37–38	483	9	18.63	297	4	13.47
39+	12	3	250.00†	10	2	200.00†
Total	14376	246	17.11	16801	265	15.77
Unknown	241	2	8.30	252	7	27.78
Grand total	14617	248	16.97	17053	272	15.95

*Excludes unknown birthweight.
†Based on less than 20 cases.

played in Figure 8–6 and Table 8–6. The rates are not greatly different for infants of both races.

The rates of children neurologically abnormal at one year, while slightly higher for whites in each category, are not strikingly different between the races (Fig. 8–7). The infants with the smallest heads at birth had, as expected, the highest rates of abnormality. There is, however, an increase in the rate for children with large heads. The children of both races with the biggest heads (those of 39 cm. and above) were few in number and are, thus, not plotted on the graph; however, the rates of abnormality among these children were very high. (Table 8–7.)

9

APGAR SCORES

Major physiological changes in the function of cardio-pulmonary systems occur at the moment of birth. The condition of the infant during this critical period is influenced by a number of intrauterine and delivery factors. An objective assessment of the condition in the moments after birth was recorded for each infant, using the Apgar Score (1).

In 1953, Dr. Virginia Apgar (2) devised a simple numerical scoring system to evaluate the condition of a newborn infant one minute after delivery. The NINCDS Collaborative Perinatal Project incorporated the Apgar scoring system into the protocol at one and five minutes and periodically thereafter if the five-minute score was below 7. The Apgar scoring system is a ten-point scale, with a high score indicating a neonate in optimal condition and a low score an infant in poor condition.

Five items are evaluated to determine the score. The five items are: heart rate, respiratory effort, muscle tone, reflex irritability, and color. For details of scoring, see PED–1, *Delivery Room Observation of the Neonate* (see Appendix), which contains a preprinted format on which the Apgar subscores are defined.

The delivery room observers, provided by the NCPP, were trained in Apgar scoring techniques and to obtain objective observations. These observers were free of other responsibilities in the delivery room and after the birth of the baby devoted full attention to the observation of the neonate. Observers were members of the NCPP team and were not administratively responsible to the obstetrician performing the delivery. The observers were instructed to evaluate the score items as closely as possible to the specified time, using a stopwatch or timer. The acceptable time range for scoring was plus or minus thirty seconds of the designated time; that is, the score was coded as a one-minute score only if the observations were made thirty to ninety seconds after delivery.

Table 9-1. One-Minute APGAR Score by Birthweight — White

| | Number* | | | | | | | |
| | Birthweight (gm) | | | | | | | |
Score	Under 1001	1001– 1500	1501– 2000	2001– 2500	2501– 3000	3001– 3500	3501+	Total
0	1	1	0	4	3	1	6	16
1	19	14	18	26	61	70	64	272
2	8	7	12	31	84	118	85	345
3	6	9	11	24	71	132	116	369
4	3	5	13	43	86	190	148	488
5	2	6	15	57	156	315	284	835
6	3	5	22	80	244	481	441	1276
7	0	7	23	87	345	679	617	1758
8	1	7	32	210	816	1682	1456	4204
9	0	4	38	284	1382	2975	2268	6951
10	0	0	0	26	120	195	137	478
Total	43	65	184	872	3368	6838	5622	16992
	Percent							
0	2.33	1.54	0	0.46	0.09	0.01	0.11	0.09
1	44.19	21.54	9.78	2.98	1.81	1.02	1.14	1.60
2	18.60	10.77	6.52	3.56	2.49	1.73	1.51	2.03
3	13.95	13.85	5.98	2.75	2.11	1.93	2.06	2.17
4	6.98	7.69	7.07	4.93	2.55	2.78	2.63	2.87
5	4.65	9.23	8.15	6.54	4.63	4.61	5.05	4.91
6	6.98	7.69	11.96	9.17	7.24	7.03	7.84	7.51
7	0	10.77	12.50	9.98	10.24	9.93	10.97	10.35
8	2.33	10.77	17.39	24.08	24.23	24.60	25.90	24.74
9	0	6.15	20.65	32.57	41.03	43.51	40.34	40.91
10	0	0	0	2.98	3.56	2.85	2.44	2.81
Total	100.00	100.00	100.00	100.00	100.00	100.00	100.00	100.00

*With known birthweight, gestation, and APGAR score.

ONE-MINUTE APGAR SCORES

Scores by race, within birthweight groups, are very similar, with black infants in low birthweight groups having slightly fewer low scores. In Tables 9–1 and 9–2 birthweight is shown in 500 gram categories, from 1000 grams and below to 3501 grams and above, and Apgar scores are shown from 0 to 10. In the birthweight groups over 2500 grams, most babies have normal scores in the 7 and above range and there is little change in the distribution of scores with increasing birthweight. However, below 2501 grams, the frequency of low Apgar scores is highest in the lowest birthweight groups. For example, 48 percent of the whites and 38 percent of the blacks, in the 1001- to 1500-gram birthweight category, have Apgar scores, at one minute, of 3 or below. By contrast, of babies weighing 3001 and 3500 grams, only 4.7 percent of whites and 4.4 percent of blacks had one-minute scores of 3 and below. In this birthweight group, over 80 percent of both white and black babies had scores of 7 and above.

As shown in these tables, more black than white babies had scores of 10. However, there is little difference between the races when scores of 8 and above are

Table 9-2. One–Minute APGAR Score by Birthweight — Black

| | Number* | | | | | | |
| | Birthweight (gm) | | | | | | |
Score	Under 1001	1001– 1500	1501– 2000	2001– 2500	2501– 3000	3001– 3500	3501+	Total
0	2	3	3	2	3	6	2	21
1	26	23	17	43	47	74	33	263
2	18	22	14	48	83	100	58	343
3	15	15	35	31	91	122	67	376
4	4	19	21	65	112	151	73	445
5	7	17	39	72	184	240	133	692
6	7	22	37	129	303	427	255	1180
7	2	13	46	169	421	541	292	1484
8	3	17	69	288	863	1234	587	3061
9	0	12	91	621	2443	3152	1272	7591
10	0	2	12	168	640	853	340	2015
Total	84	165	384	1636	5190	6900	3112	17471
	Percent						
0	2.38	1.82	0.78	0.12	0.06	0.09	0.06	0.12
1	30.95	13.94	4.43	2.63	0.91	1.07	1.06	1.51
2	21.43	13.33	3.65	2.93	1.60	1.45	1.86	1.96
3	17.86	9.09	9.11	1.89	1.75	1.77	2.15	2.15
4	4.76	11.52	5.47	3.97	2.16	2.19	2.35	2.55
5	8.33	10.30	10.16	4.40	3.55	3.48	4.27	3.96
6	8.33	13.33	9.64	7.89	5.84	6.19	8.19	6.75
7	2.38	7.88	11.98	10.33	8.11	7.84	9.38	8.49
8	3.57	10.30	17.97	17.60	16.63	17.88	18.86	17.52
9	0	7.27	23.70	37.96	47.07	45.68	40.87	43.45
10	0	1.21	3.13	10.27	12.33	12.36	10.93	11.53
Total	100.00	100.00	100.00	100.00	100.00	100.00	100.00	100.00

*With known birthweight, gestation, and APGAR score.

added together. Because of the increased skin pigment in black babies, slight degrees of localized cyanosis may be difficult to detect, which results in higher subscores for skin color.

Tables 9–3 and 9–4 show the distributions of Apgar scores under 7 by birthweight and gestational age. The data, which are somewhat difficult to interpret, show that Apgar scores below 7 are related to both birthweight and gestational age. The greatest risk of low scores is in the lowest two birthweight groups. However, in the groups of larger infants (3001 to 3500 and 3501 and above), the likelihood of scores below 7 seems increased for those with short gestation (i.e., under 34 weeks) and for those with gestation of 43 weeks and above. For low-birthweight infants (below 2001 grams), gestational age seems to add little to the effect of birthweight in the relationship to Apgar scores below 7.

As might be expected, the mean birthweight by one-minute Apgar score (Fig. 9–1 and Table 9–5) indicates the relationship between birthweight and Apgar score, discussed above. The babies with low one-minute scores have low average birthweights. The effect is clearly discerned for infants of both races. In this figure, as in others, where mean birthweights are compared, there is approximately 200 grams difference between white and black infants for each score.

Table 9-3. One-Minute APGAR Scores Under 7
by Birthweight by Gestation at Delivery — White

Number*

| Gestation (wk) | Birthweight (gm) | | | | | | | |
	Under 1001	1001–1500	1501–2000	2001–2500	2501–3000	3001–3500	3501+	Total
Under 34	41	55	65	62	62	61	28	374
34–36	1	8	55	212	237	173	104	790
37–39	1	2	41	345	1287	1802	840	4318
40–42	0	0	16	207	1487	4058	3718	9486
43+	0	0	7	46	295	744	932	2024
Total	43	65	184	872	3368	6838	5622	16992

APGAR Scores Under 7

Gestation (wk)	Under 1001	1001–1500	1501–2000	2001–2500	2501–3000	3001–3500	3501+	Total
Under 34	40	41	34	19	12	16	12	174
34–36	1	6	26	68	50	23	27	201
37–39	1	0	19	95	248	327	159	849
40–42	0	0	9	61	323	766	725	1884
43+	0	0	3	22	72	175	221	493
Total	42	47	91	265	705	1307	1144	3601

Percent Scores Under 7

Gestation (wk)	Under 1001	1001–1500	1501–2000	2001–2500	2501–3000	3001–3500	3501+	Total
Under 34	97.56	74.55	52.31	30.65	19.35	26.23	42.86	46.52
34–36	100.00†	75.00†	47.27	32.08	21.10	13.29	25.96	25.44
37–39	100.00†	0 †	46.34	27.54	19.27	18.15	18.93	19.66
40–42	–	–	56.25†	29.47	21.72	18.88	19.50	19.86
43+	–	–	42.86†	47.83	24.41	23.52	23.71	24.36
Total	97.67	72.31	49.46	30.39	20.93	19.11	20.35	21.19

*With known birthweight, gestation, and APGAR score.
†Based on less than 20 cases.

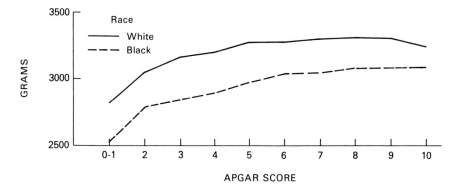

Figure 9-1. Mean Birthweight by One-Minute APGAR Score by Race

Table 9–4. One-Minute APGAR Scores Under 7 by Birthweight by Gestation at Delivery — Black

Number*

| | Birthweight (gm) | | | | | | | |
Gestation (wk)	Under 1001	1001– 1500	1501– 2000	2001– 2500	2501– 3000	3001– 3500	3501+	Total
Under 34	77	124	186	204	248	270	91	1200
34–36	5	26	113	430	611	502	162	1849
37–39	1	9	51	613	2139	2223	723	5759
40–42	1	6	24	303	1788	3195	1715	7032
43+	0	0	10	86	404	710	421	1631
Total	84	165	384	1636	5190	6900	3112	17471

APGAR Scores Under 7

Gestation (wk)	Under 1001	1001– 1500	1501– 2000	2001– 2500	2501– 3000	3001– 3500	3501+	Total
Under 34	73	94	86	55	27	47	15	397
34–36	4	20	46	101	101	78	23	373
37–39	1	3	25	144	322	333	115	943
40–42	1	4	5	70	284	515	376	1255
43+	0	0	4	20	89	147	92	352
Total	79	121	166	390	823	1120	621	3320

Percent Scores Under 7

Gestation (wk)	Under 1001	1001– 1500	1501– 2000	2001– 2500	2501– 3000	3001– 3500	3501+	Total
Under 34	94.81	75.81	46.24	26.96	10.89	17.41	16.48	33.08
34–36	80.00†	76.92	40.71	23.49	16.53	15.54	14.20	20.17
37–39	100.00†	33.33†	49.02	23.49	15.05	14.98	15.91	16.37
40–42	100.00†	66.67†	20.83	23.10	15.88	16.12	21.92	17.85
43+	–	–	40.00†	23.26	22.03	20.70	21.85	21.58
Total	94.05	73.33	43.23	23.84	15.86	16.23	19.96	19.00

*With known birthweight, gestation, and APGAR score.
†Based on less than 20 cases.

Tables 9–6 and 9–7 report the neonatal death rate by one-minute Apgar score by birthweight for whites and blacks. These tables and Figures 9–2 and 9–3 show that, in general, the lower the Apgar score, the higher the neonatal mortality rate; and that for each Apgar score, the rate for neonates under 2501 grams is remarkably higher than that for neonates over 2500 grams. Within birthweight-race groups, the lower the score the higher the neonatal death rate. The rather dramatic difference in mortality between low and high scores in the under-2501-gram group for both races is in part a reflection of birthweight differences within the group. In other words, if birthweight subgroups below 2501 grams were tabulated, the lower the birthweight the higher the frequency of low Apgar scores.

Tables 9–8 and 9–9 show the neurological abnormality rate at one year by one-minute Apgar score by race and birthweight groups. Because of small numbers, Apgar scores are grouped as 0–3, 4–6, and 7–10. Within each race-birthweight group, there is approximately a twofold difference in the rate of neurological abnormality between neonates grouped 0–3, as compared with those in the 7–10 group, suggesting a relationship between the condition of the infant at birth, as measured by the Apgar score and neurological findings at one year.

Table 9-5. Mean Birthweight by One-Minute APGAR Score by Race

Score	WHITE		BLACK	
	Livebirths with Known Birthweight	Mean Birthweight	Livebirths with Known Birthweight	Mean Birthweight
0–1	292	2824	290	2529
2	346	3051	346	2788
3	369	3164	380	2846
4	489	3198	449	2895
5	837	3275	697	2976
6	1281	3274	1187	3040
7	1768	3298	1494	3047
8	4231	3308	3078	3082
9	6996	3301	7656	3083
10	482	3239	2030	3086
Total	17091	3278	17607	3048
Unknown	1390	3194	1897	2955
Grand total	18481	3272	19504	3039

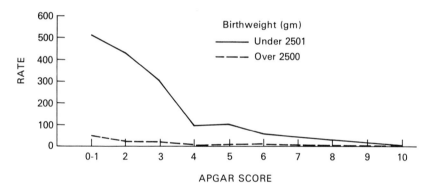

Figure 9-2. Neonatal Deaths by One-Minute APGAR Score by Birthweight — White

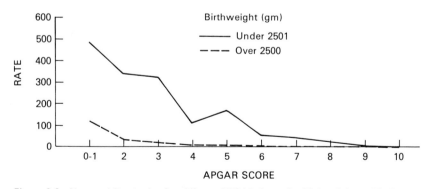

Figure 9-3. Neonatal Deaths by One-Minute APGAR Score by Birthweight — Black

Table 9-6. Neonatal Deaths by One-Minute APGAR Score by Birthweight — White

Score	Under 2501 gm			Over 2500 gm			Total		
	Livebirths	Neonatal Deaths	Rate	Livebirths	Neonatal Deaths	Rate	Livebirths	Neonatal Deaths	Rate
0-1	84	43	511.90	208	10	48.08	292	53	181.51
2	58	25	431.03	288	6	20.83	346	31	89.60
3	50	15	300.00	319	6	18.81	369	21	56.91
4	64	6	93.75	425	2	4.71	489	8	16.36
5	80	8	100.00	757	5	6.61	837	13	15.53
6	110	6	54.55	1171	9	7.69	1281	15	11.71
7	118	5	42.37	1650	4	2.42	1768	9	5.09
8	250	7	28.00	3981	12	3.01	4231	19	4.49
9	329	5	15.20	6667	12	1.80	6996	17	2.43
10	26	0	0	456	2	4.39	482	2	4.15
Total	1169	120	102.65	15922	68	4.27	17091	188	11.00
Unknown	150	27	180.00	1240	8	6.45	1390	35	25.18
Grand total	1319	147	111.45	17162	76	4.43	18481	223	12.07

Table 9-7. Neonatal Deaths by One-Minute APGAR Score by Birthweight — Black

Score	Under 2501 gm			Over 2500 gm			Total		
	Livebirths	Neonatal Deaths	Rate	Livebirths	Neonatal Deaths	Rate	Livebirths	Neonatal Deaths	Rate
0-1	122	59	483.61	168	20	119.05	290	79	272.41
2	103	35	339.81	243	8	32.92	346	43	124.28
3	96	31	322.92	284	6	21.13	380	37	97.37
4	110	12	109.09	339	3	8.85	449	15	33.41
5	137	23	167.88	560	6	10.71	697	29	41.61
6	196	11	56.12	991	7	7.06	1187	18	15.16
7	232	10	43.10	1262	2	1.58	1494	12	8.03
8	382	9	23.56	2696	12	4.45	3078	21	6.82
9	730	6	8.22	6926	22	3.18	7656	28	3.66
10	184	0	0	1846	3	1.63	2030	3	1.48
Total	2292	196	85.51	15315	89	5.81	17607	285	16.19
Unknown	325	42	129.23	1572	9	5.73	1897	51	26.88
Grand total	2617	238	90.94	16887	98	5.80	19504	336	17.23

Table 9-8. Children Neurologically Abnormal at One Year by One-Minute APGAR Score by Birthweight — White

Score	Under 2501 gm			Over 2500 gm			Total		
	One-Year Exam	Abnormals	Rate	One-Year Exam	Abnormals	Rate	One-Year Exam	Abnormals	Rate
0-3	82	7	85.37	658	20	30.40	740	27	36.49
4-6	192	8	41.67	1937	44	22.72	2129	52	24.42
7-10	564	24	42.55	10408	128	12.30	10972	152	13.85
Total	838	39	46.54	13003	192	14.77	13841	231	16.69
Unknown	83	9	108.43	693	8	11.54	776	17	21.91
Grand total	921	48	52.12	13696	200	14.60	14617	248	16.97

Table 9-9. Children Neurologically Abnormal at One Year by One-Minute APGAR Score by Birthweight — Black

Score	Under 2501 gm			Over 2500 gm			Total		
	One-Year Exam	Abnormals	Rate	One-Year Exam	Abnormals	Rate	One-Year Exam	Abnormals	Rate
0-3	165	10	60.61	579	12	20.73	744	22	29.57
4-6	354	18	50.85	1660	27	16.27	2014	45	22.34
7-10	1333	49	36.76	11405	128	11.22	12738	177	13.90
Total	1852	77	41.58	13644	167	12.24	15496	244	15.75
Unknown	240	9	37.50	1317	19	14.43	1557	28	17.98
Grand total	2092	86	41.11	14961	186	12.43	17053	272	15.95

Table 9-10. Five-Minute APGAR Score by Birthweight — White

	Number*							
	Birthweight (gm)							
Score	Under 1001	1001– 1500	1501– 2000	2001– 2500	2501– 3000	3001– 3500	3501+	Total
0	1	0	0	2	1	1	1	6
1	19	10	5	6	10	13	9	72
2	8	7	4	7	9	14	17	66
3	7	4	5	9	10	18	18	71
4	1	5	4	4	16	21	18	69
5	3	1	7	19	26	41	38	135
6	3	11	14	29	48	87	77	269
7	1	7	25	45	76	136	128	418
8	1	10	37	120	353	582	491	1594
9	0	11	70	508	2254	4823	3974	11640
10	0	1	15	124	601	1163	912	2816
Total	44	67	186	873	3404	6899	5683	17156
	Percent							
0	2.27	0	0	0.23	0.03	0.01	0.02	0.03
1	43.18	14.93	2.69	0.69	0.29	0.19	0.16	0.42
2	18.18	10.45	2.15	0.80	0.26	0.20	0.30	0.38
3	15.91	5.97	2.69	1.03	0.29	0.26	0.32	0.41
4	2.27	7.46	2.15	0.46	0.47	0.30	0.32	0.40
5	6.82	1.49	3.76	2.18	0.76	0.59	0.67	0.79
6	6.82	16.42	7.53	3.32	1.41	1.26	1.35	1.57
7	2.27	10.45	13.44	5.15	2.23	1.97	2.25	2.44
8	2.27	14.93	19.89	13.75	10.37	8.44	8.64	9.29
9	0	16.42	37.63	58.19	66.22	69.91	69.93	67.85
10	0	1.49	8.06	14.20	17.66	16.86	16.05	16.41
Total	100.00	100.00	100.00	100.00	100.00	100.00	100.00	100.00

*With known birthweight, gestation, and APGAR score.

FIVE-MINUTE APGAR SCORES

The five-minute Apgar scores, by birthweight, for whites and blacks are shown in Tables 9–10 through 9–13. The distribution of Apgar score by birthweight groups for whites and blacks is quite similar, except at the scores of 9 and 10 where the substantial difference is accounted for by the skin color subscore, as many more black infants were given a score of 2 and compared to white infants who were more often given a score of 1. When the scores of 9 and 10 were combined, 84.9 percent of blacks and 84.3 percent of whites fell into this group. For both races, there are fewer infants with low scores at five minutes than at one minute.

The neonatal death rates by five-minute Apgar scores, by birthweight and race groups, are shown in Tables 9–14 and 9–15. For both whites and blacks, and within birthweight groupings, there was a markedly higher neonatal death rate for low Apgar scores, as compared to high scores. With progressively lower Apgar scores at five minutes, the associated neonatal mortality rate is higher. Figures 9–4 and

Table 9-11. Five-Minute APGAR Score by Birthweight — Black

Number*

Score	Birthweight (gm)							
	Under 1001	1001– 1500	1501– 2000	2001– 2500	2501– 3000	3001– 3500	3501+	Total
0	1	1	1	1	2	1	0	7
1	23	12	7	7	8	22	7	86
2	19	11	8	16	15	29	13	111
3	12	14	10	10	20	28	17	111
4	11	11	12	23	30	29	13	129
5	5	20	15	18	46	37	31	172
6	10	31	28	56	96	96	47	364
7	4	12	28	69	111	138	88	450
8	5	31	61	150	326	461	239	1273
9	2	23	120	697	2294	3057	1504	7697
10	0	12	93	631	2386	3141	1253	7516
Total	92	178	383	1678	5334	7039	3212	17916

Percent

Score	Under 1001	1001– 1500	1501– 2000	2001– 2500	2501– 3000	3001– 3500	3501+	Total
0	1.09	0.56	0.26	0.06	0.04	0.01	0	0.04
1	25.00	6.74	1.83	0.42	0.15	0.31	0.22	0.48
2	20.65	6.18	2.09	0.95	0.28	0.41	0.40	0.62
3	13.04	7.87	2.61	0.60	0.37	0.40	0.53	0.62
4	11.96	6.18	3.13	1.37	0.56	0.41	0.40	0.72
5	5.43	11.24	3.92	1.07	0.86	0.53	0.97	0.96
6	10.87	17.42	7.31	3.34	1.80	1.36	1.46	2.03
7	4.34	6.74	7.31	4.11	2.08	1.96	2.74	2.51
8	5.43	17.42	15.93	8.94	6.11	6.55	7.44	7.11
9	2.17	12.92	31.33	41.54	43.01	43.43	46.82	42.97
10	0	6.74	24.28	37.60	44.73	44.62	39.01	41.95
Total	100.00	100.00	100.00	100.00	100.00	100.00	100.00	100.00

*With known birthweight, gestation, and APGAR score.

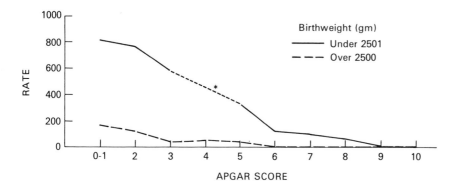

*Based on less than 20 cases.

Figure 9-4. Neonatal Deaths by Five-Minute APGAR score by Birthweight — White

Table 9-12. Five-Minute APGAR Scores Under 7 by Birthweight by Gestation at Delivery — White

	Number*							
	Birthweight (gm)							
Gestation (wk)	Under 1001	1001– 1500	1501– 2000	2001– 2500	2501– 3000	3001– 3500	3501+	Total
Under 34	43	53	68	61	58	62	28	373
34–36	1	10	55	202	237	178	105	788
37–39	0	2	40	347	1315	1813	845	4362
40–42	0	1	16	216	1495	4097	3757	9582
43+	0	1	7	47	299	749	948	2051
Total	44	67	186	873	3404	6899	5683	17156
	APGAR Scores Under 7							
Under 34	41	34	21	7	5	4	3	115
34–36	1	3	7	27	13	5	3	59
37–39	0	0	5	24	39	54	24	146
40–42	0	0	5	15	50	100	106	276
43+	0	1	1	3	13	32	42	92
Total	42	38	39	76	120	195	178	688
	Percent Scores Under 7							
Under 34	95.35	64.15	30.88	11.47	8.62	6.45	10.71	30.83
34–36	100.00†	30.00†	12.73	13.37	5.49	2.81	2.86	7.49
37–39	–	0 †	12.50	6.92	2.97	2.98	2.84	3.35
40–42	–	0 †	31.25†	6.94	3.34	2.44	2.82	2.88
43+	–	100.00†	14.29†	6.38	4.35	4.27	4.43	4.49
Total	95.45	56.72	20.97	8.71	3.53	2.83	3.13	4.01

*With known birthweight, gestation, and APGAR score.
†Based on less than 20 cases.

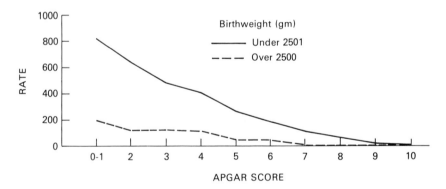

Figure 9-5. Neonatal Deaths by Five-Minute APGAR Score by Birthweight — Black

Table 9-13. Five-Minute APGAR Scores Under 7
by Birthweight by Gestation at Delivery — Black

	Number*							
	Birthweight (gm)							
Gestation (wk)	Under 1001	1001– 1500	1501– 2000	2001– 2500	2501– 3000	3001– 3500	3501+	Total
Under 34	85	135	180	209	256	270	92	1227
34–36	5	28	115	437	630	519	167	1901
37–39	1	10	53	633	2182	2264	742	5885
40–42	1	5	25	310	1852	3256	1774	7223
43+	0	0	10	89	414	730	437	1680
Total	92	178	383	1678	5334	7039	3212	17916
	APGAR Scores Under 7							
Under 34	75	83	40	22	10	6	1	237
34–36	4	11	25	35	37	10	3	125
37–39	1	3	11	47	70	63	19	214
40–42	1	3	3	22	73	127	83	312
43+	0	0	2	5	27	36	22	92
Total	81	100	81	131	217	242	128	980
	Percent Scores Under 7							
Under 34	88.24	61.48	22.22	10.53	3.91	2.22	1.09	19.32
34–36	80.00†	39.29	21.74	8.01	5.87	1.93	1.80	6.58
37–39	100.00†	30.00†	20.75	7.42	3.21	2.78	2.56	3.64
40–42	100.00†	60.00†	12.00	7.10	3.94	3.90	4.68	4.32
43+	–	–	20.00†	5.62	6.52	4.93	5.03	5.48
Total	88.04	56.18	21.15	7.81	4.07	3.44	3.99	5.47

*With known birthweight, gestation, and APGAR score.
†Based on less than 20 cases.

9–5 show that babies with lower Apgar scores at five minutes have a greater risk of mortality than those with similar scores at one minute.

The mean birthweight by five-minute Apgar score by race is shown in Table 9–18. For both whites and blacks as the mean birthweight decreased, five-minute Apgar scores also decreased (Fig. 9–6.)

Tables 9–16 and 9–17 show the rate of neurological abnormality at one year, by five-minute Apgar score, by birthweight for whites and blacks. For this table, five-minute Apgar scores have been grouped as 0–3, 4–6, and 7–10. The number of children with scores of 3 and below at five minutes is small. To be remembered is the extremely high mortality rate for neonates under 2501 grams with five-minute Apgar scores of 0–3. Among white survivors examined at one year, the neurological abnormality rate was 45.87 for children with five-minute scores of 0–3 as compared with 15.63 for those with scores of 7–10. For black infants, the low and high five-minute score groups were associated with rates of 35.71 and 14.62, respectively. The relationship between stress at birth and neurological outcome at one year, suggested by consideration of the one-minute Apgar scores, is strongly reinforced by the data on five-minute scores.

Table 9-14. Neonatal Deaths by Five-Minute APGAR Score by Birthweight — White

Score	Under 2501 gm			Over 2500 gm			Total		
	Livebirths	Neonatal Deaths	Rate	Livebirths	Neonatal Deaths	Rate	Livebirths	Neonatal Deaths	Rate
0–1	43	35	813.95	35	6	171.43	78	41	525.64
2	26	20	769.23	40	5	125.00	66	25	378.79
3	26	15	576.92	46	2	43.48	72	17	236.11
4	14	7	500.00*	56	3	53.57	70	10	142.86
5	30	10	333.33	107	5	46.73	137	15	109.49
6	57	7	122.81	212	2	9.43	269	9	33.46
7	78	8	102.56	340	4	11.76	418	12	28.71
8	168	12	71.43	1431	10	6.99	1599	22	13.76
9	592	7	11.82	11116	25	2.25	11708	32	2.73
10	141	1	7.09	2698	7	2.59	2839	8	2.82
Total	1175	122	103.83	16081	69	4.29	17256	191	11.07
Unknown	144	25	173.61	1081	7	6.48	1225	32	26.12
Grand total	1319	147	111.45	17162	76	4.43	18481	223	12.07

*Based on less than 20 cases.

Table 9-15. Neonatal Deaths by Five-Minute APGAR Score by Birthweight — Black

Score	Under 2501 gm			Over 2500 gm			Total		
	Livebirths	Neonatal Deaths	Rate	Livebirths	Neonatal Deaths	Rate	Livebirths	Neonatal Deaths	Rate
0–1	55	45	818.18	41	8	195.12	96	53	552.08
2	55	35	636.36	58	7	120.69	113	42	371.68
3	46	22	478.26	66	8	121.21	112	30	267.86
4	57	23	403.51	72	8	111.11	129	31	240.31
5	58	15	258.62	114	5	43.86	172	20	116.28
6	128	23	179.69	241	10	41.49	369	33	89.43
7	113	12	106.19	339	2	5.90	452	14	30.97
8	249	16	64.26	1032	7	6.78	1281	23	17.95
9	850	11	12.94	6907	19	2.75	7757	30	3.87
10	743	5	6.73	6831	18	2.64	7574	23	3.04
Total	2354	207	87.94	15701	92	5.86	18055	299	16.56
Unknown	263	31	117.87	1186	6	5.06	1449	37	25.53
Grand total	2617	238	90.94	16887	98	5.80	19504	336	17.23

Table 9-16. Children Neurologically Abnormal at One Year by Five-Minute APGAR Score by Birthweight — White

Score	Under 2501 gm			Over 2500 gm			Total		
	One-Year Exam	Abnormals	Rate	One-Year Exam	Abnormals	Rate	One-Year Exam	Abnormals	Rate
0–3	19	3	157.89*	90	2	22.22	109	5	45.87
4–6	57	6	105.26	299	11	36.79	356	17	47.75
7–10	766	34	44.39	12735	177	13.90	13501	211	15.63
Total	842	43	51.07	13124	190	14.48	13966	233	16.68
Unknown	79	5	63.29	572	10	17.48	651	15	23.04
Grand total	921	48	52.12	13696	200	14.60	14617	248	16.97

*Based on less than 20 cases.

Table 9-17. Children Neurologically Abnormal at One Year by Five-Minute APGAR Score by Birthweight — Black

Score	Under 2501 gm			Over 2500 gm			Total		
	One-Year Exam	Abnormals	Rate	One-Year Exam	Abnormals	Rate	One-Year Exam	Abnormals	Rate
0–3	46	1	21.74	122	5	40.98	168	6	35.71
4–6	163	14	85.89	364	8	21.98	527	22	41.75
7–10	1692	59	34.87	13492	163	12.08	15184	222	14.62
Total	1901	74	38.93	13978	176	12.59	15879	250	15.74
Unknown	191	12	62.83	983	10	10.17	1174	22	18.74
Grand total	2092	86	41.11	14961	186	12.43	17053	272	15.95

Table 9-18. Mean Birthweight by Five-Minute APGAR Score by Race

Score	WHITE Livebirths with Known Birthweight	WHITE Mean Birthweight	BLACK Livebirths with Known Birthweight	BLACK Mean Birthweight
0–1	78	2141	96	2085
2	66	2640	113	2383
3	72	2774	112	2508
4	70	2973	129	2524
5	137	3044	172	2707
6	269	3067	369	2696
7	418	3110	452	2908
8	1599	3218	1281	2995
9	11708	3214	7757	3097
10	2839	3290	7574	3097
Total	17256	3278	18055	3048
Unknown	1225	3178	1449	2931
Grand total	18481	3272	19504	3039

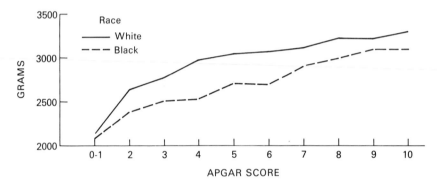

Figure 9-6. Mean Birthweight by Five-Minute APGAR Score by Race

REFERENCES

(1) J. S. Drage and H. Berendes. 1966. Apgar scores and the outcome of the newborn. *Pediatric Clinics of North America* 13: 635–43.

(2) V. Apgar. 1953. A proposal for a new method of evaluation of the newborn infant. *Current Researches in Anesthesia and Analgesia* 32: 260–67.

10

NEONATAL HEMATOCRITS

Pathological processes occurring during intrauterine life or the neonatal period may seriously affect the normal development of the red blood cells or result in their loss or premature destruction. Low hematocrit levels in the neonatal period, therefore, reflect a number of pathological conditions, including hemorrhage, shock, erythroblastosis and other hemolytic anemias, sepsis, and general immaturity. Early delivery of an immature fetus may result in a pathological outcome due to inadequacy or failure of physiological adaptation. In survivors of the immediate neonatal period, the problem may be accentuated by the very rapid increase in body size of the small immature infant during the first few weeks of extrauterine life.

Hematocrit levels, because of their suspected relationship to the quality of long-term survival were systematically recorded in the NCPP. The observations reported here are concerned with red blood cell concentration per se, as measured by the lowest hematocrit level obtained during the nursery period. While it is the effect of the lowest level that is examined, a wide spectrum of such levels from those below 40 mm. to those of 80 mm. and above were encountered.

The hematocrit or hemoglobin level, or both, were routinely assessed at forty-eight hours of age (plus or minus twelve hours). Capillary blood samples obtained by "heel stick" were used. Determinations were made at other times as clinically indicated. The data reported here are the lowest levels regardless of age. In a relatively small percentage of infants, only hemoglobin levels were available. It should be noted that no values are available for 13 percent of the white and 16 percent of the black babies. Certain biases are introduced because these data are missing in a rather large proportion of the very small immature infants who died during the first forty-eight hours of life without a blood evaluation.

The graphs and tables presented in this section show the distributions of lowest hematocrit levels observed during the neonatal period and the relationships of these levels to neonatal death, birthweight, and neurological abnormality at one year. More detailed analyses concerned with gestational age and birthweight relationships will be available in later publications.

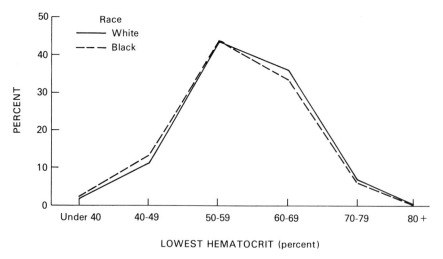

Figure 10-1. Lowest Hematocrit of Newborn by Race

DISTRIBUTION OF LOWEST HEMATOCRIT LEVELS

The distribution curves of lowest recorded levels are quite similar for both black and white babies (Fig. 10–1). The blacks have a slightly greater proportion of lower levels and a correspondingly smaller proportion of higher levels than the whites. When examined by birthweight in two groupings, 2500 grams and below, and above 2500 grams, Tables 10–1 and 10–2 clearly show that the small babies tend to have lower hematocrit levels than the larger babies; 10.13 percent of white and 11.35 percent of black babies under 2501 grams have hematocrit levels below 40 mm., whereas only 1.26 percent of the white and 1.12 percent of the black infants weighing more than 2500 grams at birth had these low levels. Furthermore, 61.18 percent of the white and 68.49 of the black babies below 2501 grams had hematocrit levels of below 60 mm., as compared with 56.36 percent of the white and 58.77 percent of the black infants above 2501 grams.

The distribution of mean birthweight for babies of each race in relation to the lowest recorded hematocrit level reveals the same trends, i.e., that smaller infants tended to have lower levels. The black babies were, on the average, smaller in each hematocrit category than the white babies. A 415-gram difference was observed in the average weight of white and black babies whose hematocrit levels were below 40 mm.; at higher hematocrit levels, the average birthweight difference was approximately 200 grams heavier in the white babies. (Fig. 10–2 and Table 10–3.)

NEONATAL DEATHS BY LOWEST HEMATOCRIT

As might be expected, the neonatal death rates were observed to be higher in babies with low hematocrit levels. In part, this was a function of the well-recognized

Table 10-1. Lowest Hematocrit of Newborn by Birthweight — White

Lowest Hematocrit (percent)	Under 2501 gm			Over 2500 gm			Total		
	Livebirths	Percent	Cumulative Percent	Livebirths	Percent	Cumulative Percent	Livebirths	Percent	Cumulative Percent
Under 40	106	10.13	10.13	189	1.26	1.26	295	1.84	1.84
40–49	172	16.44	26.58	1656	11.03	12.29	1828	11.38	13.22
50–59	362	34.61	61.18	6617	44.08	56.36	6979	43.46	56.68
60–69	320	30.59	91.77	5484	36.53	92.89	5804	36.14	92.82
70–79	81	7.74	99.52	1013	6.75	99.64	1094	6.81	99.63
80+	5	0.48	100.00	54	0.36	100.00	59	0.37	100.00
Total	1046	100.00		15013	100.00		16059	100.00	
Unknown	273	20.70		2149	12.52		2422	13.11	
Grand total	1319	100.00		17162	100.00		18481	100.00	

Table 10-2. Lowest Hematocrit of Newborn by Birthweight — Black

Lowest Hematocrit (percent)	Under 2501 gm			Over 2500 gm			Total		
	Livebirths	Percent	Cumulative Percent	Livebirths	Percent	Cumulative Percent	Livebirths	Percent	Cumulative Percent
Under 40	232	11.35	11.35	159	1.12	1.12	391	2.40	2.40
40–49	370	18.10	29.45	1813	12.73	13.85	2183	13.40	15.80
50–59	798	39.04	68.49	6398	44.92	58.77	7196	44.18	59.99
60–69	513	25.10	93.59	4975	34.93	93.79	5488	33.70	93.68
70–79	126	6.16	99.76	859	6.03	99.73	985	6.05	99.73
80+	5	0.24	100.00	39	0.27	100.00	44	0.27	100.00
Total	2044	100.00		14243	100.00		16287	100.00	
Unknown	573	21.90		2644	15.66		3217	16.49	
Grand total	2617	100.00		16887	100.00		19504	100.00	

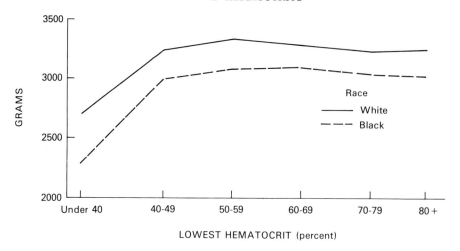

Figure 10-2. Mean Birthweight by Lowest Hematocrit of Newborn by Race

Table 10–3. Mean Birthweight by Lowest Hematocrit of Newborn by Race

Lowest Hematocrit (percent)	WHITE		BLACK	
	Livebirths	Mean Birthweight	Livebirths	Mean Birthweight
Under 40	295	2701	391	2286
40–49	1828	3237	2183	2995
50–59	6979	3329	7196	3080
60–69	5804	3283	5488	3101
70–79	1094	3231	985	3042
80+	59	3249	44	3028
Total	16059	3283	16287	3054
Unknown	2422	3194	3217	2964
Grand total	18481	3272	19504	3039

relationship between low birthweight and increased risk of neonatal death. However, examination of the data controlled on birthweight showed a small but distinct decrease in risk of neonatal death for babies weighing over 2500 grams with increasing levels of hematocrit, to levels of 70 mm. in the white babies and to 80 mm. in the black babies. (Figs. 10–3 and 10–4 and Tables 10–4 and 10–5.)

NEUROLOGICAL ABNORMALITIES AT ONE YEAR

The distribution curves of definite neurological abnormalities at one year in relation to the lowest neonatal hematocrit recorded are quite similar for babies of both races. There were high rates of abnormality for babies of both races who were

Table 10-4. Neonatal Deaths by Lowest Hematocrit of Newborn by Birthweight — White

Lowest Hematocrit (percent)	Under 2501 gm			Over 2500 gm			Total		
	Livebirths	Neonatal Deaths	Rate	Livebirths	Neonatal Deaths	Rate	Livebirths	Neonatal Deaths	Rate
Under 40	106	6	56.60	189	2	10.58	295	8	27.12
40–49	172	9	52.33	1656	11	6.64	1828	20	10.94
50–59	362	7	19.34	6617	15	2.27	6979	22	3.15
60–69	320	5	15.63	5484	8	1.46	5804	13	2.24
70–79	81	1	12.35	1013	5	4.94	1094	6	5.48
80+	5	0	0 *	54	0	0	59	0	0
Total	1046	28	26.77	15013	41	2.73	16059	69	4.30
Unknown	273	119	435.90	2149	35	16.29	2422	154	63.58
Grand total	1319	147	111.45	17162	76	4.43	18481	223	12.07

*Based on less than 20 cases.

Table 10-5. Neonatal Deaths by Lowest Hematocrit of Newborn by Birthweight — Black

Lowest Hematocrit (percent)	Under 2501 gm			Over 2500 gm			Total		
	Livebirths	Neonatal Deaths	Rate	Livebirths	Neonatal Deaths	Rate	Livebirths	Neonatal Deaths	Rate
Under 40	232	4	17.24	159	3	18.87	391	7	17.90
40–49	370	10	27.03	1813	9	4.96	2183	19	8.70
50–59	798	18	22.56	6398	20	3.13	7196	38	5.28
60–69	513	7	13.65	4975	8	1.61	5488	15	2.73
70–79	126	1	7.94	859	1	1.16	985	2	2.03
80+	5	0	0 *	39	0	0	44	0	0
Total	2044	40	19.57	14243	41	2.88	16287	81	4.97
Unknown	573	198	345.55	2644	57	21.56	3217	255	79.27
Grand total	2617	238	90.94	16887	98	5.80	19504	336	17.23

*Based on less than 20 cases.

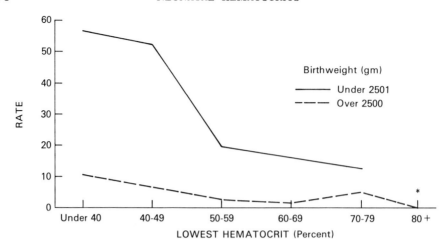

*Based on less than 20 cases.

Figure 10-3. Neonatal Deaths by Lowest Hematocrit of Newborn by Birthweight-White

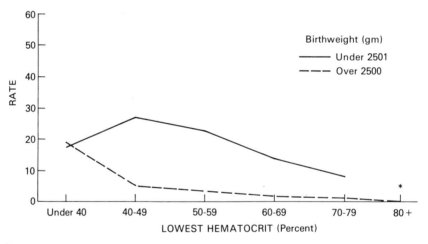

*Based on less than 20 cases.

Figure 10-4. Neonatal Deaths by Lowest Hematocrit of Newborn by Birthweight — Black

anemic, as indicated by hematocrit levels below 40 mm. The rate dropped and remained low for black babies until a level of 79 mm. was reached. There was some increase in risk for black babies with levels of 80 mm. and above. Risk of neurological abnormality was lowest for white babies whose hematocrit was between 50 and 59 mm.; the risks increased slightly to 79 mm. and rose sharply for babies whose hematocrit was 80 mm. or more. However, it should be noted that the numbers of cases are rather small. (Fig. 10–5 and Tables 10–6 and 10–7.)

Table 10-6. Children Neurologically Abnormal at One Year by Lowest Hematocrit of Newborn by Birthweight — White

Lowest Hematocrit (percent)	Under 2501 gm			Over 2500 gm			Total		
	One-Year Exam	Abnormals	Rate	One-Year Exam	Abnormals	Rate	One-Year Exam	Abnormals	Rate
Under 40	83	9	108.43	157	8	50.96	240	17	70.83
40–49	119	6	50.42	1363	22	16.14	1482	28	18.89
50–59	291	9	30.93	5495	62	11.28	5786	71	12.27
60–69	253	8	31.62	4456	68	15.26	4709	76	16.14
70–79	73	7	95.89	825	9	10.91	898	16	17.82
80+	5	2	400.00*	46	2	43.48	51	4	78.43
Total	824	41	49.76	12342	171	13.86	13166	212	16.10
Unknown	97	7	72.16	1354	29	21.42	1451	36	24.81
Grand total	921	48	52.12	13696	200	14.60	14617	248	16.97

*Based on less than 20 cases.

Table 10-7. Children Neurologically Abnormal at One Year by Lowest Hematocrit of Newborn by Birthweight — Black

Lowest Hematocrit (percent)	Under 2501 gm			Over 2500 gm			Total		
	One-Year Exam	Abnormals	Rate	One-Year Exam	Abnormals	Rate	One-Year Exam	Abnormals	Rate
Under 40	204	18	88.24	142	8	56.34	346	26	75.14
40–49	309	11	35.60	1574	20	12.71	1883	31	16.46
50–59	689	19	27.58	5719	69	12.07	6408	88	13.73
60–69	454	17	37.44	4522	52	11.50	4976	69	13.87
70–79	115	5	43.48	794	3	3.78	909	8	8.80
80+	5	1	200.00*	36	0	0	41	1	24.39
Total	1776	71	39.98	12787	152	11.89	14563	223	15.31
Unknown	316	15	47.47	2174	34	15.64	2490	49	19.68
Grand total	2092	86	41.11	14961	186	12.43	17053	272	15.95

*Based on less than 20 cases.

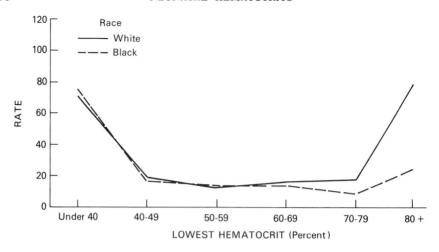

Figure 10-5. Children Neurologically Abnormal at One Year by Lowest Hematocrit of
Newborn by Race

COMMENT

There would seem to be increased risks of neonatal death and neurological abnormality at one year associated with hematocrit levels that are above or below the
normal neonatal range of 40 to 60 mm.; low levels below 40 mm. indicating anemia
and the high levels above 60 mm. indicating some degree of polycythemia or hemo-
concentration. These observations merit further study.

11

NEONATAL SERUM BILIRUBIN LEVELS, HYPERBILIRUBINEMIA, AND LATER NEUROLOGICAL DEVELOPMENT

INTRODUCTION

The neurotoxicity of free bilirubin and the causal relationship between high levels of serum bilirubin, free bilirubin in the tissues, and nerve cell damage as manifested by kernicterus and sensorineural deafness have long been recognized. During the past twenty-five years it has been accepted practice to prevent the occurrence of central nervous system injury from hyperbilirubinemia during the neonatal period by employing exchange transfusion to reduce serum bilirubin levels that have become elevated to 20 mg%, or in those cases where it was anticipated that bilirubin concentration would reach high levels.

In recent years, the validity of the cut-off point at the 20 mg% bilirubin level has been questioned, particularly in low-birthweight babies. The possibility that subtle neurological and cognitive defects might be causally related to intermediate levels of bilirubin (15–19 mg%) led to the routine determination of serum bilirubin levels among all NCPP neonates. Jaundice, while a clinical sign of hyperbilirubinemia, is an unreliable predictor of serum bilirubin level.

The NCPP provided an opportunity to examine the possible role of bilirubin neurotoxicity in the production of a spectrum of mental and neurological deficits, ranging from the overt gross motor signs characteristic of kernicterus to the subtle fine motor and intellectual abnormalities associated with the syndrome of minimal brain dysfunction (MBD). Minimal brain damage related to bilirubin toxicity has been described by Odell et al. (1), and Upadhyay (2) has reported the increased frequency of subtle neurological findings in the absence of overt motor or intellectual deficits in four- and five-year-old children with neonatal hyperbilirubinemia. Boggs, Hardy, and Frazier (3), in a preliminary study of 23,000 infants in the NCPP, found evidence of an association between neonatal hyperbilirubinemia and depression of Bayley Mental and Motor Developmental Scores at age eight months. Increasing percentages of low developmental scores were associated with increasing maximum serum bilirubin levels above 10 mg%, even when the recognized effects of birthweight and Apgar score were taken into account. These findings, through age one year, have recently been confirmed in the NCPP population by Scheidt et al. (6). The data from Johns Hopkins, presented by Hardy and Peeples (4), were in accord and showed, in addition, a relationship between neurological status at one year and neonatal bilirubin level.

The clinical observations suggesting an association between neurological deficits and levels of neonatal serum bilirubin that are only moderately elevated (15 to 19 mg%) have extended the use of exchange transfusions to some babies whose levels peak below 20 mg%. However, this procedure is not without risk. In recent years, phototherapy (5) has been introduced as an adjunct therapy and to prevent the occurrence of high levels. Phototherapy was not used during the period of the NCPP nursery phase, therefore no information is available from this study as to its possible effect in reducing serum bilirubin levels or in preventing the occurrence of elevated levels. However, in view of the controversy surrounding its possible benefits and hazards, it was important to examine possible associations, which may be present within the large body of NCPP data, between bilirubin levels and later outcome.

In order to investigate possible bilirubin neurotoxicity, it is necessary to make allowance for the presence of other variables, such as low birthweight and short gestation, which themselves are associated with increased rates of neurological abnormality.

The data presented here pertain to the possible long-range effects of various levels of neonatal hyperbilirubinemia, recognized through the first year of life. Definition of longer-range effects through age seven years and more detailed clinical relationships, while not possible here, are the subject of an intensive investigation that is under way (6). The data presented here represent a definition of the scope of the problem through one year of age. As almost 8 percent of white infants and 6 percent of black infants have levels above 12 mg% during the neonatal period, hyperbilirubinemia is potentially a problem of considerable magnitude. It is important to define more precisely the potential risk from hyperbilirubinemia in order that optimal clinical management required to prevent neurological injury can be instituted.

Serum bilirubin determinations (direct, indirect, and total) were made on all infants as clinically indicated for the medical care of the baby and became part of the NCPP record. In addition, a routine determination was made on each study infant at 48 hours (± 12 hours) as part of the NCPP protocol. If the total level was 10 mg% or above, the determination was repeated in 24 hours and, if still above 10 mg%, again at four to five days. If the infant's birthweight was below

2250 grams (5 lbs.), three determinations were required, one at 48 hours, a second 24 hours later, and a third at four to five days of age.

The determinations considered here are the *maximum total* serum levels recorded during the neonatal period for each infant, regardless of the age at the time the serum sample was obtained.

Because of variability between institutions during the early months of the study, in both bilirubin methodology and accuracy of results, measures were taken to assure the quality of the data. The procedures and methodology were standardized by a committee of which Dr. Milton Westphal was chairman. This group monitored the quality and reproducibility of the bilirubin determinations by providing "unknown" samples to each institution periodically throughout the course of the study. These quality control procedures, which proved effective, have been described by Westphal et al. (7). The quality control methods in the NCPP were unique and have not generally been available for the many published reports on the effects of hyperbilirubinemia, making comparisons among them difficult.

As the first routine determination of bilirubin level was not required until 48 hours of age, and as determinations were not made at other times unless clinical indications were present, the bilirubin level of many of the infants who died during the first 24 to 48 hours was not determined. As 90 percent of neonatal deaths occurred prior to 48 hours, there are a number of missing observations in the bilirubin data accounted for by early neonatal deaths.

The tables and graphs that accompany this section display the distributions of various maximum total serum bilirubin levels by race, birthweight, and gestational age.

RACE

Distributions of maximum levels reported in Figure 11–1 were very similar by race; over 70 percent of the infants of both races had levels of 7 mg% or less; 21

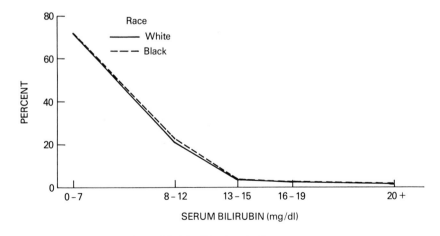

Figure 11-1. Highest Total Serum Bilirubin of Newborn by Race

Table 11-1. Highest Total Serum Bilirubin of Newborn by Birthweight — White

mg/dl	Under 2501 gm			Over 2500 gm			Total		
	Livebirths	Percent	Cumulative Percent	Livebirths	Percent	Cumulative Percent	Livebirths	Percent	Cumulative Percent
0–7	488	42.73	100.00	11908	73.73	100.00	12396	71.69	100.00
8–12	336	29.42	57.27	3243	20.08	26.27	3579	20.70	28.31
13–15	128	11.21	27.85	531	3.29	6.19	659	3.81	7.62
16–19	114	9.98	16.64	315	1.95	2.90	429	2.48	3.81
20+	76	6.65	6.65	153	0.95	0.95	229	1.32	1.32
Total	1142	100.00		16150	100.00		17292	100.00	
Unknown	177	13.42		1012	5.90		1189	6.43	
Grand total	1319	100.00		17162	100.00		18481	100.00	

Table 11-2. Highest Total Serum Bilirubin of Newborn by Birthweight — Black

mg/dl	Under 2501 gm			Over 2500 gm			Total		
	Livebirths	Percent	Cumulative Percent	Livebirths	Percent	Cumulative Percent	Livebirths	Percent	Cumulative Percent
0–7	1137	50.29	100.00	11734	74.48	100.00	12871	71.45	100.00
8–12	719	31.80	49.71	3309	21.00	25.52	4028	22.36	28.55
13–15	225	9.95	17.91	412	2.62	4.51	637	3.54	6.19
16–19	113	5.00	7.96	202	1.28	1.90	315	1.75	2.66
20+	67	2.96	2.96	97	0.62	0.62	164	0.91	0.91
Total	2261	100.00		15754	100.00		18015	100.00	
Unknown	356	13.60		1133	6.71		1489	7.63	
Grand total	2617	100.00		16887	100.00		19504	100.00	

percent of the whites and 22 percent of the blacks had levels in the range of 8 to 12 mg%. Slightly larger percentages of white infants than blacks had levels above 15 mg%; 3.80 as compared with 2.66 percent. This small difference may reflect the increased frequency of Rh blood group incompatibility among the whites. While the overall distributions by race were similar, there were substantial differences between the low-weight black and white infants.

BIRTHWEIGHT

When examined by birthweight a striking difference in bilirubin distributions is noted between the low-birthweight infants and those above 2500 grams (Tables 11–1 and 11–2). Among low-birthweight infants, only 43 percent of the white and 50 percent of the black infants had maximum bilirubin levels of 7 mg% or below, as compared with 74 percent of both white and black infants above 2500 grams. Almost 17 percent of the white and 8 percent of the black low-birthweight infants had levels above 15 mg%, as compared with 2.9 percent of white, and 1.9 percent of black babies weighing over 2500 grams at birth.

When bilirubin distributions are examined within 500-gram birthweight categories, extending from 1001 to 1500 grams through 3001 grams and above, the association with birthweight is more precisely demonstrated (Figs. 11–2 and 11–3 and Tables 11–3 and 11–4). The proportion of high bilirubin levels (16–19 and 20 mg% and above) generally decreases sharply with each increment of birthweight. Among white infants of 1001–1500 grams, 32 percent, and among blacks, 19 percent had bilirubin levels over 15 mg%, as compared with 2.7 percent of the whites and 1.7 percent of the blacks weighing 3001 to 3500 grams.

The distributions of mean birthweight by bilirubin and by race (Fig. 11–4 and Table 11–5) show that the average birthweight was progressively lower as the maximum bilirubin level recorded increased, with a difference of over 500 grams between white infants with levels that did not exceed 7 mg% and those with levels of 20 mg% or above. The difference in birthweight for blacks with the lowest and highest levels was almost 400 grams.

BIRTHWEIGHT AND GESTATIONAL AGE

The relationships between the birthweight and gestational age and maximum bilirubin level are shown in two ways in Figures 11–5 through 11–8. When the mean bilirubin level is graphed for each grouping of birthweight and gestational age, it is clear that the smallest infants within each gestational age grouping tended to have the highest average bilirubin levels. Within all birthweight categories, even those above 3000 grams, the least mature infants (i.e., those with the shortest gestational age) had higher levels than those of longer gestation.

When the distributions of infants with levels above 15 mg% were examined by gestational age and birthweight, similar findings were obtained, though birthweight above 2500 grams seemed to have a lesser effect than the gestational age category of the infant.

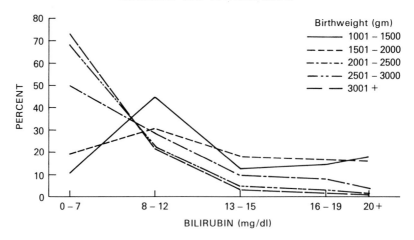

Figure 11-2. Highest Total Serum Bilirubin of Newborn by Birthweight — White

Table 11-3. Highest Total Serum Bilirubin of Newborn by Birthweight (500 gm Intervals) — White

	Livebirths with Known Birthweight							
	Birthweight (gm)							
mg/dl	Under 1001	1001– 1500	1501– 2000	2001– 2500	2501– 3000	3001– 3500	3501+	Total
0–7	2	6	36	444	2345	5089	4474	12396
8–12	1	25	57	253	771	1484	988	3579
13–15	2	7	34	85	162	221	148	659
16–19	3	8	31	72	105	129	81	429
20+	1	10	30	35	55	58	40	229
Total	9	56	188	889	3438	6981	5731	17292
Unknown	52	25	35	65	215	443	354	1189
Grand total	61	81	223	954	3653	7424	6085	18481
Mean	13.11	13.89	12.74	8.52	6.44	5.76	5.24	5.97
Percent								
0–7	22.22*	10.71	19.15	49.94	68.21	72.90	78.07	71.69
8–12	11.11*	44.64	30.32	28.46	22.43	21.26	17.24	20.70
13–15	22.22*	12.50	18.09	9.56	4.71	3.17	2.58	3.81
16–19	33.33*	14.29	16.49	8.10	3.05	1.85	1.41	2.48
20+	11.11*	17.86	15.96	3.94	1.60	0.83	0.70	1.32
Total	100.00	100.00	100.00	100.00	100.00	100.00	100.00	100.00
Unknown	85.25	30.86	15.70	6.81	5.89	5.97	5.82	6.43
Grand total	100.00	100.00	100.00	100.00	100.00	100.00	100.00	100.00
Percent over 15	44.44*	32.14	32.45	12.04	4.65	2.68	2.11	3.81

*Based on less than 20 cases.

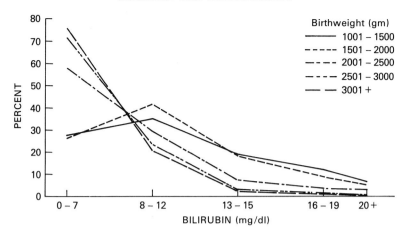

Figure 11-3. Highest Total Serum Bilirubin of Newborn by Birthweight — Black

Table 11-4. Highest Total Serum Bilirubin of Newborn by Birthweight (500 gm Intervals) — Black

				Livebirths with Known Birthweight				
				Birthweight (gm)				
mg/dl	Under 1001	1001– 1500	1501– 2000	2001– 2500	2501– 3000	3001– 3500	3501+	Total
0–7	4	37	101	995	3840	5405	2489	12871
8–12	8	47	162	502	1262	1458	589	4028
13–15	5	25	70	125	175	171	66	637
16–19	0	16	35	62	88	81	33	315
20+	1	9	21	36	29	42	26	164
Total	18	134	389	1720	5394	7157	3203	18015
Unknown	101	69	51	135	423	472	238	1489
Grand total	119	203	440	1855	5817	7629	3441	19504
Mean	10.54	11.18	10.74	7.43	6.02	5.60	5.29	6.00
				Percent				
0–7	22.22*	27.61	25.96	57.85	71.19	75.52	77.71	71.45
8–12	44.44*	35.07	41.65	29.19	23.40	20.37	18.39	22.36
13–15	27.78*	18.66	17.99	7.27	3.24	2.39	2.06	3.54
16–19	0 *	11.94	9.00	3.60	1.63	1.13	1.03	1.75
20+	5.56*	6.72	5.40	2.09	0.54	0.59	0.81	0.91
Total	100.00	100.00	100.00	100.00	100.00	100.00	100.00	100.00
Unknown	84.87	33.99	11.59	7.28	7.27	6.19	6.92	7.63
Grand total	100.00	100.00	100.00	100.00	100.00	100.00	100.00	100.00
Percent over 15	5.56*	18.66	14.40	5.70	2.17	1.72	1.84	2.66

*Based on less than 20 cases.

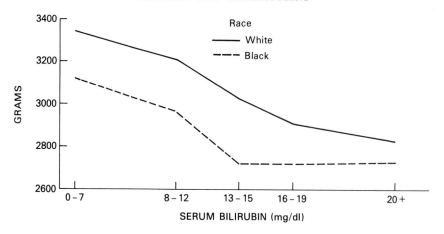

Figure 11-4. Mean Birthweight by Highest Serum Bilirubin of Newborn by Race

Table 11-5. Mean Birthweight
by Highest Total Serum Bilirubin of Newborn by Race

mg/dl	WHITE Livebirths with Known Birthweight	WHITE Mean Birthweight	BLACK Livebirths with Known Birthweight	BLACK Mean Birthweight
0–7	12396	3341	12871	3119
8–12	3579	3208	4028	2963
13–15	659	3025	637	2719
16–19	429	2908	315	2717
20+	229	2825	164	2726
Total	17292	3284	18015	3060
Unknown	1189	3095	1489	2795
Grand total	18481	3272	19504	3039

Thus, the most mature infants, as evidenced by birthweight and gestational age, tended, as one would expect, to be those with lowest maximum bilirubin levels. (See Tables 11–6 and 11–7.)

NEONATAL DEATHS

Among whites, 155 of 223 and among blacks, 263 of 336 neonatal deaths had no bilirubin level reported. In general, these infants were those dying very soon after birth, without medical indication for bilirubin determination, who did not live long enough for routine bilirubin study at forty-eight hours. Because of the relatively small numbers of neonatal deaths where bilirubin information was available, these data are not shown.

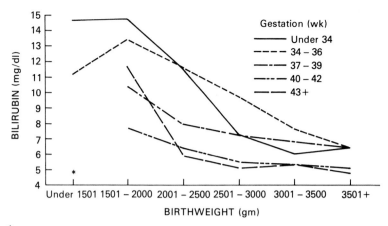

* Based on less than 20 cases.

Figure 11-5. Mean Highest Total Serum Bilirubin of Newborn by Birthweight by Gestation at Delivery — White

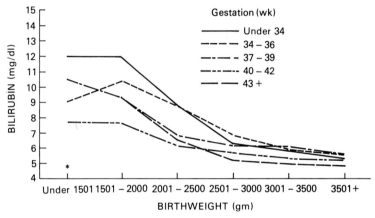

* Based on less than 20 cases.

Figure 11-6. Mean Highest Total Serum Bilirubin of Newborn by Birthweight by Gestation at Delivery — Black

NEUROLOGICAL ABNORMALITIES AT ONE YEAR

Generally speaking, increasing frequencies of definite neurological abnormalities at one year were observed with increasing maximum bilirubin levels above 12 mg%. (Tables 11–8 and 11–9.) These relationships are of such importance that they are the focus of a special, more detailed study that has been reported separately (6).

ERYTHROBLASTOSIS

This clinical diagnosis was based on the presence of Rh or major blood group incompatibility between mother and infant, with isoimmunization, accompanied

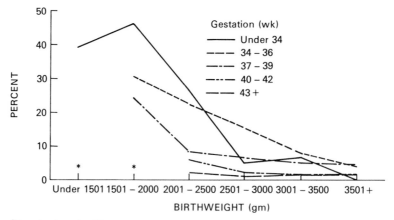

* Based on less than 20 cases.

Figure 11-7. Highest Total Serum Bilirubin of Newborn over 15 by
Birthweight by Gestation at Delivery — White

Table 11-6. Highest Total Serum Bilirubin of Newborn by Birthweight by Gestation at Delivery — White

			Number			
			Birthweight (gm)			
Gestation (wk)	Under 1501	1501– 2000	2001– 2500	2501– 3000	3001– 3500	3501+
Number						
Under 34	51	65	60	61	61	28
34–36	10	62	205	234	165	105
37–39	2	41	354	1318	1829	856
40–42	1	14	219	1509	4135	3758
43+	1	6	46	299	755	945
Mean Bilirubin						
Under 34	14.67	14.74	11.53	7.30	6.02	6.39
34–36	11.20	13.42	11.60	9.73	7.65	6.38
37–39	12.00*	10.41	7.95	7.22	6.81	6.38
40–42	6.00*	7.71	6.36	5.47	5.31	5.07
43+	18.00*	11.67	5.89	5.09	5.31	4.74
Number over 15						
Under 34	20	30	16	3	4	0
34–36	1	19	46	36	13	4
37–39	0	10	30	86	90	38
40–42	0	1	13	31	69	63
43+	1	1	1	3	11	16
Percent over 15						
Under 34	39.22	46.15	26.67	4.92	6.56	0
34–36	10.00†	30.65	22.44	15.38	7.88	3.81
37–39	0 †	24.39	8.47	6.53	4.92	4.44
40–42	0 †	7.14†	5.94	2.05	1.67	1.68
43+	100.00†	16.67†	2.17	1.00	1.46	1.69

*Based on less than 5 cases.
†Based on less than 20 cases.

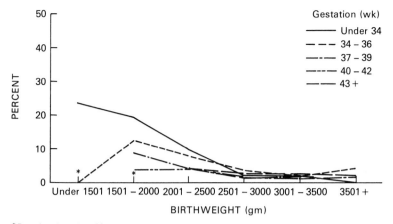

*Based on less than 20 cases.

Figure 11-8. Highest Total Serum Bilirubin of Newborn over 15 by
Birthweight by Gestation at Delivery — Black

Table 11-7. Highest Total Serum Bilirubin of Newborn by Birthweight by Gestation at Delivery — Black

Number

Gestation (wk)	Under 1501	1501– 2000	2001– 2500	2501– 3000	3001– 3500	3501+
Under 34	106	181	212	264	283	96
34–36	27	113	435	629	534	165
37–39	10	57	650	2193	2283	747
40–42	7	26	317	1846	3283	1741
43+	1	9	90	411	729	435

Mean Bilirubin

Gestation (wk)	Under 1501	1501– 2000	2001– 2500	2501– 3000	3001– 3500	3501+
Under 34	11.99	11.97	8.84	6.30	5.83	5.31
34–36	9.04	10.42	8.76	6.87	5.95	5.57
37–39	10.50	9.32	6.83	6.16	6.09	5.65
40–42	7.71	7.65	6.14	5.69	5.33	5.22
43+	7.00*	9.33	6.54	5.22	4.98	4.84

Number over 15

Gestation (wk)	Under 1501	1501– 2000	2001– 2500	2501– 3000	3001– 3500	3501+
Under 34	25	35	21	6	6	0
34–36	0	14	34	23	11	7
37–39	1	5	26	50	60	13
40–42	0	1	12	31	38	31
43+	0	1	4	5	8	8

Percent over 15

Gestation (wk)	Under 1501	1501– 2000	2001– 2500	2501– 3000	3001– 3500	3501+
Under 34	23.58	19.34	9.91	2.27	2.12	0
34–36	0	12.39	7.82	3.66	2.06	4.24
37–39	10.00†	8.77	4.00	2.28	2.63	1.74
40–42	0 †	3.85	3.79	1.68	1.16	1.78
43+	0 †	11.11†	4.44	1.22	1.10	1.84

*Based on less than 5 cases.
†Based on less than 20 cases.

Table 11-8. Children Neurologically Abnormal at One Year
by Highest Total Serum Bilirubin of Newborn by Birthweight — White

mg/dl	Under 2501 gm			Over 2500 gm			Total		
	One-Year Exam	Abnormals	Rate	One-Year Exam	Abnormals	Rate	One-Year Exam	Abnormals	Rate
0–7	388	17	43.81	9757	135	13.84	10145	152	14.98
8–12	262	10	38.17	2614	35	13.39	2876	45	15.65
13–15	97	6	61.86	426	7	16.43	523	13	24.86
16–19	85	5	58.82	266	8	30.08	351	13	37.04
20+	59	6	101.69	122	3	24.59	181	9	49.72
Total	891	44	49.38	13185	188	14.26	14076	232	16.48
Unknown	30	4	133.33	511	12	23.48	541	16	29.57
Grand total	921	48	52.12	13696	200	14.60	14617	248	16.97

Table 11-9. Children Neurologically Abnormal at One Year
by Highest Total Serum Bilirubin of Newborn by Birthweight — Black

mg/dl	Under 2501 gm			Over 2500 gm			Total		
	One-Year Exam	Abnormals	Rate	One-Year Exam	Abnormals	Rate	One-Year Exam	Abnormals	Rate
0–7	1005	35	34.83	10494	126	12.01	11499	161	14.00
8–12	618	22	35.60	2967	35	11.80	3585	57	15.90
13–15	186	7	37.63	366	7	19.13	552	14	25.36
16–19	99	8	80.81	181	1	5.52	280	9	32.14
20+	59	6	101.69	90	5	55.56	149	11	73.83
Total	1967	78	39.65	14098	174	12.34	16065	252	15.69
Unknown	125	8	64.00	863	12	13.90	988	20	20.24
Grand total	2092	86	41.11	14961	186	12.43	17053	272	15.95

Table 11-10. Erythroblastosis — Rh — Newborn

Birthweight (gm)	WHITE			BLACK		
	Livebirths with Newborn Exam (number)	With Condition		Livebirths with Newborn Exam (number)	With Condition	
		(number)	(percent)		(number)	(percent)
Under 2501	1287	26	2.02	2570	8	0.31
Over 2500	16742	87	0.52	16689	24	0.14
Total	18029	113	0.63	19259	32	0.17

Neonatal Deaths

	Livebirths with Newborn Exam (number)	Neonatal Deaths		Livebirths with Newborn Exam (number)	Neonatal Deaths	
		(number)	(rate)		(number)	(rate)
With condition						
Under 2501	26	6	230.77	8	1	125.00†
Over 2500	87	4	45.98	24	0	0
Total	113	10	88.50	32	1	31.25
Without condition						
Under 2501	1226*	126	102.77	2480*	217	87.50
Over 2500	16578*	65	3.92	16564*	90	5.43
Total	17804*	191	10.73	19044*	307	16.12

Neurologically Abnormal at One Year

	One-Year Exam (number)	Neurologically Abnormal		One-Year Exam (number)	Neurologically Abnormal	
		(number)	(rate)		(number)	(rate)
With condition						
Under 2501	19	0	0 †	6	0	0 †
Over 2500	70	0	0	23	1	43.48
Total	89	0	0	29	1	34.48
Without condition						
Under 2501	870	43	49.43	2007	78	38.86
Over 2500	13475	193	14.32	14769	183	12.39
Total	14345	236	16.45	16776	261	15.56

Mean birthweight (gm): White — with condition: 2888   Without condition: 3276
                        Black — with condition: 2840   Without condition: 3046

*Excludes cases with other abnormalities within the system.
†Based on less than 20 cases.

by clinical symptoms. In Rh incompatibility, a positive Coombs' test was required for the diagnosis of erythroblastosis.

A total of 113 cases of Rh erythroblastosis were reported among white neonates, a frequency of occurrence of 0.63 percent. Of these babies, almost 25 percent weighed less than 2501 grams, more than a threefold increase in low birthweight. Some increase in neonatal deaths was noted, but not in neurological abnormalities at one year. (Table 11–10.)

Among blacks, 32 cases of Rh erythroblastosis were reported (0.17 percent). Twenty-five percent were of low birthweight. There were too few cases to make any judgments about risks of neonatal death or neurological abnormality.

Table 11-11. Direct Coombs' Test — Newborn

Birthweight	WHITE			BLACK		
	Livebirths Tested	Positive Tests		Livebirths Tested	Positive Tests	
		No.	%		No.	%
Under 2501 gm	1205	47	3.90	2361	32	1.36
Over 2500 gm	16292	490	3.01	15990	252	1.58
Total	17497	537	3.07	18351	284	1.55

Forty-three cases of ABO erythroblastosis were reported in white infants and 63 among black infants. The rate of low birthweight was not significantly increased and the mean birthweight was 3132 for white children with the condition, as compared with 3276 for those without. Comparable birthweights for blacks were 2940 and 3046, respectively. (See Tables 12–88 and 12–89.)

COOMBS' TEST

Major blood grouping and Rh typing and a direct Coombs' test for the presence of antibody absorbed onto the surface of red cells was carried out on cord blood from each infant. The Coombs' test, when positive, was helpful in the diagnosis of Rh isoimmunization and in making a diagnosis of Rh erythroblastosis. Table 11–11 shows the frequency of positive Coombs' tests observed in white and black babies. Approximately 3 percent of the white and 1.55 percent of the black babies had positive tests.

EXCHANGE TRANSFUSIONS

One or more exchange transfusions were carried out for 172 white and 136 black infants. These figures give the frequency of this procedure in this population. (See Tables 12–98 and 12–99, Chapter 12, for information regarding mortality and neurological outcome.)

REFERENCES

(1) G. B. Odell, G. N. B. Storey, and L. A. Rosenberg. 1970. Studies in kernicterus. III. The saturation of serum proteins with bilirubin during neonatal life and its relationship to brain damage at five years. *Journal of Pediatrics* 76: 12–21.

(2) Y. Upadhyay. 1971. A longitudinal study of full-term neonates with hyperbilirubinemia to four years of age. *Johns Hopkins Medical Journal* 128: 273–77.

(3) T. R. Boggs, J. B. Hardy, and T. M. Frazier. 1967. Correlation of neonatal serum total bilirubin concentrations and developmental status at age eight months. *Journal of Pediatrics* 71: 553–60.

(4) J. B. Hardy and M. O. Peeples. 1971. Serum bilirubin levels in newborn infants. Distributions and associations with neurological abnormalities during the first year of life. *Johns Hopkins Medical Journal* 128: 265–72.

(5) J. F. Lucey. 1973. The effects of light on the newly born infant. *Journal of Perinatal Medicine* 1: 1–6.

(6) P. C. Scheidt, E. D. Mellits, J. B. Hardy, J. S. Drage, and T. R. Boggs. 1977. Toxicity to bilirubin in neonates: Infant development during first year in relation to maximum neonatal bilirubin concentration. *Journal of Pediatrics* 91/2: 292–97.

(7) M. Westphal, E. Viergiver, and R. Roth. 1962. Analysis of a bilirubin survey. *Pediatrics* 30: 12–16.

12

SPECIFIC NEONATAL
DIAGNOSES

INTRODUCTION

This chapter is concerned with a description of selected conditions and procedures reported during the newborn period and their possible relationship to subsequent abnormality. As the risks of neonatal death and neurological abnormality are strongly related to the infant's weight at birth, the risk is examined, for each condition, in two birthweight groups, above 2500 grams and 2500 grams and below.

The data presented in this chapter are diverse and detailed. The basic diagnostic summary tables are presented for white and black infants separately and within each race. They are to be found at the end of the chapter (see Tables 12–62 through 12–99). They include: (1) the frequency with which the various definite diagnoses and conditions were reported in infants in the two birthweight groups; (2) the risk of neonatal death, expressed as rate per 1000 livebirths; (3) the risk of definite neurological abnormality at one year of age, expressed as rate per 1000 children examined; and (4) the average birthweight for the group of babies with each diagnosis. For comparative purposes, similar information is given in each table for all those children without any specific diagnoses within the organ system presented.

In perusing the summary tables, it must be remembered that as each organ system is reported independently, the "none" or no abnormality category pertains only to that specific organ system under consideration, and a child may have had an abnormality reported under another system. Also, the opportunity for multiple diagnoses existed and therefore a child may have been tallied in more than one diagnostic category within a system. For example, it will be noted that 6 percent of both white and black infants were resuscitated during the first five minutes of life; some of these will have been infants with respiratory distress, others may have had primary apnea, and still others both distress and apnea; these tabulations do not tell us how many of the infants resuscitated fell into each category.

The diagnostic summary tables are, as indicated, arranged by organ system. Two systems are discussed in considerable detail. Because of the particular importance of neurological development in the NCPP, the data pertaining to certain aspects of neurological function have been examined in greater detail and the results are presented in the section dealing with neurological diagnoses. Similarly, because of the important role of respiratory malfunction in neonatal mortality and morbidity, the analyses in the section on respiratory diagnoses have also been extended by additional detail, discussion, and interpretation. In this section, it was possible to include an examination of the role of gestational age, in addition to that of birthweight, in relation to adverse outcome.

With few exceptions, the data for other systems are presented in tabular form, without additional comment. An interpretive summary is included at the end of the chapter.

The Newborn Diagnostic Summary

As already described in Chapter 3, the PED–8, *Newborn Diagnostic Summary,* was completed for each neonate upon hospital discharge or death prior to discharge. The length of nursery stay is discussed in Chapter 3. This summary was developed to provide systematic documentation of medical observations, diagnoses, and procedures. The diagnoses were recorded on the basis of specific criteria defined in the manual. They were recorded as "definite" in the presence of clear-cut clinical, biochemical, radiological, and/or pathological evidence, or as "suspect" when the diagnosis appeared likely, but was not clear-cut. The data presented here are retricted to those cases where the diagnoses was "definite"; those with "suspect" diagnoses have been included with the large group of infants who were considered normal. It should be pointed out that for some major diagnostic categories there were few, if any, "suspect" cases, while for other conditions, where diagnostic criteria are less clear-cut, the "suspect" cases were more numerous.

The data have been reviewed for interinstitutional differences. In only a few instances, unusual interinstitutional variation was noted (e.g., the frequency of preauricular sinuses at one institution); such variation pertained to minor findings and reflected an unusual interest of a specific examiner. In addition, as can be seen in the tables, the frequencies of the various major diagnoses by race were quite similar. Exceptions were those few conditions, such as Rh erythroblastosis and polydactyly, where racial differences were expected and observed. This similarity by race supports the pooling of data from the institutions in this report.

The diagnostic information, as outlined above, is presented in the extensive tables that follow, for the 18,029 white and 19,259 black live, singleborn infants, with known birthweight, who received the newborn examination. These tables are based on the diagnoses reported on the PED–8, *Newborn Diagnostic Summary,* by the collaborating institutions, at the time of the infant's discharge from the hospital nursery. Listed under the appropriate organ system are those congenital malformations reported during the newborn hospital stay, or on the post-mortem examination if the child died during this period. As would be expected, only a portion of all congenital malformations was identified in the nursery. A comparison of the malformations reported during the nursery period and by one year of age is presented in Chapter 16, and a specific report of congenital malformations in the NCPP has been published elsewhere (1).

NEUROLOGICAL ABNORMALITIES AND BIRTH INJURIES

Brain Abnormality

Brain abnormality was a summary diagnosis based on evidence of abnormal neurological function observed during the nursery stay and thought to reflect an abnormality of brain function. Abnormalities of cranial and peripheral nerves and of the spinal cord were reported separately.

In order to arrive at the diagnosis, three steps were required. First, a decision had to be made as to whether the abnormality was clear-cut and *definite* or was merely *suspected*. Second, the significant manifestations that reflected the brain abnormality were reported individually as definite or suspect. Third, the duration of the abnormality was reported as transient or persistent throughout the nursery stay. In order for an overall diagnosis of brain abnormality to be made, it was necessary that one or more of the individual manifestations be present. It should be noted that some of the manifestations were observed in babies who were not considered, on the basis of all the evidence available, to be sufficiently affected to warrant an overall diagnosis of definite brain abnormality; these babies were diagnosed as suspect. For example, there were 137 white infants (approximately 0.8 percent) who were reported to have a definite abnormality of brain function, while there were 237 who were reported to manifest definite jitteriness or tremulousness and 324 who were definitely hypotonic. Some of these infants were reported as suspect for brain abnormality. As has been the general practice in this report, the presentation of data has been restricted to those diagnoses considered definite. Children with suspected diagnoses were included with the large group considered normal.

As indicated in the accompanying tables and graphs, a diagnosis of definite brain abnormality was not frequent in the newborn period. It was made in 137 white babies (0.8 percent) and 192 black babies (1 percent). A striking difference existed in the frequency of the condition in babies weighing 2500 grams or below, as compared with babies weighing more than that. It will be noted that the slightly higher overall rate for all black infants is largely accounted for by the greater frequency of low-weight babies among the blacks. (Table 12–1.)

The greatly increased rates of neonatal death and neurological abnormality at one year of age, associated with definite brain abnormality in the newborn period, are clearly seen for babies of both birthweight groups in both races.

Seizures. Seizures were coded as definitely present only if observed by a reliable observer. A suspect diagnosis was not changed to a definite one on the basis of electroencephalographic changes alone.

Seizures in the newborn period were not of common occurrence. This diagnosis

Table 12-1. Brain Abnormality — Newborn

Birthweight (gm)	WHITE			BLACK		
	Livebirths with Newborn Exam (number)	With Condition		Livebirths with Newborn Exam (number)	With Condition	
		(number)	(percent)		(number)	(percent)
Under 2501	1287	52	4.04	2570	89	3.46
Over 2500	16742	85	0.51	16689	103	0.62
Total	18029	137	0.76	19259	192	1.00

Neonatal Deaths

	Livebirths with Newborn Exam (number)	Neonatal Deaths		Livebirths with Newborn Exam (number)	Neonatal Deaths	
		(number)	(rate)		(number)	(rate)
With condition						
Under 2501	52	31	596.15	89	60	674.16
Over 2500	85	25	294.12	103	31	300.97
Total	137	56	408.76	192	91	473.96
Without condition						
Under 2501	915*	58	63.39	1998*	97	48.55
Over 2500	14845*	32	2.16	14976*	45	3.00
Total	15760*	90	5.71	16974*	142	8.37

Neurologically Abnormal at One Year

	One-Year Exam (number)	Neurologically Abnormal		One-Year Exam (number)	Neurologically Abnormal	
		(number)	(rate)		(number)	(rate)
With condition						
Under 2501	14	3	214.29†	20	6	300.00
Over 2500	52	21	403.85	60	10	166.67
Total	66	24	363.64	80	16	200.00
Without condition						
Under 2501	694	24	34.58	1695	50	29.50
Over 2500	12122	134	11.05	13405	132	9.85
Total	12816	158	12.33	15100	182	12.05

Mean birthweight (gm): White — with condition: 2638   Without condition: 3293
Black — with condition: 2384   Without condition: 3064

*Excludes cases with other abnormalities within the system.
†Based on less than 20 cases.

was reported in Table 12–2 for 46 white (0.26 percent) and 62 black (0.32 percent) infants. The mean birthweight was slightly less for babies of both races with seizures, and rates of neonatal death and neurological abnormality were markedly increased, as compared with babies without any abnormal brain function reported.

Seizure disorders observed in the NCPP are being investigated in depth and will be the subject of a separate report.

Jitteriness. The presence of jitteriness or tremulousness was reported on the basis of observations during multiple pediatric and neurological examinations. The report depended on the presence of excessive tremulous movement occurring spontaneously or in response to an external stimulus. These movements, which tended to

Table 12-2. Seizures — Newborn

Birthweight (gm)	WHITE			BLACK		
	Livebirths with Newborn Exam (number)	With Condition (number)	With Condition (percent)	Livebirths with Newborn Exam (number)	With Condition (number)	With Condition (percent)
Under 2501	1287	12	0.93	2570	20	0.78
Over 2500	16742	34	0.20	16689	42	0.25
Total	18029	46	0.26	19259	62	0.32

Neonatal Deaths

	Livebirths with Newborn Exam (number)	Neonatal Deaths (number)	Neonatal Deaths (rate)	Livebirths with Newborn Exam (number)	Neonatal Deaths (number)	Neonatal Deaths (rate)
With condition						
Under 2501	12	2	166.67†	20	10	500.00
Over 2500	34	9	264.71	42	15	357.14
Total	46	11	239.13	62	25	403.23
Without condition						
Under 2501	915*	58	63.39	1998*	97	48.55
Over 2500	14845*	32	2.16	14976*	45	3.00
Total	15760*	90	5.71	16974*	142	8.37

Neurologically Abnormal at One Year

	One-Year Exam (number)	Neurologically Abnormal (number)	Neurologically Abnormal (rate)	One-Year Exam (number)	Neurologically Abnormal (number)	Neurologically Abnormal (rate)
With condition						
Under 2501	6	0	0 †	7	1	142.86†
Over 2500	21	4	190.48	24	5	208.33
Total	27	4	148.15	31	6	193.55
Without condition						
Under 2501	694	24	34.58	1695	50	29.50
Over 2500	12122	134	11.05	13405	132	9.85
Total	12816	158	12.33	15100	182	12.05

Mean birthweight (gm): White — with condition: 3003   Without condition: 3293
Black — with condition: 2736   Without condition: 3064

*Excludes cases with other abnormalities within the system.
†Based on less than 20 cases.

occur in repeated bursts, were noted particularly in the upper extremities and were distinguished from coarse myoclonic jerks.

A twofold increase in frequency was observed in low-birthweight babies, and the mean birthweight was slightly less in jittery babies of both races (Table 12–3). The neonatal death rate and the rate of neurological abnormalities at one year were also higher for babies of both races exhibiting jitteriness in the neonatal period and who were diagnosed as having suspect or definite brain abnormality. Neonatologists have long speculated about the long-range outcome for jittery babies. Jittery babies had at least a threefold increase in neurological abnormalities at one year in both races and for both low-weight and larger babies.

Table 12-3. Jitteriness — Newborn

Birthweight (gm)	WHITE			BLACK		
	Livebirths with Newborn Exam (number)	With Condition		Livebirths with Newborn Exam (number)	With Condition	
		(number)	(percent)		(number)	(percent)
Under 2501	1287	31	2.41	2570	91	3.54
Over 2500	16742	206	1.23	16689	307	1.84
Total	18029	237	1.31	19259	398	2.07

Neonatal Deaths

	Livebirths with Newborn Exam (number)	Neonatal Deaths		Livebirths with Newborn Exam (number)	Neonatal Deaths	
		(number)	(rate)		(number)	(rate)
With condition						
Under 2501	31	0	0	91	6	65.93
Over 2500	206	4	19.42	307	3	9.77
Total	237	4	16.88	398	9	22.61
Without condition						
Under 2501	915*	58	63.39	1998*	97	48.55
Over 2500	14845*	32	2.16	14976*	45	3.00
Total	15760*	90	5.71	16974*	142	8.37

Neurologically Abnormal at One Year

	One-Year Exam (number)	Neurologically Abnormal		One-Year Exam (number)	Neurologically Abnormal	
		(number)	(rate)		(number)	(rate)
With condition						
Under 2501	27	4	148.15	75	7	93.33
Over 2500	177	7	39.55	274	10	36.50
Total	204	11	53.92	349	17	48.71
Without condition						
Under 2501	694	24	34.58	1695	50	29.50
Over 2500	12122	134	11.05	13405	132	9.85
Total	12816	158	12.33	15100	182	12.05

Mean birthweight (gm): White — with condition: 3172   Without condition: 3293
Black — with condition: 2906   Without condition: 3064

*Excludes cases with other abnormalities within the system.

Hypertonia. Muscle tone was evaluated on a number of occasions during the newborn period in the PED–2, *Neonatal Examination*, and in the PED–6, *Neonatal Neurological Examination*, at 48 hours (± 12 hours). The examiner was instructed to consider the maturity of the baby in assessing the tone. (Table 12–4.)

Hypertonia included rigidity, spasticity, and increased muscle tone. As may be seen in the accompanying graphs and tables, this condition was of relatively infrequent occurrence in low-birthweight babies. The average birthweight, for both races, was 500 to 600 grams greater for babies with hypertonia than for babies diagnosed as having abnormal brain function in general; nevertheless, babies of both races with hypertonia had significantly higher rates of neonatal death and

Table 12-4. Hypertonia — Newborn

Birthweight (gm)	WHITE Livebirths with Newborn Exam (number)	With Condition (number)	With Condition (percent)	BLACK Livebirths with Newborn Exam (number)	With Condition (number)	With Condition (percent)
Under 2501	1287	10	0.78	2570	35	1.36
Over 2500	16742	82	0.49	16689	121	0.73
Total	18029	92	0.51	19259	156	0.81

Neonatal Deaths

	Livebirths with Newborn Exam (number)	Neonatal Deaths (number)	Neonatal Deaths (rate)	Livebirths with Newborn Exam (number)	Neonatal Deaths (number)	Neonatal Deaths (rate)
With condition						
Under 2501	10	1	100.00†	35	1	28.57
Over 2500	82	5	60.98	121	10	82.64
Total	92	6	65.22	156	11	70.51
Without condition						
Under 2501	915*	58	63.39	1998*	97	48.55
Over 2500	14845*	32	2.16	14976*	45	3.00
Total	15760*	90	5.71	16974*	142	8.37

Neurologically Abnormal at One Year

	One-Year Exam (number)	Neurologically Abnormal (number)	Neurologically Abnormal (rate)	One-Year Exam (number)	Neurologically Abnormal (number)	Neurologically Abnormal (rate)
With condition						
Under 2501	8	1	125.00†	28	1	35.71
Over 2500	63	8	126.98	103	5	48.54
Total	71	9	126.76	131	6	45.80
Without condition						
Under 2501	694	24	34.58	1695	50	29.50
Over 2500	12122	134	11.05	13405	132	9.85
Total	12816	158	12.33	15100	182	12.05

Mean birthweight (gm): White — with condition: 3151   Without condition: 3293
Black — with condition: 2915   Without condition: 3064

*Excludes cases with other abnormalities within the system.
†Based on less than 20 cases.

neurological abnormality at one year than babies with normal muscle tone. The frequency of this finding was minimally higher in black infants; this seemed to be related to the higher frequency of affected low-birthweight infants in this racial group. Hypertonia was thought to reflect suspect or definite brain abnormality in 92 (0.51 percent) white and in 156 (0.81 percent) black infants.

Hypotonia. Among infants with suspect or definite brain abnormality, the diagnosis of reduced muscle tone was made with some frequency in both races: in 324 (1.8 percent) white and 415 (2.2 percent) black infants. The small racial difference reflected the increased frequency of low birthweight among the blacks (Table 12–5). Hypotonia was prevalent among small babies; a markedly lower mean

Table 12-5. Hypotonia — Newborn

Birthweight (gm)	WHITE			BLACK		
	Livebirths with Newborn Exam (number)	With Condition		Livebirths with Newborn Exam (number)	With Condition	
		(number)	(percent)		(number)	(percent)
Under 2501	1287	116	9.01	2570	189	7.35
Over 2500	16742	208	1.24	16689	226	1.35
Total	18029	324	1.80	19259	415	2.15

Neonatal Deaths

	Livebirths with Newborn Exam (number)	Neonatal Deaths		Livebirths with Newborn Exam (number)	Neonatal Deaths	
		(number)	(rate)		(number)	(rate)
With condition						
Under 2501	116	48	413.79	189	75	396.83
Over 2500	208	22	105.77	226	28	123.89
Total	324	70	216.05	415	103	248.19
Without condition						
Under 2501	915*	58	63.39	1998*	97	48.55
Over 2500	14845*	32	2.16	14976*	45	3.00
Total	15760*	90	5.71	16974*	142	8.37

Neurologically Abnormal at One Year

	One-Year Exam (number)	Neurologically Abnormal		One-Year Exam (number)	Neurologically Abnormal	
		(number)	(rate)		(number)	(rate)
With condition						
Under 2501	51	12	235.29	97	17	175.26
Over 2500	160	25	156.25	178	21	117.98
Total	211	37	175.36	275	38	138.18
Without condition						
Under 2501	694	24	34.58	1695	50	29.50
Over 2500	12122	134	11.05	13405	132	9.85
Total	12816	158	12.33	15100	182	12.05

Mean birthweight (gm): White — with condition: 2747 Without condition: 3293
Black — with condition: 2468 Without condition: 3064

*Excludes cases with other abnormalities within the system.

birthweight (over 500 grams less for both whites and blacks) was noted for those with reduced muscle tone. Not only was this finding associated with an increased frequency of low birthweight and reduced mean birthweight, but it was also accompanied by a high risk of neonatal death and residual neurological damage. Hypotonia occurred with almost three times the frequency of hypertonia. Hypotonia was strongly related to low birthweight, whereas hypertonia was not.

Hypoactivity. This condition referred to paucity of spontaneous body movement as a reflection of brain abnormality (suspect or definite) at various times during the hospital stay. It, too, depended on subjective impression and the examiner's experience in diagnosis. Like hypotonia, it was noted to be of high frequency in low-

Table 12-6. Hypoactivity — Newborn

Birthweight (gm)	WHITE			BLACK		
	Livebirths with Newborn Exam (number)	With Condition		Livebirths with Newborn Exam (number)	With Condition	
		(number)	(percent)		(number)	(percent)
Under 2501	1287	66	5.13	2570	129	5.02
Over 2500	16742	85	0.51	16689	158	0.95
Total	18029	151	0.84	19259	287	1.49

Neonatal Deaths

	Livebirths with Newborn Exam (number)	Neonatal Deaths		Livebirths with Newborn Exam (number)	Neonatal Deaths	
		(number)	(rate)		(number)	(rate)
With condition						
Under 2501	66	37	560.61	129	59	457.36
Over 2500	85	17	200.00	158	23	145.57
Total	151	54	357.62	287	82	285.71
Without condition						
Under 2501	915*	58	63.39	1998*	97	48.55
Over 2500	14845*	32	2.16	14976*	45	3.00
Total	15760*	90	5.71	16974*	142	8.37

Neurologically Abnormal at One Year

	One-Year Exam (number)	Neurologically Abnormal		One-Year Exam (number)	Neurologically Abnormal	
		(number)	(rate)		(number)	(rate)
With condition						
Under 2501	24	6	250.00	62	6	96.77
Over 2500	57	9	157.89	120	10	83.33
Total	81	15	185.19	182	16	87.91
Without condition						
Under 2501	694	24	34.58	1695	50	29.50
Over 2500	12122	134	11.05	13405	132	9.85
Total	12816	158	12.33	15100	182	12.05

Mean birthweight (gm): White — with condition: 2546   Without condition: 3293
                                    Black — with condition: 2490   Without condition: 3064

*Excludes cases with other abnormalities within the system.

birthweight infants. It was observed with somewhat greater frequency in black (1.5 percent) than white (0.8 percent) babies. Also, like hypotonia, it was strongly associated with increased rates of neonatal death and of neurological abnormality at one year of age in both white and black infants. (Table 12–6.)

Hyperactivity. Very few babies were noted to be hyperactive as a reflection of brain abnormality: only 9 white and 23 black babies. These tended to be large babies. There was no associated mortality or residual neurological damage. (See Tables 12–62 and 12–63.)

Lethargy. This diagnosis also depended on a subjective impression, referring to a marked depression in the apparent state of consciousness or awareness as dis-

Table 12-7. Lethargy — Newborn

Birthweight (gm)	WHITE			BLACK		
	Livebirths with Newborn Exam (number)	With Condition		Livebirths with Newborn Exam (number)	With Condition	
		(number)	(percent)		(number)	(percent)
Under 2501	1287	50	3.89	2570	62	2.41
Over 2500	16742	79	0.47	16689	91	0.55
Total	18029	129	0.72	19259	153	0.79

Neonatal Deaths

	Livebirths with Newborn Exam (number)	Neonatal Deaths		Livebirths with Newborn Exam (number)	Neonatal Deaths	
		(number)	(rate)		(number)	(rate)
With condition						
Under 2501	50	27	540.00	62	27	435.48
Over 2500	79	13	164.56	91	10	109.89
Total	129	40	310.08	153	37	241.83
Without condition						
Under 2501	915*	58	63.39	1998*	97	48.55
Over 2500	14845*	32	2.16	14976*	45	3.00
Total	15760*	90	5.71	16974*	142	8.37

Neurologically Abnormal at One Year

	One-Year Exam (number)	Neurologically Abnormal		One-Year Exam (number)	Neurologically Abnormal	
		(number)	(rate)		(number)	(rate)
With condition						
Under 2501	19	1	52.63†	31	4	129.03
Over 2500	57	6	105.26	73	3	41.10
Total	76	7	92.11	104	7	67.31
Without condition						
Under 2501	694	24	34.58	1695	50	29.50
Over 2500	12122	134	11.05	13405	132	9.85
Total	12816	158	12.33	15100	182	12.05

Mean birthweight (gm): White — with condition: 2614   Without condition: 3293
Black — with condition: 2508   Without condition: 3064

*Excludes cases with other abnormalities within the system.
†Based on less than 20 cases.

tinguished from a reduction in gross motor activity. Lethargy, in babies diagnosed to have a brain abnormality, was associated with low birthweight and with increased rates of neonatal mortality and neurological abnormality at one year. (Table 12–7.)

Symmetrical but Abnormal Deep Tendon Reflexes. Abnormality of reflexes was another reflection of brain abnormality. Reported in Table 12–8 are all symmetrical but abnormal or absent reflexes or automatisms, with the exception of abnormal Moro responses, which are reported separately. The frequency of reflex abnormalities was about three times higher in babies weighing less than 2500 grams at birth. Abnormal reflexes were associated with high rates of neonatal death and neurological abnormality at one year. Among white neonates, 113 (0.63 percent)

Table 12-8. Symmetrical, but Abnormal Reflexes — Newborn

Birthweight (gm)	WHITE Livebirths with Newborn Exam (number)	With Condition (number)	With Condition (percent)	BLACK Livebirths with Newborn Exam (number)	With Condition (number)	With Condition (percent)
Under 2501	1287	34	2.64	2570	63	2.45
Over 2500	16742	79	0.47	16689	126	0.75
Total	18029	113	0.63	19259	189	0.98

Neonatal Deaths

	Livebirths with Newborn Exam (number)	Neonatal Deaths (number)	Neonatal Deaths (rate)	Livebirths with Newborn Exam (number)	Neonatal Deaths (number)	Neonatal Deaths (rate)
With condition						
Under 2501	34	10	294.12	63	14	222.22
Over 2500	79	8	101.27	126	13	103.17
Total	113	18	159.29	189	27	142.86
Without condition						
Under 2501	915*	58	63.39	1998*	97	48.55
Over 2500	14845*	32	2.16	14976*	45	3.00
Total	15760*	90	5.71	16974*	142	8.37

Neurologically Abnormal at One Year

	One-Year Exam (number)	Neurologically Abnormal (number)	Neurologically Abnormal (rate)	One-Year Exam (number)	Neurologically Abnormal (number)	Neurologically Abnormal (rate)
With condition						
Under 2501	17	4	235.29†	42	5	119.05
Over 2500	62	10	161.29	103	9	87.38
Total	79	14	177.22	145	14	96.55
Without condition						
Under 2501	694	24	34.58	1695	50	29.50
Over 2500	12122	134	11.05	13405	132	9.85
Total	12816	158	12.33	15100	182	12.05

Mean birthweight (gm): White — with condition: 2880   Without condition: 3293
Black — with condition: 2727   Without condition: 3064

*Excludes cases with other abnormalities within the system.
†Based on less than 20 cases.

exhibited symmetrical but abnormal reflexes; among blacks, the condition occurred in 189 (0.98 percent).

Asymmetry of Reflexes or Tone. This abnormality was observed less frequently than symmetrical abnormality; it was reported in 31 white and 73 black babies. This was predominantly a condition of larger babies; the average birthweight of the whites was 3350 grams, an increase of 57 grams over those without brain abnormality. There was some increase in residual neurological damage in babies of both races, and increased mortality in blacks. (See Tables 12–62 and 12–63.)

Abnormal Moro. The Moro response was elicited by holding the baby face up, inclined in a semisitting position. The back of the head was supported in one of the examiner's hands. The neck was extended and the head suddenly allowed to drop

Table 12-9. Abnormal Moro — Newborn

Birthweight (gm)	WHITE			BLACK		
	Livebirths with Newborn Exam (number)	With Condition		Livebirths with Newborn Exam (number)	With Condition	
		(number)	(percent)		(number)	(percent)
Under 2501	1287	56	4.35	2570	126	4.90
Over 2500	16742	94	0.56	16689	217	1.30
Total	18029	150	0.83	19259	343	1.78

Neonatal Deaths

	Livebirths with Newborn Exam (number)	Neonatal Deaths		Livebirths with Newborn Exam (number)	Neonatal Deaths	
		(number)	(rate)		(number)	(rate)
With condition						
Under 2501	56	23	410.71	126	48	380.95
Over 2500	94	15	159.57	217	22	101.38
Total	150	38	253.33	343	70	204.08
Without condition						
Under 2501	915*	58	63.39	1998*	97	48.55
Over 2500	14845*	32	2.16	14976*	45	3.00
Total	15760*	90	5.71	16974*	142	8.37

Neurologically Abnormal at One Year

	One-Year Exam (number)	Neurologically Abnormal		One-Year Exam (number)	Neurologically Abnormal	
		(number)	(rate)		(number)	(rate)
With condition						
Under 2501	24	6	250.00	68	14	205.88
Over 2500	67	11	164.18	179	12	67.04
Total	91	17	186.81	247	26	105.26
Without condition						
Under 2501	694	24	34.58	1695	50	29.50
Over 2500	12122	134	11.05	13405	132	9.85
Total	12816	158	12.33	15100	182	12.05

Mean birthweight (gm): White — with condition: 2749   Without condition: 3293
Black — with condition: 2619   Without condition: 3064

*Excludes cases with other abnormalities within the system.

back approximately 30 degrees. The normal response included abduction and extension of the arms followed by flexion in an embracing motion, accompanied by flexion of the legs. The stimulus-response sequence was repeated three times in making a final evaluation. Absent, generally depressed or asymmetrical responses were considered to be abnormal. However, failure of response on the basis of a suspected brachial plexus injury or a fractured clavicle was not coded as abnormal in the category of brain abnormality.

Among babies with evidence of abnormal brain function, abnormal Moro reflexes were reported about twice as frequently among the black babies as the white. Table 12–9 shows that they occurred in 343 (1.78 percent) of black and 150 (0.83 percent) of white babies. They were found more frequently in those of low weight;

Table 12-10. Abnormal Cry — Newborn

Birthweight (gm)	WHITE			BLACK		
	Livebirths with Newborn Exam (number)	With Condition		Livebirths with Newborn Exam (number)	With Condition	
		(number)	(percent)		(number)	(percent)
Under 2501	1287	43	3.34	2570	124	4.82
Over 2500	16742	110	0.66	16689	126	0.75
Total	18029	153	0.85	19259	250	1.30

Neonatal Deaths

	Livebirths with Newborn Exam (number)	Neonatal Deaths		Livebirths with Newborn Exam (number)	Neonatal Deaths	
		(number)	(rate)		(number)	(rate)
With condition						
Under 2501	43	17	395.35	124	54	435.48
Over 2500	110	15	136.36	126	22	174.60
Total	153	32	209.15	250	76	304.00
Without condition						
Under 2501	915*	58	63.39	1998*	97	48.55
Over 2500	14845*	32	2.16	14976*	45	3.00
Total	15760*	90	5.71	16974*	142	8.37

Neurologically Abnormal at One Year

	One-Year Exam (number)	Neurologically Abnormal		One-Year Exam (number)	Neurologically Abnormal	
		(number)	(rate)		(number)	(rate)
With condition						
Under 2501	22	3	136.36	60	10	166.67
Over 2500	76	10	131.58	92	11	119.57
Total	98	13	132.65	152	21	138.16
Without condition						
Under 2501	694	24	34.58	1695	50	29.50
Over 2500	12122	134	11.05	13405	132	9.85
Total	12816	158	12.33	15100	182	12.05

Mean birthweight (gm): White — with condition: 2799   Without condition: 3293
Black — with condition: 2407   Without condition: 3064

*Excludes cases with other abnormalities within the system.

the mean birthweight was lower by almost 550 grams in the white and by about 450 grams in the black babies. Rates of neonatal death and of residual neurological abnormality were very high for infants of both races with abnormal Moro responses.

Abnormal Cry. The quality of infant cry, normal or high pitched, stridulous, incessant, etc., was evaluated throughout the nursery stay. The cry was also considered abnormal if it could not be elicited by considerable painful stimulation. In infants with evidence of brain abnormality, approximately 1 percent of both white and black babies exhibited abnormalities of cry (Table 12–10). As with other neurological findings, the low-weight babies were more frequently abnormal, exhibiting rates of abnormality approximately four times as high as babies weighing more than 2500 grams at birth. Abnormal cry was accompanied by high rates of neonatal death and neurological abnormality at one year for babies of both races. Abnormal cry was diagnosed in 153 (0.85 percent) white and 250 (1.30 percent) black babies.

Abnormal Suck. The sucking reflex was examined by placing a sterile nipple or similar object in the mouth of an infant who had not been recently fed. If there was no spontaneous response, the intensity of the stimulus was increased by moving or slowly withdrawing the nipple. If sucking was absent when initially tested, a further attempt was made later in the examination before making a final judgment.

In babies with evidence of brain abnormality, absence of the sucking reflex was related to low birthweight. It was infrequently absent in babies of more than 2500 grams. Absence was indicative of high risks of neonatal mortality and residual neurological damage for babies in both racial groups. The diagnosis was made in 91 (0.50 percent) white and 144 (0.75 percent) black babies. (Table 12–11.)

Cranial and Peripheral Nerve Abnormalities and Selected Birth Injuries

The diagnoses considered in this section included a group of conditions frequently, but not invariably, thought to be associated with trauma during the birth process.

Ocular Nerve Abnormality. This abnormality was reported on the basis of the the presence of strabismus or ptosis. It occurred infrequently; 21 cases were observed in the white (0.12 percent) and 26 cases in the black babies (0.14 percent). The mean birthweight of those infants with the condition differed only slightly from those without. As the number of cases was small, the association with risk could not be assessed meaningfully. (Table 12–12.)

Facial Nerve Abnormality. Babies with either definite paralysis or weakness due to facial nerve injury or abnormality were included in this category. In the reporting process, no attempt was made to distinguish between paralysis of the upper and lower motor neuron types. Like ocular nerve and brachial plexus injuries, facial nerve palsies were infrequent (Table 12–13). Facial palsy was observed in 62 (0.34 percent) of the white and 45 (0.23 percent) of the black babies. Such palsies were not associated with low birthweight, in fact there was an increase of 45 grams in the average birthweight of white infants, and an increase of 264 grams in black infants with the condition, as compared to those without. The average birthweight of the affected black babies was only 10 grams less than the affected whites, instead of the usual average difference of approximately 200 grams.

No increase in the neonatal death rate was observed, but there was some increase in the rate of neurological abnormality at one year among babies noted to have facial palsy during the newborn period.

Brachial Plexus Abnormality. Injury or abnormality of the brachial plexus resulting in definite palsy was an infrequent finding. Table 12–14 reported it in only 15 white babies, 14 of whom weighed over 2500 grams at birth. Their average birthweight was increased more than 400 grams. There were no neonatal deaths and two babies were neurologically abnormal at one year. The findings among black babies were similar, but with some increase in frequency. There were 32 cases, no deaths, and two infants were neurologically abnormal.

Table 12-11. Abnormal Suck — Newborn

Birthweight (gm)	WHITE			BLACK		
	Livebirths with Newborn Exam (number)	With Condition		Livebirths with Newborn Exam (number)	With Condition	
		(number)	(percent)		(number)	(percent)
Under 2501	1287	34	2.64	2570	85	3.31
Over 2500	16742	57	0.34	16689	59	0.35
Total	18029	91	0.50	19259	144	0.75

Neonatal Deaths

	Livebirths with Newborn Exam (number)	Neonatal Deaths		Livebirths with Newborn Exam (number)	Neonatal Deaths	
		(number)	(rate)		(number)	(rate)
With condition						
Under 2501	34	12	352.94	85	36	423.53
Over 2500	57	12	210.53	59	15	254.24
Total	91	24	263.74	144	51	354.17
Without condition						
Under 2501	915*	58	63.39	1998*	97	48.55
Over 2500	14845*	32	2.16	14976*	45	3.00
Total	15760*	90	5.71	16974*	142	8.37

Neurologically Abnormal at One Year

	One-Year Exam (number)	Neurologically Abnormal		One-Year Exam (number)	Neurologically Abnormal	
		(number)	(rate)		(number)	(rate)
With condition						
Under 2501	15	3	200.00†	43	5	116.28
Over 2500	37	8	216.22	38	6	157.89
Total	52	11	211.54	81	11	135.80
Without condition						
Under 2501	694	24	34.58	1695	50	29.50
Over 2500	12122	134	11.05	13405	132	9.85
Total	12816	158	12.33	15100	182	12.05

Mean birthweight (gm):   White — with condition: 2694   Without condition: 3293
                         Black — with condition: 2238   Without condition: 3064

*Excludes cases with other abnormalities within the system.
†Based on less than 20 cases.

Gordon et al. (2) have reported a four-year follow-up on NCPP babies with bracial plexus injury and indicate that most cases improve to the point where residua of injury are no longer evident.

Fractured Clavicle. Fracture of the clavicle was reported in 24 white infants; all weighed over 2500 grams at birth, with an average of 3796 grams. There were no deaths and no neurological abnormalities reported for the group. Twenty-eight black infants were reported to have a fracture of the clavicle; all but one weighed above 2500 grams. The average birthweight of 3123 showed an increase of less than 100 grams, as compared with the whites, where an increase of more than 500 grams was observed. The data pertaining to fracture of the clavicle are displayed with other abnormalities of the musculoskeletal system in Tables 12–66 and 12–67.

Table 12-12. Ocular Nerve Abnormality — Newborn

Birthweight (gm)	WHITE Livebirths with Newborn Exam (number)	With Condition (number)	With Condition (percent)	BLACK Livebirths with Newborn Exam (number)	With Condition (number)	With Condition (percent)
Under 2501	1287	2	0.16	2570	2	0.08
Over 2500	16742	19	0.11	16689	24	0.14
Total	18029	21	0.12	19259	26	0.14

Neonatal Deaths

	Livebirths with Newborn Exam (number)	Neonatal Deaths (number)	Neonatal Deaths (rate)	Livebirths with Newborn Exam (number)	Neonatal Deaths (number)	Neonatal Deaths (rate)
With condition						
Under 2501	2	0	0 †	2	1	500.00†
Over 2500	19	0	0 †	24	0	0
Total	21	0	0	26	1	38.46
Without condition						
Under 2501	915*	58	63.39	1998*	97	48.55
Over 2500	14845*	32	2.16	14976*	45	3.00
Total	15760*	90	5.71	16974*	142	8.37

Neurologically Abnormal at One Year

	One-Year Exam (number)	Neurologically Abnormal (number)	Neurologically Abnormal (rate)	One-Year Exam (number)	Neurologically Abnormal (number)	Neurologically Abnormal (rate)
With condition						
Under 2501	1	0	0 †	1	1	1000.00†
Over 2500	16	3	187.50†	23	0	0
Total	17	3	176.47†	24	1	41.67
Without condition						
Under 2501	694	24	34.58	1695	50	29.50
Over 2500	12122	134	11.05	13405	132	9.85
Total	12816	158	12.33	15100	182	12.05

Mean birthweight (gm): White — with condition: 3237   Without condition: 3293
Black — with condition: 3128   Without condition: 3064

*Excludes cases with other abnormalities within the system.
†Based on less than 20 cases.

Cephalhematoma. This diagnostic category included only those babies thought to have definite cephalhematoma, as distinguished from caput succedaneum. The condition was quite frequent, occurring in 251 cases (1.39 percent) among the white and 127 (0.66 percent) among the black babies (Table 12–15).

It is interesting to note the rather striking difference in frequency by race. The condition occurred more than twice as often in white babies as compared with blacks. Body weight had an important relationship to the condition, for example, only 10 of the 251 white infants weighed 2500 grams or less. Primigravidity did not seem to be an important factor, as only 40 percent of white and 34 percent of blacks whose babies had the condition were primipara.*

* Unpublished data.

Table 12-13. Facial Nerve Abnormality — Newborn

Birthweight (gm)	WHITE Livebirths with Newborn Exam (number)	WHITE With Condition (number)	WHITE With Condition (percent)	BLACK Livebirths with Newborn Exam (number)	BLACK With Condition (number)	BLACK With Condition (percent)
Under 2501	1287	7	0.54	2570	1	0.04
Over 2500	16742	55	0.33	16689	44	0.26
Total	18029	62	0.34	19259	45	0.23

Neonatal Deaths

	Livebirths with Newborn Exam (number)	Neonatal Deaths (number)	Neonatal Deaths (rate)	Livebirths with Newborn Exam (number)	Neonatal Deaths (number)	Neonatal Deaths (rate)
With condition						
Under 2501	7	0	0 †	1	0	0 †
Over 2500	55	0	0	44	0	0
Total	62	0	0	45	0	0
Without condition						
Under 2501	915*	58	63.39	1998*	97	48.55
Over 2500	14845*	32	2.16	14976*	45	3.00
Total	15760*	90	5.71	16974*	142	8.37

Neurologically Abnormal at One Year

	One-Year Exam (number)	Neurologically Abnormal (number)	Neurologically Abnormal (rate)	One-Year Exam (number)	Neurologically Abnormal (number)	Neurologically Abnormal (rate)
With condition						
Under 2501	6	0	0 †	1	0	0 †
Over 2500	47	7	148.94	41	6	146.34
Total	53	7	132.08	42	6	142.86
Without condition						
Under 2501	694	24	34.58	1695	50	29.50
Over 2500	12122	134	11.05	13405	132	9.85
Total	12816	158	12.33	15100	182	12.05

Mean birthweight (gm): White — with condition: 3338   Without condition: 3293
                        Black — with condition: 3328   Without condition: 3064

*Excludes cases with other abnormalities within the system.
†Based on less than 20 cases.

While there was perhaps some increase in the neonatal death rate for white babies with cephalhematoma, the number of cases was small. In blacks, the increased rate was clear. There was no increase in neurological abnormalities at one year in whites; possibly a slight increase in blacks.

Skull Fractures. Skull fractures were reported in only 7 white and 5 black neonates. This injury was associated with large birthweight and presumably large head size. The black babies averaged 500 grams and the whites 200 grams above the mean birthweight of those without abnormality in the central nervous system. (See Tables 12–62 and 12–63.)

Intracranial Hemorrhage. Included were subdural, subarachnoid, and intra-

Table 12-14. Brachial Plexus Abnormality — Newborn

Birthweight (gm)	WHITE Livebirths with Newborn Exam (number)	With Condition (number)	With Condition (percent)	BLACK Livebirths with Newborn Exam (number)	With Condition (number)	With Condition (percent)
Under 2501	1287	1	0.08	2570	2	0.08
Over 2500	16742	14	0.08	16689	30	0.18
Total	18029	15	0.08	19259	32	0.17

Neonatal Deaths

	Livebirths with Newborn Exam (number)	Neonatal Deaths (number)	Neonatal Deaths (rate)	Livebirths with Newborn Exam (number)	Neonatal Deaths (number)	Neonatal Deaths (rate)
With condition						
Under 2501	1	0	0 †	2	0	0 †
Over 2500	14	0	0 †	30	0	0
Total	15	0	0 †	32	0	0
Without condition						
Under 2501	915*	58	63.39	1998*	97	48.55
Over 2500	14845*	32	2.16	14976*	45	3.00
Total	15760*	90	5.71	16974*	142	8.37

Neurologically Abnormal at One Year

	One-Year Exam (number)	Neurologically Abnormal (number)	Neurologically Abnormal (rate)	One-Year Exam (number)	Neurologically Abnormal (number)	Neurologically Abnormal (rate)
With condition						
Under 2501	0	0	—	2	0	0 †
Over 2500	12	2	166.67†	27	2	74.07
Total	12	2	166.67†	29	2	68.97
Without condition						
Under 2501	694	24	34.58	1695	50	29.50
Over 2500	12122	134	11.05	13405	132	9.85
Total	12816	158	12.33	15100	182	12.05

Mean birthweight (gm): White — with condition: 3719   Without condition: 3293
Black — with condition: 3638   Without condition: 3064

*Excludes cases with other abnormalities within the system.
†Based on less than 20 cases.

ventricular hemorrhages. The diagnosis depended upon autopsy findings, or ventricular, subdural, or lumbar spinal puncture. This condition occurred primarily in low-weight babies (27 of the 39 whites, and 43 of the 61 blacks were less than 2500 grams). The mean birthweight of babies with the condition (1828 grams in whites and 1843 in blacks) was about half of those without. The death rate from intracranial hemorrhage was very high; all the 61 black babies, and 35 of the 39 white babies died. Two of the three surviving whites examined at one year were neurologically abnormal. The relative infrequency of the condition in this study may be related to the fact that most babies received vitamin K shortly after delivery as a preventive measure for hemorrhagic disease of the newborn (Table 12–16.)

Table 12-15. Cephalhematoma — Newborn

Birthweight (gm)	WHITE			BLACK		
	Livebirths with Newborn Exam (number)	With Condition		Livebirths with Newborn Exam (number)	With Condition	
		(number)	(percent)		(number)	(percent)
Under 2501	1287	10	0.78	2570	16	0.62
Over 2500	16742	241	1.44	16689	111	0.67
Total	18029	251	1.39	19259	127	0.66

Neonatal Deaths

	Livebirths with Newborn Exam (number)	Neonatal Deaths		Livebirths with Newborn Exam (number)	Neonatal Deaths	
		(number)	(rate)		(number)	(rate)
With condition						
Under 2501	10	2	200.00†	16	8	500.00†
Over 2500	241	2	8.30	111	2	18.02
Total	251	4	15.94	127	10	78.74
Without condition						
Under 2501	915*	58	63.39	1998*	97	48.55
Over 2500	14845*	32	2.16	14976*	45	3.00
Total	15760*	90	5.71	16974*	142	8.37

Neurologically Abnormal at One Year

	One-Year Exam (number)	Neurologically Abnormal		One-Year Exam (number)	Neurologically Abnormal	
		(number)	(rate)		(number)	(rate)
With condition						
Under 2501	7	0	0 †	8	0	0 †
Over 2500	199	1	5.03	104	3	28.85
Total	206	1	4.85	112	3	26.79
Without condition						
Under 2501	694	24	34.58	1695	50	29.50
Over 2500	12122	134	11.05	13405	132	9.85
Total	12816	158	12.33	15100	182	12.05

Mean birthweight (gm):   White — with condition: 3378   Without condition: 3293
                       Black — with condition: 3024   Without condition: 3064

*Excludes cases with other abnormalities within the system.
†Based on less than 20 cases.

RESPIRATORY ABNORMALITY

A number of conditions considered to be causing or contributing to respiratory abnormality are reported in this section. In general, before a definite diagnosis was made there was documentation of the condition by X-ray, laboratory, or autopsy findings. These conditions were not mutually exclusive and more than one could be reported for a given infant. The 16,195 white and 17,358 black children without respiratory abnormality are used as the comparison groups, but it should be realized that these children may have had abnormalities affecting other organ systems.

The importance of respiratory abnormalities is clearly demonstrated by examina-

Table 12-16. Intracranial Hemorrhage — Newborn

Birthweight (gm)	WHITE Livebirths with Newborn Exam (number)	WHITE With Condition (number)	WHITE With Condition (percent)	BLACK Livebirths with Newborn Exam (number)	BLACK With Condition (number)	BLACK With Condition (percent)
Under 2501	1287	27	2.10	2570	43	1.67
Over 2500	16742	12	0.07	16689	18	0.11
Total	18029	39	0.22	19259	61	0.32

Neonatal Deaths

	Livebirths with Newborn Exam (number)	Neonatal Deaths (number)	Neonatal Deaths (rate)	Livebirths with Newborn Exam (number)	Neonatal Deaths (number)	Neonatal Deaths (rate)
With condition						
Under 2501	27	27	1000.00	43	43	1000.00
Over 2500	12	8	666.67†	18	18	1000.00†
Total	39	35	897.44	61	61	1000.00
Without condition						
Under 2501	915*	58	63.39	1998*	97	48.55
Over 2500	14845*	32	2.16	14976*	45	3.00
Total	15760*	90	5.71	16974*	142	8.37

Neurologically Abnormal at One Year

	One-Year Exam (number)	Neurologically Abnormal (number)	Neurologically Abnormal (rate)	One-Year Exam (number)	Neurologically Abnormal (number)	Neurologically Abnormal (rate)
With condition						
Under 2501	0	0	–	0	0	–
Over 2500	3	2	666.67†	0	0	–
Total	3	2	666.67†	0	0	–
Without condition						
Under 2501	694	24	34.58	1695	50	29.50
Over 2500	12122	134	11.05	13405	132	9.85
Total	12816	158	12.33	15100	182	12.05

Mean birthweight (gm): White — with condition: 1828   Without condition: 3293
Black — with condition: 1843   Without condition: 3064

*Excludes cases with other abnormalities within the system.
†Based on less than 20 cases.

tion of their relationship with neonatal mortality. The risk of death increased markedly in the presence of respiratory problems. Although respiratory abnormalities were more frequent in low-weight infants, the risk of death for infants with respiratory symptoms was increased in both birthweight groups (2500 grams and below, and above 2500 grams). The impact of respiratory problems on the neonatal death rate is clearly seen by comparing the overall rates of 13.6 for whites and 19.7 for blacks for *all* conditions, with the rates of only 2.1 for white infants and 1.6 for blacks when respiratory abnormalities are excluded.

As is the case with other problems, respiratory abnormalities during the neonatal period may reflect the presence of a number of maternal conditions, both prenatal and perinatal. The long-term outcome for children with respiratory abnormalities depends not only on the damage related to the respiratory malfunction itself (hypoxia, metabolic imbalance) but also on a number of underlying and possibly related conditions, such as immaturity, infection, cardiac and CNS pathology, and residual lung damage of iatrogenic origin.

The data are presented separately for infants weighing above 2500 and below 2501 grams, so that a judgment can be made as to the strength of the association observed with low birthweight. Recent advances in the understanding of neonatal respiratory problems have indicated the important role of gestational age as an index of fetal maturity; both the frequency and outcome of respiratory problems may be influenced by gestational age at delivery. Therefore, in addition to birthweight, in this section the data have also been developed for gestational age to show relationships between respiratory problems and birthweight-gestational age categories.

Primary Apnea

The diagnosis of primary apnea was made if there was no spontaneous onset of respiration for more than two minutes after delivery (complete expulsion of the infant). Table 12–17 shows that the condition was observed in 158 white babies (0.88 percent) and 376 black babies (1.95 percent). This difference in frequency cannot readily be explained. There was essentially no difference in fresh stillbirth rates (i.e., deaths presumably occurring during labor and delivery), where the rate was 10.5 for whites and 12.2 for blacks. Furthermore, low birthweight, which is more frequent in black infants, is not the explanation either, as primary apnea occurred more often in black than white babies in both birthweight groups. The condition was associated with low birthweight, a marked increase in neonatal deaths, and a doubling of the rate of neurological abnormalities at one year of age.

Resuscitation

Resuscitation during First Five Minutes after Birth. Procedures for resuscitation included the administration of oxygen under positive pressure, trachial intubation, trachial suction, cardiac massage, and artificial or assisted respiration. However, the use of an increased concentration of oxygen in the ambient air and painful stimuli were not included under this heading. Table 12–18 indicates that resuscitative procedures were used with considerable frequency; 1089 white babies (6.04 percent) and 1146 black babies (5.95 percent) were resuscitated during the first five minutes. In Table 12–20 and some of the following tables, those who were resuscitated both during the first five minutes and at a later time are each considered separately; for whites, 4.2 percent were resuscitated only in the first period, 0.8 percent only after five minutes, and 1.9 percent during both periods. The percentages for blacks were 3.7, 1.0, and 2.2, respectively.

As would be expected, the procedures were used more frequently for low-birthweight infants, for approximately 14 percent of such infants of each race. While, on a percentage basis, babies of low birthweight required resuscitation more

Table 12-17. Primary Apnea — Newborn

Birthweight (gm)	WHITE			BLACK		
	Livebirths with Newborn Exam (number)	With Condition		Livebirths with Newborn Exam (number)	With Condition	
		(number)	(percent)		(number)	(percent)
Under 2501	1287	43	3.34	2570	137	5.33
Over 2500	16742	115	0.69	16689	239	1.43
Total	18029	158	0.88	19259	376	1.95

Neonatal Deaths

	Livebirths with Newborn Exam (number)	Neonatal Deaths		Livebirths with Newborn Exam (number)	Neonatal Deaths	
		(number)	(rate)		(number)	(rate)
With condition						
Under 2501	43	27	627.91	137	67	489.05
Over 2500	115	4	34.78	239	22	92.05
Total	158	31	196.20	376	89	236.70
Without condition						
Under 2501	857*	9	10.50	1854*	5	2.70
Over 2500	15338*	25	1.63	15504*	23	1.48
Total	16195*	34	2.10	17358*	28	1.61

Neurologically Abnormal at One Year

	One-Year Exam (number)	Neurologically Abnormal		One-Year Exam (number)	Neurologically Abnormal	
		(number)	(rate)		(number)	(rate)
With condition						
Under 2501	14	1	71.43†	62	3	48.39
Over 2500	91	3	32.97	195	5	25.64
Total	105	4	38.10	257	8	31.13
Without condition						
Under 2501	675	25	37.04	1656	56	33.82
Over 2500	12501	167	13.36	13892	166	11.95
Total	13176	192	14.57	15548	222	14.28

Mean birthweight (gm): White — with condition: 2856   Without condition: 3304
Black — with condition: 2582   Without condition: 3085

*Excludes cases with other abnormalities within the system.
†Based on less than 20 cases.

than twice as frequently as babies over 2500 grams, it should be noted that approximately 5 percent of the bigger babies also were resuscitated. Thus, it was not entirely a phenomenon of low birthweight.

Babies requiring resuscitation to establish or maintain respiration during the first five minutes after birth exhibited increased rates of neonatal death. The rate of neurological abnormality at one year for black infants needing resuscitation was approximately twice that of those who did not; in whites there was an almost threefold difference.

Resuscitation after the First Five Minutes after Birth. The same definition of procedures for resuscitation pertained as in the preceding section. However, this

Table 12–18. Resuscitation During First 5 Minutes of Life — Newborn

Birthweight (gm)	WHITE Livebirths with Newborn Exam (number)	With Condition (number)	With Condition (percent)	BLACK Livebirths with Newborn Exam (number)	With Condition (number)	With Condition (percent)
Under 2501	1287	185	14.37	2570	358	13.93
Over 2500	16742	904	5.40	16689	788	4.72
Total	18029	1089	6.04	19259	1146	5.95

Neonatal Deaths

	Livebirths with Newborn Exam (number)	Neonatal Deaths (number)	Neonatal Deaths (rate)	Livebirths with Newborn Exam (number)	Neonatal Deaths (number)	Neonatal Deaths (rate)
With condition						
Under 2501	185	56	302.70	358	109	304.47
Over 2500	904	20	22.12	788	40	50.76
Total	1089	76	69.79	1146	149	130.02
Without condition						
Under 2501	857*	9	10.50	1854*	5	2.70
Over 2500	15338*	25	1.63	15504*	23	1.48
Total	16195*	34	2.10	17358*	28	1.61

Neurologically Abnormal at One Year

	One-Year Exam (number)	Neurologically Abnormal (number)	Neurologically Abnormal (rate)	One-Year Exam (number)	Neurologically Abnormal (number)	Neurologically Abnormal (rate)
With condition						
Under 2501	105	12	114.29	210	12	57.14
Over 2500	740	22	29.73	657	13	19.79
Total	845	34	40.24	867	25	28.84
Without condition						
Under 2501	675	25	37.04	1656	56	33.82
Over 2500	12501	167	13.36	13892	166	11.95
Total	13176	192	14.57	15548	222	14.28

Mean birthweight (gm): White — with condition: 3074   Without condition: 3304
Black — with condition: 2771   Without condition: 3085

*Excludes cases with other abnormalities within the system.

category included infants in whom the procedure was reported after a lapse of five minutes, or more, from the time of birth. Included also are those babies who required resuscitation because of apnea at any later time during their nursery stay. Obviously, as a baby requiring assistance to establish or maintain respiration in the period immediately after birth may also have required resuscitation later, there is some overlap with the previous section. The extent of the overlap may be judged from Tables 12–19 through 12–26 (which also show the relationship with birthweight and gestational age). Table 12–19 indicates that later assistance in maintaining satisfactory respiration was required by 484 white and 626 black babies, about half the number requiring assistance during the five minutes following birth. Approximately 10 percent of the low-weight babies needed help and slightly over

Table 12-19. Resuscitation After First 5 Minutes of Life — Newborn

Birthweight (gm)	WHITE			BLACK		
	Livebirths with Newborn Exam (number)	With Condition		Livebirths with Newborn Exam (number)	With Condition	
		(number)	(percent)		(number)	(percent)
Under 2501	1287	141	10.96	2570	269	10.47
Over 2500	16742	343	2.05	16689	357	2.14
Total	18029	484	2.68	19259	626	3.25

Neonatal Deaths

	Livebirths with Newborn Exam (number)	Neonatal Deaths		Livebirths with Newborn Exam (number)	Neonatal Deaths	
		(number)	(rate)		(number)	(rate)
With condition						
Under 2501	141	75	531.91	269	134	498.14
Over 2500	343	26	75.80	357	44	123.25
Total	484	101	208.68	626	178	284.35
Without condition						
Under 2501	857*	9	10.50	1854*	5	2.70
Over 2500	15338*	25	1.63	15504*	23	1.48
Total	16195*	34	2.10	17358*	28	1.61

Neurologically Abnormal at One Year

	One-Year Exam (number)	Neurologically Abnormal		One-Year Exam (number)	Neurologically Abnormal	
		(number)	(rate)		(number)	(rate)
With condition						
Under 2501	54	4	74.07	117	9	76.92
Over 2500	253	5	19.76	279	7	25.09
Total	307	9	29.32	396	16	40.40
Without condition						
Under 2501	675	25	37.04	1656	56	33.82
Over 2500	12501	167	13.36	13892	166	11.95
Total	13176	192	14.57	15548	222	14.28

Mean birthweight (gm): White — with condition: 2854   Without condition: 3304
Black — with condition: 2486   Without condition: 3085

*Excludes cases with other abnormalities within the system.

2 percent of the larger infants. Again, a substantial association with neonatal death and residual abnormality was noted. The neonatal mortality rates for babies of both races requiring resuscitation after the first five minutes were considerably higher than for those requiring only initial help.

Resuscitation and Neonatal Findings: Neonatal Deaths by Time of Resuscitation. The rates of neonatal death are compared in the graph and tables that follow for those infants resuscitated: (1) during the first five minutes of life only; (2) after the first five minutes only; (3) during both periods; and (4) those not resuscitated. The group at greatest risk is that in which resuscitation was performed only after the first five minutes. (See Fig. 12–1 and Table 12–20.)

The higher neonatal death rates for black infants in each resuscitation period

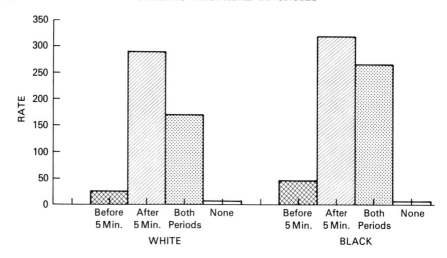

Figure 12-1. Neonatal Deaths by Resuscitation by Race

Table 12-20. Neonatal Deaths by Resuscitation by Race

	WHITE			BLACK		
Resuscitation	Livebirths with Newborn Exam*	Neonatal Deaths	Rate	Livebirths with Newborn Exam*	Neonatal Deaths	Rate
Before 5 min. only	753	19	25.23	709	32	45.13
After 5 min. only	148	43	290.54	194	62	319.59
In both periods	335	57	170.15	426	114	267.61
None	16703	95	5.69	17820	110	6.17
Total	17939	214	11.93	19149	318	16.61

*With known birthweight and gestation.

are quite apparent. The tables that follow explore this relationship in terms of birthweight and gestation.

Neonatal Deaths and Resuscitation by Birthweight. Tables 12–21 through 12–24 show time of resuscitation by birthweight. A clear association was observed, the smallest babies being resuscitated most often; of those weighing 1500 grams and below, only 51 percent of the whites and 46 percent of the blacks were not resuscitated. Among babies of both races weighing over 3000 grams, 94 percent were not resuscitated. The smallest babies of both races experienced the highest death rates, and those requiring resuscitation had rates somewhat higher than those who were not resuscitated.

Neonatal Deaths, Resuscitation, and Gestational Age. Tables 12–25 and 12–26 show the relationship observed between gestational age, neonatal death rate, and resuscitation. As expected, the risks of mortality were much higher in both races for infants in each gestational age category reported to have been resuscitated than for those who were not. The relationship between mortality and gestational age

Table 12-21. Resuscitation by Birthweight — White

Birthweight (gm)	Livebirths with Newborn Exam*					Percent				
	Resusc. Before 5 Min. Only	Resusc. After 5 Min. Only	Resusc. Both Periods	Not Resusc.	Total	Resusc. Before 5 Min. Only	Resusc. After 5 Min. Only	Resusc. Both Periods	Not Resusc.	Total
Under 1501	18	14	35	69	136	13.24	10.29	25.74	50.74	100.00
1501–2000	24	12	16	157	209	11.48	5.74	7.66	75.12	100.00
2001–2500	52	23	40	820	935	5.56	2.46	4.28	87.70	100.00
2501–3000	179	31	64	3281	3555	5.04	.87	1.80	92.29	100.00
3001+	480	68	180	12376	13104	3.66	.52	1.37	94.44	100.00
Total	753	148	335	16703	17939	4.20	.83	1.87	93.11	100.00

*With known birthweight and gestation.

Table 12-22. Resuscitation by Birthweight — Black

Birthweight (gm)	Livebirths with Newborn Exam*					Percent				
	Resusc. Before 5 Min. Only	Resusc. After 5 Min. Only	Resusc. Both Periods	Not Resusc.	Total	Resusc. Before 5 Min. Only	Resusc. After 5 Min. Only	Resusc. Both Periods	Not Resusc.	Total
Under 1501	33	50	82	138	303	10.89	16.50	27.06	45.54	100.00
1501–2000	40	20	53	316	429	9.32	4.66	12.35	73.66	100.00
2001–2500	105	21	40	1651	1817	5.78	1.16	2.20	90.86	100.00
2501–3000	169	44	80	5406	5699	2.97	0.77	1.40	94.86	100.00
3001+	362	59	171	10309	10901	3.32	0.54	1.57	94.57	100.00
Total	709	194	426	17820	19149	3.70	1.01	2.22	93.06	100.00

*With known birthweight and gestation.

followed similar patterns, however, whether the children were resuscitated or not. It must be remembered that resuscitation is employed to alleviate certain severe respiratory problems. The higher death rates for children resuscitated reflect the underlying pathology present rather than the adverse effects of resuscitation per se. As this was not a controlled study, it was not possible to determine the success rate of the resuscitation procedures.

Aspiration before, during, or after Delivery. This diagnosis was made when there was evidence of aspiration of amniotic debris, blood, or meconium into the lower respiratory tract. The diagnosis of aspiration before or during delivery was made in slightly over 1 percent of both black and white infants of low birthweight and in approximately 0.2 percent of larger babies. The condition is associated with high rates of mortality.

Aspiration after delivery was diagnosed in only 10 white (0.06 percent) and 17 black (0.09 percent) babies. This condition occurred with much greater frequency in low-weight babies as compared with those over 2500 grams; 0.31 percent compared with 0.04 percent in white, and 0.27 percent as compared with 0.06 percent in black babies. The numbers of cases observed were too small to permit meaning-

Table 12-23. Neonatal Deaths by Resuscitation by Birthweight — White

Birthweight (gm)	With Resuscitation			Without Resuscitation			Total		
	Livebirths with Newborn Exam*	Neonatal Deaths	Rate	Livebirths with Newborn Exam*	Neonatal Deaths	Rate	Livebirths with Newborn Exam*	Neonatal Deaths	Rate
Under 1501	67	47	701.49	69	40	579.71	136	87	639.71
1501–2000	52	15	288.46	157	10	63.69	209	25	119.62
2001–2500	115	23	200.00	820	6	7.32	935	29	31.02
2501–3000	274	15	54.74	3281	16	4.88	3555	31	8.72
3001+	728	19	26.10	12376	23	1.86	13104	42	3.21
Total	1236	119	96.28	16703	95	5.69	17939	214	11.93

*With known birthweight and gestation.

Table 12-24. Neonatal Deaths by Resuscitation by Birthweight — Black

Birthweight (gm)	With Resuscitation			Without Resuscitation			Total		
	Livebirths with Newborn Exam*	Neonatal Deaths	Rate	Livebirths with Newborn Exam*	Neonatal Deaths	Rate	Livebirths with Newborn Exam*	Neonatal Deaths	Rate
Under 1501	165	114	690.91	138	51	369.57	303	165	544.55
1501–2000	113	24	212.39	316	8	25.32	429	32	74.59
2001–2500	166	16	96.39	1651	9	5.45	1817	25	13.76
2501–3000	293	23	78.50	5406	17	3.14	5699	40	7.02
3001+	592	31	52.36	10309	25	2.43	10901	56	5.14
Total	1329	208	156.51	17820	110	6.17	19149	318	16.61

*With known birthweight and gestation.

Table 12-25. Neonatal Deaths by Resuscitation by Gestation at Delivery — White

Gestation (wk)	With Resuscitation			Without Resuscitation			Total		
	Livebirths with Newborn Exam*	Neonatal Deaths	Rate	Livebirths with Newborn Exam*	Neonatal Deaths	Rate	Livebirths with Newborn Exam*	Neonatal Deaths	Rate
Under 34	115	63	547.83	310	42	135.48	425	105	247.06
34–36	91	19	208.79	746	7	9.38	837	26	31.06
37–39	304	16	52.63	4256	14	3.29	4560	30	6.58
40–42	575	15	26.09	9393	22	2.34	9968	37	3.71
43+	151	6	39.74	1998	10	5.01	2149	16	7.45
Total	1236	119	96.28	16703	95	5.69	17939	214	11.93

*With known birthweight and gestation.

Table 12-26. Neonatal Deaths by Resuscitation by Gestation at Delivery — Black

Gestation (wk)	With Resuscitation			Without Resuscitation			Total		
	Livebirths with Newborn Exam*	Neonatal Deaths	Rate	Livebirths with Newborn Exam*	Neonatal Deaths	Rate	Livebirths with Newborn Exam*	Neonatal Deaths	Rate
Under 34	256	125	488.28	1104	63	57.07	1360	188	138.24
34–36	156	26	166.67	1885	7	3.71	2041	33	16.17
37–39	354	20	56.50	5969	19	3.18	6323	39	6.17
40–42	424	24	56.60	7232	16	2.21	7656	40	5.22
43+	139	13	93.53	1630	5	3.07	1769	18	10.18
Total	1329	208	156.51	17820	110	6.17	19149	318	16.61

*With known birthweight and gestation.

Table 12-27. Aspiration before or during Delivery — Newborn

Birthweight (gm)	WHITE Livebirths with Newborn Exam (number)	With Condition (number)	With Condition (percent)	BLACK Livebirths with Newborn Exam (number)	With Condition (number)	With Condition (percent)
Under 2501	1287	17	1.32	2570	29	1.13
Over 2500	16742	27	0.16	16689	30	0.18
Total	18029	44	0.24	19259	59	0.31

Neonatal Deaths

	Livebirths with Newborn Exam (number)	Neonatal Deaths (number)	Neonatal Deaths (rate)	Livebirths with Newborn Exam (number)	Neonatal Deaths (number)	Neonatal Deaths (rate)
With condition						
Under 2501	17	13	764.71†	29	27	931.03
Over 2500	27	5	185.19	30	14	466.67
Total	44	18	409.09	59	41	694.92
Without condition						
Under 2501	857*	9	10.50	1854*	5	2.70
Over 2500	15338*	25	1.63	15504*	23	1.48
Total	16195*	34	2.10	17358*	28	1.61

Neurologically Abnormal at One Year

	One-Year Exam (number)	Neurologically Abnormal (number)	Neurologically Abnormal (rate)	One-Year Exam (number)	Neurologically Abnormal (number)	Neurologically Abnormal (rate)
With condition						
Under 2501	4	0	0 †	2	0	0 †
Over 2500	18	2	111.11†	14	1	71.43†
Total	22	2	90.91	16	1	62.50†
Without condition						
Under 2501	675	25	37.04	1656	56	33.82
Over 2500	12501	167	13.36	13892	166	11.95
Total	13176	192	14.57	15548	222	14.28

Mean birthweight (gm): White — with condition: 2636   Without condition: 3304
Black — with condition: 2237   Without condition: 3085

*Excludes cases with other abnormalities within the system.
†Based on less than 20 cases.

ful evaluation of outcome other than mortality, which was high. (Tables 12–27 and 12–28.)

Summary. Active intervention to initiate and/or maintain spontaneous respiration was required with considerable frequency, both in the immediate period after birth (6 percent of all infants and 14 percent of those with low birthweight) and later (3 percent of all and 11 percent of low-weight babies).

As high rates of mortality and residual neurological abnormality may result from the conditions underlying apnea, or from the anoxic injury resulting from respiratory failure, the need for trained personnel and proper equipment to deal with this emergency is obvious. However, in spite of efforts to initiate and maintain respira-

Table 12–28. Aspiration after Delivery — Newborn

Birthweight (gm)	WHITE			BLACK		
	Livebirths with Newborn Exam (number)	With Condition		Livebirths with Newborn Exam (number)	With Condition	
		(number)	(percent)		(number)	(percent)
Under 2501	1287	4	0.31	2570	7	0.27
Over 2500	16742	6	0.04	16689	10	0.06
Total	18029	10	0.06	19259	17	0.09

Neonatal Deaths

	Livebirths with Newborn Exam (number)	Neonatal Deaths		Livebirths with Newborn Exam (number)	Neonatal Deaths	
		(number)	(rate)		(number)	(rate)
With condition						
Under 2501	4	0	0 †	7	4	571.43†
Over 2500	6	1	166.67†	10	2	200.00†
Total	10	1	100.00†	17	6	352.94†
Without condition						
Under 2501	857*	9	10.50	1854*	5	2.70
Over 2500	15338*	25	1.63	15504*	23	1.48
Total	16195*	34	2.10	17358*	28	1.61

Neurologically Abnormal at One Year

	One-Year Exam (number)	Neurologically Abnormal		One-Year Exam (number)	Neurologically Abnormal	
		(number)	(rate)		(number)	(rate)
With condition						
Under 2501	3	1	333.33†	2	0	0 †
Over 2500	4	0	0 †	6	0	0 †
Total	7	1	142.86†	8	0	0 †
Without condition						
Under 2501	675	25	37.04	1656	56	33.82
Over 2500	12501	167	13.36	13892	166	11.95
Total	13176	192	14.57	15548	222	14.28

Mean birthweight (gm): White — with condition: 2444   Without condition: 3304
Black — with condition: 2628   Without condition: 3085

*Excludes cases with other abnormalities within the system.
†Based on less than 20 cases.

tion, many of these resuscitated infants die. While some of these deaths occur in nonviable infants with marked degrees of immaturity or severe congenital malformations, other infants die as the result of less obvious causes. There is need for further investigation in this area.

Respiratory Distress

Introduction. The respiratory distress syndrome (RDS) contributed significantly to overall mortality and morbidity in low-weight infants. As may be seen in the tables and graphs presented, the effect was greater for those with both low birthweight and shorter gestational ages. Although modern techniques for respiratory support (3) have substantially improved the likelihood for survival, the problem remains one of the most serious in neonatal pediatrics.

Babies in whom a diagnosis of primary atelectasis and/or hyaline membrane disease (HMD) was reported are included in the group considered to have RDS. These conditions were reported separately in the NCPP as the basic similarity in the underlying pathophysiological mechanisms was not appreciated at the time the project was begun. In this discussion, the clinical observations are first considered separately for each condition. The conditions were then combined in order that the larger number of infants could provide for a more meaningful examination of birthweight-gestational age relationships, perinatal mortality, and the possible role of delivery by Cesarean section in the causation of RDS.

Primary Atelectasis. This diagnosis was made when there was evidence (clinical, radiological, and/or pathological) of incomplete expansion of a lung or of a significant portion of a lung. The designation "primary" implies the failure of alveolar expansion that normally begins with the first introduction of air into the lungs with the first breath and is rapidly and largely completed with the first vigorous cry. A minimal degree of atelectasis, however, is probably physiological during the first few days, as lung function studies suggest progressive expansion over the first 72 hours. Atelectasis occurs when the infant fails to achieve adequate pulmonary expansion. It is due in most instances to immaturity of lung structure and to inadequate amounts of surfactant material, which together lead to the requirement for high opening air pressures to overcome pulmonary resistance to alveolar expansion (4,5,6).

Other contributing factors may be inadequate respiratory effort due to feeble thoracic muscular activity, and lack of rigidity of the thoracic cage, which reflects immaturity. Fetal respiratory depression from oversedation during maternal analgesia and anesthesia; severe illness; major malformations of the respiratory system, heart, or diaphragm; and malfunction of the neurophysiological control of respiration are less common additional factors that must be considered in the individual case.

Primary atelectasis occurred with similar frequency in white and black infants (Table 12–29). There were 74 cases (0.41 percent) reported among the white and 111 cases (0.58 percent) among the black infants. As might be expected, the frequency was high among the low-birthweight babies; 3.73 percent for whites and 3.50 percent for blacks. The mean birthweight of babies with the condition was markedly below that of those without the condition; 2066 grams, as compared with an average of 3304 grams in white babies, and 1561 grams, as compared with 3085 grams in black babies without the condition. The marked difference (500 grams) between the average birthweight of white and black babies with atelectasis is intriguing. The larger average birthweight of white babies with atelectasis probably reflects the greater maturity at similar birthweights of low-weight black babies, as compared with white babies. (See Chapter 7.)

Primary atelectasis was associated with extremely high rates of neonatal mortality. However, among few survivors who were examined at one year, none were found to be neurologically abnormal.

Table 12-29. Primary Atelectasis — Newborn

Birthweight (gm)	WHITE Livebirths with Newborn Exam (number)	With Condition (number)	With Condition (percent)	BLACK Livebirths with Newborn Exam (number)	With Condition (number)	With Condition (percent)
Under 2501	1287	48	3.73	2570	90	3.50
Over 2500	16742	26	0.16	16689	21	0.13
Total	18029	74	0.41	19259	111	0.58

Neonatal Deaths

	Livebirths with Newborn Exam (number)	Neonatal Deaths (number)	Neonatal Deaths (rate)	Livebirths with Newborn Exam (number)	Neonatal Deaths (number)	Neonatal Deaths (rate)
With condition						
Under 2501	48	40	833.33	90	85	944.44
Over 2500	26	9	346.15	21	13	619.05
Total	74	49	662.16	111	98	882.88
Without condition						
Under 2501	857*	9	10.50	1854*	5	2.70
Over 2500	15338*	25	1.63	15504*	23	1.48
Total	16195*	34	2.10	17358*	28	1.61

Neurologically Abnormal at One Year

	One-Year Exam (number)	Neurologically Abnormal (number)	Neurologically Abnormal (rate)	One-Year Exam (number)	Neurologically Abnormal (number)	Neurologically Abnormal (rate)
With condition						
Under 2501	7	0	0 †	3	0	0 †
Over 2500	12	0	0 †	5	0	0 †
Total	19	0	0 †	8	0	0 †
Without condition						
Under 2501	675	25	37.04	1656	56	33.82
Over 2500	12501	167	13.36	13892	166	11.95
Total	13176	192	14.57	15548	222	14.28

Mean birthweight (gm): White — with condition: 2066   Without condition: 3304
Black — with condition: 1561   Without condition: 3085

*Excludes cases with other abnormalities within the system.
†Based on less than 20 cases.

Hyaline Membrane Disease (HMD). This diagnosis was coded on the basis of characteristic clinical observations supported by compatible findings on radiologic examination and/or on the basis of the microscopic examination of autopsy material. In some infants, respiratory distress was clinically evident from birth, in others, the onset of respiratory symptoms was noted soon after birth. In many instances, the specific diagnosis was made only at autopsy.

As one might have expected, the distributions of hyaline membrane disease are not essentially different from those of primary atelectasis. (Table 12–30.) The mean birthweights of infants with each condition are very similar. Eighty-one white infants (0.45 percent) and 86 black infants (0.45 percent) were reported as having

Table 12-30. Hyaline Membrane Disease — Newborn

Birthweight (gm)	WHITE Livebirths with Newborn Exam (number)	WHITE With Condition (number)	WHITE With Condition (percent)	BLACK Livebirths with Newborn Exam (number)	BLACK With Condition (number)	BLACK With Condition (percent)
Under 2501	1287	60	4.66	2570	74	2.88
Over 2500	16742	21	0.13	16689	12	0.07
Total	18029	81	0.45	19259	86	0.45

Neonatal Deaths

	Livebirths with Newborn Exam (number)	Neonatal Deaths (number)	Neonatal Deaths (rate)	Livebirths with Newborn Exam (number)	Neonatal Deaths (number)	Neonatal Deaths (rate)
With condition						
Under 2501	60	39	650.00	74	48	648.65
Over 2500	21	10	476.19	12	7	583.33†
Total	81	49	604.94	86	55	639.53
Without condition						
Under 2501	857*	9	10.50	1854*	5	2.70
Over 2500	15338*	25	1.63	15504*	23	1.48
Total	16195*	34	2.10	17358*	28	1.61

Neurologically Abnormal at One Year

	One-Year Exam (number)	Neurologically Abnormal (number)	Neurologically Abnormal (rate)	One-Year Exam (number)	Neurologically Abnormal (number)	Neurologically Abnormal (rate)
With condition						
Under 2501	15	0	0 †	22	7	318.18
Over 2500	10	1	100.00†	5	2	400.00†
Total	25	1	40.00	27	9	333.33
Without condition						
Under 2501	675	25	37.04	1656	56	33.82
Over 2500	12501	167	13.36	13892	166	11.95
Total	13176	192	14.57	15548	222	14.28

Mean birthweight (gm): White — with condition: 2042   Without condition: 3304
Black — with condition: 1695   Without condition: 3085

*Excludes cases with other abnormalities within the system.
†Based on less than 20 cases.

HMD. While the overall frequency is the same for black and white babies, 4.66 percent (60 cases) among white babies with low birthweight had HMD, as compared with 2.88 percent (74 cases) among blacks, again probably reflecting the lesser degrees of maturity among low-weight white babies, as compared with blacks.

As with primary atelectasis, the neonatal mortality rates were markedly increased, even among babies weighing over 2500 grams. The rate of neurological abnormalities at twelve months also appears increased, particularly in black babies, but the small number of survivors makes evaluation difficult. Similar findings have been reported by Fisch, et al. (7,8) from this study. However, Stahlman et al. (9) have found no residual impairment in survivors of HMD treated with vigorous intensive care, as compared with controls of similar birthweight.

Respiratory Distress Syndrome (RDS). When the diagnostic categories of primary atelectasis and hyaline membrane disease were combined as RDS, records were available for 149 white and 183 black single, liveborn infants of known gestational age and birthweight, for whom newborn examinations were done. As may be seen from the tables included in this section, race, sex, birthweight, gestational age, and type of delivery are variables, each of which influence the frequency and outcome of RDS.

Race and Sex. As may be seen in Tables 12–31 through 12–34, RDS occurred more frequently in males than in females; among whites, in 97 males and 52 females—a ratio of almost 2 to 1. In the blacks there were 103 males and 80 females. As shown in the accompanying graphs and tables, white males in every birthweight category had a greater frequency of RDS than females. The frequency of RDS within the various gestational age groupings also was generally higher in white males than in females. The sex differences in RDS by birthweight in black babies were generally similar to those in the white, but less. With respect to gestational age, for blacks there was very little sex difference at thirty-four weeks and over.

The neonatal death rates for babies with RDS were very high for infants of both races and were not appreciably different by sex.

Birthweight. Regardless of the type of delivery, low-weight infants had higher frequencies of RDS than larger children. The frequency of RDS increased progressively with decreasing birthweight (Figs. 12–2 and 12–3).

In white babies, RDS was diagnosed in 20 percent of the babies of 2000 grams or less (69 cases). The diagnosis was made in 3.5 percent (33 cases) of those weighing between 2001 and 2500 grams and in 0.6 percent (22 cases) of those between 2501 and 3000 grams birthweight. The frequency was 0.2 percent (25 cases) among the 13,104 babies weighing over 3000 grams. While RDS is primarily a syndrome of low-birthweight babies, it should be appreciated that a number of larger babies also have RDS. Over half of the white babies with RDS (53.7 percent) weighed in excess of 2000 grams at birth, and 25 of the 149 were over 3000 grams; and, as may be seen from Tables 12–31 and 12–32, the findings were similar but less marked for the blacks.

Gestational Age. When the data were examined by gestational age at delivery, a striking relationship between RDS and gestational age was apparent in the white babies. (Figs. 12–4 and 12–5 and Tables 12–33 and 12–34.) A similar relationship was present but less marked in black infants, again attesting to their greater maturity, as compared with whites. In the whites, almost 17 percent of all babies of less than 34-weeks gestation had a diagnosis of RDS. Four percent of white infants of 34- through 36-weeks gestation had RDS, and above 36 weeks the percentages of affected babies declined sharply to 0.17 percent for gestations of 40- through 42-weeks duration. For white babies of 43 weeks and above, the frequency was 0.47 percent; a slight increase, which was also observed for the blacks. These

Table 12-31. Respiratory Distress by Birthweight by Sex — White

Birthweight (gm)	Male			Female			Total		
	Livebirths with Newborn Exam*	With RDS	Percent	Livebirths with Newborn Exam*	With RDS	Percent	Livebirths with Newborn Exam*	With RDS	Percent
Under 1501	84	30	35.71	52	15	28.85	136	45	33.09
1501–2000	101	16	15.84	108	8	7.41	209	24	11.48
2001–2500	387	19	4.91	548	14	2.55	935	33	3.53
2501–3000	1570	17	1.08	1985	5	0.25	3555	22	0.62
3001+	7152	15	0.21	5952	10	0.17	13104	25	0.19
Total	9294	97	1.04	8645	52	0.60	17939	149	0.83

*With known birthweight and gestation.

Table 12-32. Respiratory Distress by Birthweight by Sex — Black

Birthweight (gm)	Male			Female			Total*		
	Livebirths with Newborn Exam†	With RDS	Percent	Livebirths with Newborn Exam†	With RDS	Percent	Livebirths with Newborn Exam†	With RDS	Percent
Under 1501	151	60	39.74	152	44	28.95	303	104	34.32
1501–2000	198	14	7.07	231	12	5.19	429	26	6.06
2001–2500	793	12	1.51	1024	8	0.78	1817	20	1.10
2501–3000	2522	7	0.28	3177	4	0.13	5699	11	0.19
3001+	5926	10	0.17	4974	12	0.24	10901	22	0.20
Total	9590	103	1.07	9558	80	0.84	19149	183	0.96

* Includes unknown sex.
†With known birthweight and gestation.

Table 12–33. Respiratory Distress by Gestation at Delivery by Sex — White

Gestation (wk)	Male			Female			Total		
	Livebirths with Newborn Exam*	With RDS	Percent	Livebirths with Newborn Exam*	With RDS	Percent	Livebirths with Newborn Exam*	With RDS	Percent
Under 34	226	46	20.35	199	25	12.56	425	71	16.71
34–36	463	21	4.54	374	13	3.48	837	34	4.06
37–39	2449	8	0.33	2111	9	0.43	4560	17	0.37
40–42	5062	14	0.28	4906	3	0.06	9968	17	0.17
43+	1094	8	0.73	1055	2	0.19	2149	10	0.47
Total	9294	97	1.04	8645	52	0.60	17939	149	0.83

*With known birthweight and gestation.

Table 12–34. Respiratory Distress by Gestation at Delivery by Sex — Black

Gestation (wk)	Male			Female			Total*		
	Livebirths with Newborn Exam†	With RDS	Percent	Livebirths with Newborn Exam†	With RDS	Percent	Livebirths with Newborn Exam†	With RDS	Percent
Under 34	704	72	10.23	656	50	7.62	1360	122	8.97
34–36	1047	13	1.24	994	8	0.80	2041	21	1.03
37–39	3236	6	0.19	3087	9	0.29	6323	15	0.24
40–42	3732	10	0.27	3923	8	0.20	7656	18	0.24
43+	871	2	0.23	898	5	0.56	1769	7	0.40
Total	9590	103	1.07	9558	80	0.84	19149	183	0.96

*Includes unknown sex.
†With known birthweight and gestation.

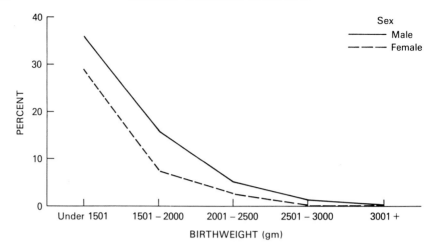

Figure 12-2. Respiratory Distress by Birthweight by Sex — White

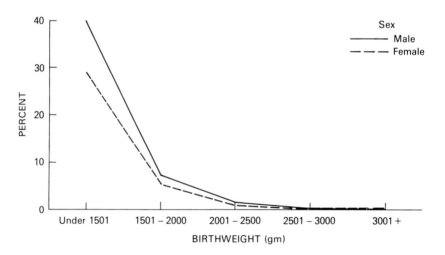

Figure 12-3. Respiratory Distress by Birthweight by Sex — Black

mature infants may have had fetal aspiration syndrome, with signs and symptoms indistinguishable from hyaline membrane disease. Relationships between birthweight, gestational age, and respiratory distress are shown in Tables 12–35 and 12–36. As expected, the highest rates are among the smallest and most immature infants, but the disease is not limited to them.

The mean birthweight is shown for babies with and without RDS by gestational age in Tables 12–37 and 12–38. In the lowest gestational age groups, there was little difference in mean birthweight between the weight of those infants who died whether or not they had RDS. In whites, from 37-weeks gestation and over, the babies who died had lower average birthweight than survivors, and children with

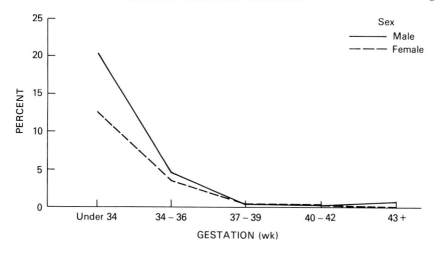

Figure 12-4. Respiratory Distress by Gestation at Delivery by Sex — White

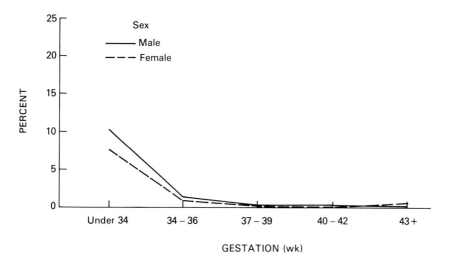

Figure 12-5. Respiratory Distress by Gestation at Delivery by Sex — Black

RDS weighed less than those without this diagnosis. In blacks, this relationship was not observed.

Neonatal Deaths. Mortality rates were high for all babies with RDS. As may be seen from Table 12–40, *only two of 45 white babies under 1500 grams birthweight with the diagnosis survived,* and almost one-third of the white infants above 3000 grams with RDS died. Similar results were found in blacks. Neonatal death rates within the various birthweight and gestational age subgroups are summarized in Tables 12–39 through 12–43 for babies with and without RDS.

In considering these very high mortality rates from RDS, it must be remembered that these babies were born between 1959 and 1966. While they were cared for in

Table 12-35. Respiratory Distress by Birthweight by Gestation at Delivery — White

Birthweight (gm)	Gestation (wk)											
	Under 34			34–36			37–39			40+		
	Livebirths with Newborn Exam*	With RDS	Rate	Livebirths with Newborn Exam*	With RDS	Rate	Livebirths with Newborn Exam*	With RDS	Rate	Livebirths with Newborn Exam*	With RDS	Rate
Under 1501	119	43	361.34	12	1	83.33†	3	1	333.33†	2	0	0†
1501–2000	73	16	219.18	66	3	45.45	47	2	42.55	23	3	130.43
2001–2500	71	11	154.93	220	17	77.27	367	5	13.62	277	0	0
2501–3000	66	0	0	247	10	40.49	1366	4	2.93	1876	8	4.26
3001+	96	1	10.42	292	3	10.27	2777	5	1.80	9939	16	1.61

*With known birthweight and gestation.
†Based on less than 20 cases.

Table 12-36. Respiratory Distress by Birthweight by Gestation at Delivery — Black

Birthweight (gm)	Gestation (wk)											
	Under 34			34–36			37–39			40+		
	Livebirths with Newborn Exam*	With RDS	Rate	Livebirths with Newborn Exam*	With RDS	Rate	Livebirths with Newborn Exam*	With RDS	Rate	Livebirths with Newborn Exam*	With RDS	Rate
Under 1501	248	94	379.03	36	9	250.00	11	1	90.91†	8	0	0†
1501–2000	206	17	82.52	124	5	40.32	61	3	49.18	38	1	26.32
2001–2500	229	9	39.30	468	5	10.68	691	3	4.34	429	3	6.99
2501–3000	278	1	3.60	675	1	1.48	2347	3	1.28	2399	6	2.50
3001+	399	1	2.51	738	1	1.36	3213	5	1.56	6551	15	2.29

*With known birthweight and gestation.
†Based on less than 20 cases.

Table 12-37. Mean Birthweight by Mortality
by Respiratory Distress by Gestation at Delivery — White

	With RDS				Without RDS			
	Livebirths with Newborn Exam*		Neonatal Deaths		Livebirths with Newborn Exam*		Neonatal Deaths	
Gestation (wk)	No.	Mean Birthweight	No.	Mean Birthweight	No.	Mean Birthweight	No.	Mean Birthweight
Under 34	71	1386	54	1218	354	2328	51	1154
34–36	34	2440	15	2351	803	2786	11	2343
37–39	17	2630	9	2394	4543	3116	21	2603
40–42	17	3250	8	2761	9951	3392	29	3142
43+	10	2937	6	2755	2139	3460	10	3371
Total	149	2085	92	1752	17790	3281	122	2156

*With known birthweight and gestation.

university-affiliated nurseries, substantial progress has been made during the intervening years in intensive care and multiphasic monitoring. While mortality under optimal care is considerably lower today, nevertheless, it remains substantial among babies with this diagnosis.

Type of Delivery. As mentioned, the type of delivery was also observed to be related to the frequency of RDS. The association between increased risk of RDS and delivery by Cesarean section is well known. The data in the British perinatal study (10), particularly those developed by Gruenwald (11), suggest that the risk of death from HMD was greatly increased when the baby was delivered by section, and that babies delivered by this method prior to the onset of labor, whether spontaneous or induced, were at even greater risk than those of mothers sectioned after labor had begun. As may be seen from Tables 12–44 through 12–47, in the NCPP, the diagnosis of RDS was made in 37 white and 30 black infants delivered by section. Fourteen of the white and 16 of the black babies with RDS were delivered after a trial of labor. Twenty-two whites and 12 blacks without labor developed RDS. The proportion developing RDS was essentially the same, whether or not labor had begun. Thus, effect of labor seems insignificant. The difference between these observations and those of Gruenwald may reflect that his series contained only 5 cases with labor prior to surgical extraction of the baby; furthermore, his risk figures were based on population estimates, not actual observations. The question is of considerable interest because it has been postulated that manufacture of pulmonary surfactant is triggered by the increase in maternal cortico-steroid level (12) that occurs shortly before the onset of labor. The data presented here, while not directly applicable, do not lend support to the hypothesis that labor is in some way protective against RDS. Before any definite statement can be made more detailed analyses are required.

It should be noted that in these large groups of infants it is the breech deliveries that have the highest risk of RDS. Thirty-one of 535 white babies (5.79 percent) and 31 of 395 black babies (7.85 percent) delivered as a breech were reported to

Table 12-38. Mean Birthweight by Mortality by Respiratory Distress by Gestation at Delivery — Black

Gestation (wk)	With RDS Livebirths with Newborn Exam* No.	Mean Birthweight	Neonatal Deaths No.	Mean Birthweight	Without RDS Livebirths with Newborn Exam* No.	Mean Birthweight	Neonatal Deaths No.	Mean Birthweight
Under 34	122	1237	104	1182	1238	2492	84	1085
34-36	21	1776	13	1609	2020	2789	20	2104
37-39	15	2487	8	2785	6308	3008	31	2854
40-42	18	3103	7	3005	7638	3218	33	3130
43+	7	2916	7	2915	1762	3218	11	3175
Total	183	1648	139	1494	18966	3055	179	1991

*With known birthweight and gestation.

Table 12-39. Neonatal Deaths by Respiratory Distress by Race and by Sex

Race	With RDS Livebirths with Newborn Exam*	Neonatal Deaths	Rate	Without RDS Livebirths with Newborn Exam*	Neonatal Deaths	Rate	Total Livebirths with Newborn Exam*	Neonatal Deaths	Rate
WHITE									
Male	97	60	618.56	9197	67	7.28	9294	127	13.66
Female	52	32	615.38	8593	55	6.40	8645	87	10.06
BLACK									
Male	103	77	747.57	9487	98	10.33	9590	175	18.25
Female	80	62	775.00	9478	81	8.55	9558	143	14.96

*With known birthweight and gestation.

Table 12-40. Neonatal Deaths by Respiratory Distress by Birthweight — White

Birthweight (gm)	With RDS			Without RDS			Total		
	Livebirths with Newborn Exam*	Neonatal Deaths	Rate	Livebirths with Newborn Exam*	Neonatal Deaths	Rate	Livebirths with Newborn Exam*	Neonatal Deaths	Rate
Under 1501	45	43	955.56	91	44	483.52	136	87	639.71
1501–2000	24	13	541.67	185	12	64.86	209	25	119.62
2001–2500	33	17	515.15	902	12	13.30	935	29	31.02
2501–3000	22	11	500.00	3533	20	5.66	3555	31	8.72
3001+	25	8	320.00	13079	34	2.60	13104	42	3.21
Total	149	92	617.45	17790	122	6.86	17939	214	11.93

*With known birthweight and gestation.

Table 12-41. Neonatal Deaths by Respiratory Distress by Birthweight — Black

Birthweight (gm)	With RDS			Without RDS			Total		
	Livebirths with Newborn Exam*	Neonatal Deaths	Rate	Livebirths with Newborn Exam*	Neonatal Deaths	Rate	Livebirths with Newborn Exam*	Neonatal Deaths	Rate
Under 1501	104	92	884.62	199	73	366.83	303	165	544.55
1501–2000	26	17	653.85	403	15	37.22	429	32	74.59
2001–2500	20	10	500.00	1797	15	8.35	1817	25	13.76
2501–3000	11	6	545.45†	5688	34	5.98	5699	40	7.02
3001+	22	14	636.36	10879	42	3.86	10901	56	5.14
Total	183	139	759.56	18966	179	9.44	19149	318	16.61

*With known birthweight and gestation.
†Based on less than 20 cases.

Table 12-42. Neonatal Deaths by Respiratory Distress by Gestation at Delivery — White

Gestation (wk)	With RDS			Without RDS			Total		
	Livebirths with Newborn Exam*	Neonatal Deaths	Rate	Livebirths with Newborn Exam*	Neonatal Deaths	Rate	Livebirths with Newborn Exam*	Neonatal Deaths	Rate
Under 34	71	54	760.56	354	51	144.07	425	105	247.06
34–36	34	15	441.18	803	11	13.70	837	26	31.06
37–39	17	9	529.41†	4543	21	4.62	4560	30	6.58
40–42	17	8	470.59†	9951	29	2.91	9968	37	3.71
43+	10	6	600.00†	2139	10	4.68	2149	16	7.45
Total	149	92	617.45	17790	122	6.86	17939	214	11.93

*With known birthweight and gestation.
†Based on less than 20 cases.

Table 12-43. Neonatal Deaths by Respiratory Distress by Gestation at Delivery — Black

Gestation (wk)	With RDS			Without RDS			Total		
	Livebirths with Newborn Exam*	Neonatal Deaths	Rate	Livebirths with Newborn Exam*	Neonatal Deaths	Rate	Livebirths with Newborn Exam*	Neonatal Deaths	Rate
Under 34	122	104	852.46	1238	84	67.85	1360	188	138.24
34–36	21	13	619.05	2020	20	9.90	2041	33	16.17
37–39	15	8	533.33†	6308	31	4.91	6323	39	6.17
40–42	18	7	388.89†	7638	33	4.32	7656	40	5.22
43+	7	7	1000.00†	1762	11	6.24	1769	18	10.18
Total	183	139	759.56	18966	179	9.44	19149	318	16.61

*With known birthweight and gestation.
†Based on less than 20 cases.

have RDS. Most were very immature; 26 of the whites and 27 of the black babies were of less than 34-weeks gestation. The relationship may in part reflect low birth-weight and extreme immaturity, rather than the method of delivery; however, for each birthweight grouping in the whites, the percent is higher for breech than for vaginal vertex deliveries. The percentage of occurrence is next highest among babies delivered by Cesarean section: 4.23 for whites and 3.14 for blacks. Among the 149 white infants with RDS, only 31 (21 percent) were breech deliveries, while other vaginal deliveries contributed 81 (54 percent) and Cesarean sections 37 (25 percent) of the total. In the blacks, of the 181 babies with RDS, 30 (17 percent) were delivered by Cesarean section.

Relationships between respiratory distress, birthweight, gestational age, and type of delivery are shown in Tables 12–48 and 12–49.

Pneumonia

Seventy-five white (0.42 percent) and 101 black (0.52 percent) babies received a definite diagnosis of pneumonia during the nursery period (Table 12–50). Be-cause of the stringent diagnostic criteria, requiring X-ray or pathological evidence of the condition, this undoubtedly represents an underestimate of the frequency of pneumonia.

The frequency of the condition was not essentially different by race. Newborns with pneumonia were noted to have slightly lower mean birthweight. Mortality rates were high for babies weighing both above and below 2500 grams; in fact, more than one-fourth of the black babies weighing over 3000 grams with pneumonia died.

The frequency of pneumonia varied by both birthweight and gestational age. The condition occurred most often among the smallest infants (Figs. 12–6 through 12–9). It was noted in 11 percent of the white and 9 percent of black infants under 1501 grams, as compared with 0.2 percent of both races weighing 3000 grams and above. Similarly, babies of the lowest gestational age, those below 34 weeks, had the highest frequency, 4.5 percent for whites and 2.9 percent for blacks. With in-creasing gestational age, the frequency progressively decreased, reaching 0.15 per-cent at 40 to 42 weeks in whites, and 0.22 at 37 to 39 weeks in blacks. The rates increased somewhat for longer gestational ages in each race. (See Tables 12–51 through 12–55.)

It is interesting to note that while the frequency of pneumonia was not different by sex overall, among the babies weighing less than 1501 grams the condition occurred more frequently among females of both races. Similarly, among babies in the shortest gestational age group, below 34 weeks, pneumonia was more frequently observed in girls.

Tables 12–56 and 12–57 showing the frequency of neonatal pneumonia by type of delivery are of interest because a clear association with labor is demonstrated. Only two of the 368 black babies delivered by Cesarean section prior to the onset of labor had pneumonia. Of babies vaginally delivered, the diagnosis occurred with greatest frequency (9 percent) in the smallest babies, those 1500 grams or below.

Table 12-44. Respiratory Distress by Birthweight by Type of Delivery — White

Birthweight (gm)	Cesarean Section			Vaginal Vertex			Breech	Total
	With Labor	Without Labor	Total*	Spontaneous	Other	Total		Livebirths with Newborn Exam†
Under 1501								
With RDS	3	1	5	14	5	19	21	45
Total	6	5	13	48	25	73	49	135
Percent	50.00‡	20.00‡	38.46‡	29.17	20.00	26.03	42.86	33.33
1501–2000								
With RDS	2	1	3	12	5	17	4	24
Total	9	10	19	80	85	165	25	209
Percent	22.22†	10.00†	15.79‡	15.00	5.88	10.30	16.00	11.48
2001–2500								
With RDS	3	11	14	10	6	16	3	33
Total	31	59	95	353	438	791	49	935
Percent	9.68	18.64	14.74	2.83	1.37	2.02	6.12	3.53
2501–3000								
With RDS	4	6	10	5	5	10	2	22
Total	69	148	235	1302	1876	3178	138	3551
Percent	5.80	4.05	4.26	0.38	0.27	0.31	1.45	0.62
3001+								
With RDS	2	3	5	11	8	19	1	25
Total	224	277	513	5019	7283	12302	274	13089
Percent	0.89	1.08	0.97	0.22	0.11	0.15	0.36	0.19
Total								
With RDS	14	22	37	52	29	81	31	149
Total	339	499	875	6802	9707	16509	535	17919
Percent	4.13	4.41	4.23	0.76	0.30	0.49	5.79	0.83

*Includes unknown labor.
†With known birthweight, gestation, and type of delivery.
‡Based on less than 20 cases.

SPECIFIC NEONATAL DIAGNOSES 161

Table 12–45. Respiratory Distress by Birthweight by Type of Delivery — Black

Birthweight (gm)	Cesarean Section			Vaginal Vertex			Breech	Total
	With Labor	Without Labor	Total*	Spontaneous	Other	Total		Livebirths with Newborn Exam†
Under 1501								
With RDS	5	4	10	54	11	65	29	104
Total	11	6	18	158	57	215	68	301
Percent	45.45†	66.67†	55.56†	34.18	19.30	30.23	42.65	34.55
1501–2000								
With RDS	5	2	7	14	3	17	1	25
Total	22	13	38	253	102	355	32	425
Percent	22.73	15.38†	18.42	5.53	2.94	4.79	3.13	5.88
2001–2500								
With RDS	2	0	2	15	3	18	0	20
Total	72	41	120	1099	544	1643	51	1814
Percent	2.78	0	1.67	1.36	0.55	1.10	0	1.10
2501–3000								
With RDS	1	2	4	4	2	6	1	11
Total	142	115	263	3425	1912	5337	88	5688
Percent	0.70	1.74	1.52	0.12	0.10	0.11	1.14	0.19
3001+								
With RDS	3	4	7	9	5	14	0	21
Total	309	193	517	6787	3419	10206	156	10879
Percent	0.97	2.07	1.35	0.13	0.15	0.14	0	0.19
Total								
With RDS	16	12	30	96	24	120	31	181
Total	556	368	956	11722	6034	17756	395	19107
Percent	2.88	3.26	3.14	0.82	0.40	0.68	7.85	0.95

*Includes unknown labor.
†With known birthweight, gestation, and type of delivery.
‡Based on less than 20 cases.

Table 12-46. Respiratory Distress by Gestation at Delivery by Type of Delivery — White

Gestation (wk)	Cesarean Section			Vaginal Vertex			Breech	Total
	With Labor	Without Labor	Total*	Spontaneous	Other	Total		Livebirths with Newborn Exam†
Under 34								
With RDS	3	3	7	28	10	38	26	71
Total	13	17	34	176	146	322	68	424
Percent	23.08‡	17.65‡	20.59	15.91	6.85	11.80	38.24	16.75
34–36								
With RDS	6	12	18	6	8	14	2	34
Total	28	61	92	314	394	708	36	836
Percent	21.43	19.67	19.57	1.91	2.03	1.98	5.56	4.07
37–39								
With RDS	3	4	7	4	4	8	2	17
Total	92	270	378	1690	2365	4055	123	4556
Percent	3.26	1.48	1.85	0.24	0.17	0.20	1.63	0.37
40–42								
With RDS	1	1	2	8	6	14	1	17
Total	157	128	295	3729	5696	9425	238	9958
Percent	0.64	0.78	0.68	0.21	0.11	0.15	0.42	0.17
43+								
With RDS	1	2	3	6	1	7	0	10
Total	49	23	76	893	1106	1999	70	2145
Percent	2.04	8.70	3.95	0.67	0.09	0.35	0	0.47
Total								
With RDS	14	22	37	52	29	81	31	149
Total	339	499	875	6802	9707	16509	535	17919
Percent	4.13	4.41	4.23	0.76	0.30	0.49	5.79	0.83

*Includes unknown labor.
†With known birthweight, gestation, and type of delivery.
‡Based on less than 20 cases.

Table 12–47. Respiratory Distress by Gestation at Delivery by Type of Delivery — Black

Gestation (wk)	Cesarean Section			Vaginal Vertex			Breech	Total
	With Labor	Without Labor	Total*	Spontaneous	Other	Total		Livebirths with Newborn Exam†
Under 34								
With RDS	7	5	13	65	15	80	27	120
Total	42	18	62	815	375	1190	98	1350
Percent	16.67	27.78‡	20.97	7.98	4.00	6.72	27.55	8.89
34–36								
With RDS	4	1	5	12	3	15	1	21
Total	64	31	98	1281	608	1889	47	2034
Percent	6.25	3.23	5.10	0.94	0.49	0.79	2.13	1.03
37–39								
With RDS	2	2	4	6	2	8	3	15
Total	178	208	400	3806	2007	5813	98	6311
Percent	1.12	0.96	1.00	0.16	0.10	0.14	3.06	0.24
40–42								
With RDS	1	3	5	10	3	13	0	18
Total	204	85	300	4770	2452	7222	123	7645
Percent	0.49	3.53	1.67	0.21	0.12	0.18	0	0.24
43+								
With RDS	2	1	3	3	1	4	0	7
Total	68	26	96	1050	592	1642	29	1767
Percent	2.96	3.85	3.13	0.29	0.17	0.24	0	0.40
Total								
With RDS	16	12	30	96	24	120	31	181
Total	556	368	956	11722	6034	17756	395	19107
Percent	2.88	3.26	3.14	0.82	0.40	0.68	7.85	0.95

*Includes unknown labor.
†With known birthweight, gestation, and type of delivery.
‡Based on less than 20 cases.

Table 12–48. Respiratory Distress by Birthweight, by Gestation at Delivery, and by Type of Delivery — White

Birthweight (gm) and Type of Delivery	Gestation (wk)								
	Under 37			37+			Total		
	Livebirths with Newborn Exam*	With RDS	Rate	Livebirths with Newborn Exam*	With RDS	Rate	Livebirths with Newborn Exam*	With RDS	Rate
Under 2001									
Cesarean section	26	7	269.23	6	1	166.67†	32	8	250.00
Vaginal vertex	178	31	174.16	60	5	83.33	238	36	151.26
Breech	65	25	384.62	9	0	0 †	74	25	337.84
2001–2500									
Cesarean section	45	12	266.67	50	2	40.00	95	14	147.37
Vaginal vertex	224	13	58.04	567	3	5.29	791	16	20.23
Breech	22	3	136.36	27	0	0	49	3	61.22
2501+									
Cesarean section	55	6	109.09	693	9	12.99	748	15	20.05
Vaginal vertex	628	8	12.74	14852	21	1.41	15480	29	1.87
Breech	17	0	0 †	395	3	7.59	412	3	7.28
Total									
Cesarean section	126	25	198.41	749	12	16.02	875	37	42.29
Vaginal vertex	1030	52	50.49	15479	29	1.87	16509	81	4.91
Breech	104	28	269.23	431	3	6.96	535	31	57.94

*With known birthweight, gestation, and type of delivery.
†Based on less than 20 cases.

Table 12–49. Respiratory Distress by Birthweight, by Gestation at Delivery, and by Type of Delivery — Black

Birthweight (gm) and Type of Delivery	Gestation (wk)								
	Under 37			37+			Total		
	Livebirths with Newborn Exam*	With RDS	Rate	Livebirths with Newborn Exam*	With RDS	Rate	Livebirths with Newborn Exam*	With RDS	Rate
Under 2001									
Cesarean section	47	16	340.43	9	1	111.11†	56	17	303.57
Vaginal vertex	469	80	170.58	101	2	19.80	570	82	143.86
Breech	92	28	304.35	8	2	250.00†	100	30	300.00
2001–2500									
Cesarean section	39	2	51.28	81	0	0	120	2	16.67
Vaginal vertex	634	12	18.93	1009	6	5.95	1643	18	10.96
Breech	23	0	0	28	0	0	51	0	0
2501+									
Cesarean section	74	0	0	706	11	15.58	780	11	14.10
Vaginal vertex	1976	3	1.52	13567	17	1.25	15543	20	1.29
Breech	30	0	0	214	1	4.67	244	1	4.10
Total									
Cesarean section	160	18	112.50	796	12	15.08	956	30	31.38
Vaginal vertex	3079	95	30.85	14677	25	1.70	17756	120	6.76
Breech	145	28	193.10	250	3	12.00	395	31	78.48

*With known birthweight, gestation, and type of delivery.
†Based on less than 20 cases.

Table 12-50. Pneumonia — Newborn

Birthweight (gm)	WHITE			BLACK		
	Livebirths with Newborn Exam (number)	With Condition		Livebirths with Newborn Exam (number)	With Condition	
		(number)	(percent)		(number)	(percent)
Under 2501	1287	35	2.72	2570	61	2.37
Over 2500	16742	40	0.24	16689	40	0.24
Total	18029	75	0.42	19259	101	0.52

Neonatal Deaths

	Livebirths with Newborn Exam (number)	Neonatal Deaths		Livebirths with Newborn Exam (number)	Neonatal Deaths	
		(number)	(rate)		(number)	(rate)
With condition						
Under 2501	35	15	428.57	61	41	672.13
Over 2500	40	9	225.00	40	20	500.00
Total	75	24	320.00	101	61	603.96
Without condition						
Under 2501	857*	9	10.50	1854*	5	2.70
Over 2500	15338*	25	1.63	15504*	23	1.48
Total	16195*	34	2.10	17358*	28	1.61

Neurologically Abnormal at One Year

	One-Year Exam (number)	Neurologically Abnormal		One-Year Exam (number)	Neurologically Abnormal	
		(number)	(rate)		(number)	(rate)
With condition						
Under 2501	17	2	117.65†	18	1	55.56†
Over 2500	22	1	45.45	19	0	0 †
Total	39	3	76.92	37	1	27.03
Without condition						
Under 2501	675	25	37.04	1656	56	33.82
Over 2500	12501	167	13.36	13892	166	11.95
Total	13176	192	14.57	15548	222	14.28

Mean birthweight (gm): White — with condition: 2537 　　Without condition: 3304
　　　　　　　　　　　　Black — with condition: 2212 　　Without condition: 3085

*Excludes cases with other abnormalities within the system.
†Based on less than 20 cases.

This was also true of breech deliveries, where even for the larger babies the frequency was slightly higher than for other deliveries.

For infants of both races, there are interesting relationships between the occurrence of pneumonia and the type of delivery. As one would expect, among infants delivered by Cesarean section, the rate of pneumonia with prior labor appears higher than for those where labor did not occur. Overall, the rate of pneumonia among babies delivered by Cesarean section without labor was higher than one might expect and comparable to those delivered by vaginal vertex. The breech deliveries also showed a higher frequency of pneumonia. However, in both Cesarean

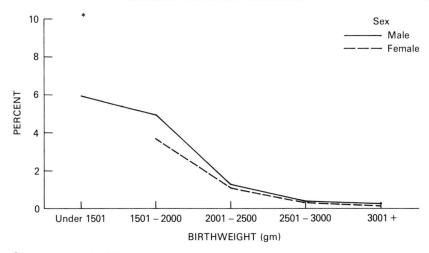

*Unplotted percent is 19.23.

Figure 12-6. Pneumonia by Birthweight by Sex — White

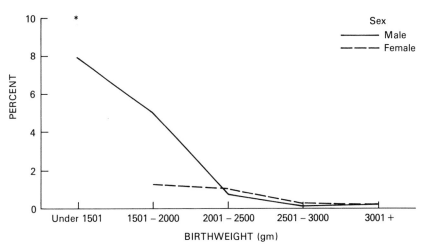

*Unplotted percent is 10.53.

Figure 12-7. Pneumonia by Birthweight by Sex — Black

section with labor and breech deliveries there was a relationship to birthweight, with pneumonia being more frequent among the low-weight babies. In infants of both races, neonatal mortality rates were markedly higher for children with pneumonia in most birthweight groups. (Tables 12–58 and 12–59.)

The need for further in depth analyses of the complex relationships suggested by this initial review is apparent and additional study of the clinical aspects of the problem is indicated.

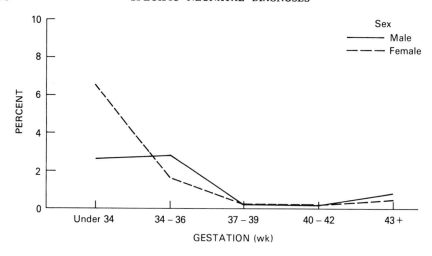

Figure 12-8. Pneumonia by Gestation at Delivery by Sex — White

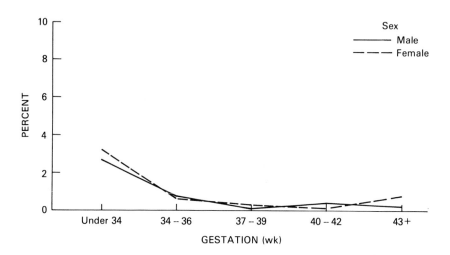

Figure 12-9. Pneumonia by Gestation at Delivery by Sex — Black

Respiratory Distress on a Cardiac Basis

There were infrequent occasions when respiratory distress was ascribed to con-
comitant cardiac abnormalities (Table 12–60). In 15 white (0.08 percent) and
16 (0.08 percent) black babies, cardiac conditions were thought to be causal or
contributory to the abnormality of respiratory function observed. These babies
were, on the average, somewhat smaller than the controls. They suffered high rates
of neonatal death. The small number of survivors exhibited no evidence of residual
neurological damage at one year of age.

Table 12-51. Pneumonia by Birthweight by Sex — White

Birthweight (gm)	Male			Female			Total		
	Livebirths with Newborn Exam*	With Pneumonia	Percent	Livebirths with Newborn Exam*	With Pneumonia	Percent	Livebirths with Newborn Exam*	With Pneumonia	Percent
Under 1501	84	5	5.95	52	10	19.23	136	15	11.03
1501–2000	101	5	4.95	108	4	3.70	209	9	4.31
2001–2500	387	5	1.29	548	6	1.09	935	11	1.18
2501–3000	1570	6	.38	1985	6	.30	3555	12	.34
3001+	7152	19	.27	5952	9	.15	13104	28	.21
Total	9294	40	.43	8645	35	.40	17939	75	.42

*With known birthweight and gestation.

Table 12-52. Pneumonia by Birthweight by Sex — Black

Birthweight (gm)	Male			Female			Total*		
	Livebirths with Newborn Exam†	With Pneumonia	Percent	Livebirths with Newborn Exam†	With Pneumonia	Percent	Livebirths with Newborn Exam†	With Pneumonia	Percent
Under 1501	151	12	7.95	152	16	10.53	303	28	9.24
1501–2000	198	10	5.05	231	3	1.30	429	13	3.03
2001–2500	793	6	.76	1024	11	1.07	1817	17	.94
2501–3000	2522	4	.16	3177	10	.31	5699	14	.25
3001+	5926	16	.27	4974	10	.20	10901	26	.24
Total	9590	48	.50	9558	50	.52	19149	98	.51

*Includes unknown sex.
†With known birthweight and gestation.

Table 12-53. Pneumonia by Gestation at Delivery by Sex — White

Gestation (wk)	Male			Female			Total		
	Livebirths with Newborn Exam*	With Pneumonia	Percent	Livebirths with Newborn Exam*	With Pneumonia	Percent	Livebirths with Newborn Exam*	With Pneumonia	Percent
Under 34	226	6	2.65	199	13	6.53	425	19	4.47
34–36	463	13	2.81	374	6	1.60	837	19	2.27
37–39	2449	4	.16	2111	4	.19	4560	8	.18
40–42	5062	8	.16	4906	7	.14	9968	15	.15
43+	1094	9	.82	1055	5	.47	2149	14	.65
Total	9294	40	.43	8645	35	.40	17939	75	.42

*With known birthweight and gestation.

Table 12-54. Pneumonia by Gestation at Delivery by Sex — Black

Gestation (wk)	Male			Female			Total*		
	Livebirths with Newborn Exam†	With Pneumonia	Percent	Livebirths with Newborn Exam†	With Pneumonia	Percent	Livebirths with Newborn Exam†	With Pneumonia	Percent
Under 34	704	19	2.70	656	21	3.20	1360	40	2.94
34–36	1047	8	.76	994	6	.60	2041	14	.69
37–39	3236	4	.12	3087	10	.32	6323	14	.22
40–42	3732	15	.40	3923	6	.15	7656	21	.27
43+	871	2	.23	898	7	.78	1769	9	.52
Total	9590	48	.50	9558	50	.52	19149	98	.51

*Includes unknown sex.
†With known birthweight and gestation.

Table 12-55. Pneumonia by Birthweight by Gestation at Delivery by Race

Birthweight (gm) and Race	Gestation (wk)					
	Under 37			37+		
	Livebirths with Newborn Exam*	With Pneumonia	Rate	Livebirths with Newborn Exam*	With Pneumonia	Rate
WHITE						
Under 2501	561	29	51.69	719	6	8.34
2501+	701	9	12.84	15958	31	1.94
BLACK						
Under 2501	1311	52	39.66	1238	6	4.85
2501+	2090	2	0.96	14510	38	2.62

*With known birthweight and gestation.

Respiratory Abnormality Associated with Central Nervous System Abnormality

A small number of infants had abnormal respiratory function attributed to abnormalities of the central nervous system. This diagnosis was made in 23 white and 34 black babies (Table 12–61). The mean birthweight of affected babies was lower than for other infants; the condition, while relatively more frequent in low-weight infants, was not limited to them. It carried a high risk of mortality for the larger as well as the smaller babies. There were too few survivors for sound judgment about residual neurological damage.

Infectious Processes

Included in Summary Tables 12–92 and 12–93 is a brief tabulation by race and birthweight of the definite neonatal infections (i.e., those documented by culture or other laboratory study, reported during the nursery stay). While, in terms of overall numbers, the infectious processes were rather infrequent (e.g., 17 cases of septicemia among the 18,000 white infants, and 31 cases among the 19,000 black infants), they were of higher frequency among the blacks than the whites and among the low-birthweight babies of both races.

Extensive studies of the role of maternal infection in relation to perinatal mortality and the long-range neurological and intellectual deficits of survivors have been under way by the Infectious Diseases Branch, NINCDS, under the direction of Dr. John L. Sever, and in some of the collaborating institutions. A number of publications have resulted from this work, several of which are referenced (13 to 19).

SUMMARY AND INTERPRETATION

Two major observations emerge from review of the data presented in this chapter. First, the risk of death increased markedly in the presence of respiratory abnormalities and, second, although a great diversity of life-threatening conditions was reported, each was relatively infrequent.

Table 12-56. Pneumonia by Birthweight by Type of Delivery — White

Birthweight (gm)	Cesarean Section				Vaginal Vertex			Breech	Total
	With Labor	Without Labor	Unknown	Total	Spontaneous	Other	Total		Livebirths with Newborn Exam*
Under 1501									
With pneumonia	1	1	0	2	5	1	6	7	15
Total	6	5	2	13	48	25	73	49	135
Percent	16.67†	20.00†	0†	15.38†	10.42	4.00	8.22	14.29	11.11
1501-2000									
With pneumonia	1	0	0	1	3	3	6	2	9
Total	9	10	0	19	80	85	165	25	209
Percent	11.11†	0	—	5.26†	3.75	3.53	3.64	8.00	4.31
2001-2500									
With pneumonia	1	0	0	1	5	4	9	1	11
Total	31	59	5	95	353	438	791	49	935
Percent	3.23	0	0†	1.05	1.42	0.91	1.14	2.04	1.18
2501-3000									
With pneumonia	2	0	1	3	3	4	7	2	12
Total	69	148	18	235	1302	1876	3178	138	3551
Percent	2.90	0	5.56†	1.28	0.23	0.21	0.22	1.45	0.34
3001+									
With pneumonia	2	2	0	4	8	15	23	1	28
Total	224	277	12	513	5019	7283	12302	274	13089
Percent	0.89	0.72	0†	0.78	0.16	0.21	0.19	0.36	0.21
Total									
With pneumonia	7	3	1	11	24	27	51	13	75
Total	339	499	37	875	6802	9707	16509	535	17919
Percent	2.06	0.60	2.70	1.26	0.35	0.28	0.31	2.43	0.42

*Excludes unknown type of delivery, birthweight, or gestation
†Based on less than 20 cases.

Table 12-57. Pneumonia by Birthweight by Type of Delivery — Black

Birthweight (gm)	Cesarean Section				Vaginal Vertex			Breech	Total
	With Labor	Without Labor	Unknown	Total	Spontaneous	Other	Total		Livebirths with Newborn Exam*
Under 1501									
With pneumonia	0	0	0	0	12	8	20	7	27
Total	11	6	1	18	158	57	215	68	301
Percent	0	0	†	†	7.59	14.04	9.30	10.29	8.97
1501–2000									
With pneumonia	0	0	0	0	11	1	12	0	12
Total	22	13	3	38	253	102	355	32	425
Percent	0	0	†	0	4.35	0.98	3.38	0	2.82
2001–2500									
With pneumonia	2	1	0	3	9	5	14	0	17
Total	72	41	7	120	1099	544	1643	51	1814
Percent	2.78	2.44	†	2.50	0.82	0.92	0.85	0	0.94
2501–3000									
With pneumonia	3	0	0	3	7	3	10	1	14
Total	142	115	6	263	3425	1912	5337	88	5688
Percent	2.11	0	†	1.14	0.20	0.16	0.19	1.14	0.25
3001+									
With pneumonia	2	1	0	3	16	5	21	2	26
Total	309	193	15	517	6787	3419	10206	156	10879
Percent	0.65	0.52	†	0.58	0.24	0.15	0.21	1.28	0.24
Total									
With pneumonia	7	2	0	9	55	22	77	10	96
Total	556	368	32	956	11722	6034	17756	395	19107
Percent	1.26	0.54	0	0.94	0.47	0.36	0.43	2.53	0.50

*Excludes unknown type of delivery, birthweight, or gestation
†Based on less than 20 cases.

Table 12-58. Neonatal Deaths by Pneumonia by Birthweight — White

Birthweight (gm)	With Pneumonia			Without Pneumonia			Total		
	Livebirths with Newborn Exam*	Neonatal Deaths	Rate	Livebirths with Newborn Exam*	Neonatal Deaths	Rate	Livebirths with Newborn Exam*	Neonatal Deaths	Rate
Under 1501	15	12	800.00†	121	75	619.83	136	87	639.71
1501–2000	9	1	111.11†	200	24	120.00	209	25	119.62
2001–2500	11	2	181.82†	924	27	29.22	935	29	31.02
2501–3000	12	2	166.67†	3543	29	8.19	3555	31	8.72
3001+	28	7	250.00	13076	35	2.68	13104	42	3.21
Total	75	24	320.00	17864	190	10.64	17939	214	11.93

*With known birthweight and gestation.
†Based on less than 20 cases.

Table 12-59. Neonatal Deaths by Pneumonia by Birthweight — Black

Birthweight (gm)	With Pneumonia			Without Pneumonia			Total		
	Livebirths with Newborn Exam*	Neonatal Deaths	Rate	Livebirths with Newborn Exam*	Neonatal Deaths	Rate	Livebirths with Newborn Exam*	Neonatal Deaths	Rate
Under 1501	28	25	892.86	275	140	509.09	303	165	544.55
1501–2000	13	8	615.38†	416	24	57.69	429	32	74.59
2001–2500	17	5	294.12†	1800	20	11.11	1817	25	13.76
2501–3000	14	10	714.29†	5685	30	5.28	5699	40	7.02
3001+	26	10	384.62	10875	46	4.23	10901	56	5.14
Total	98	58	591.84	19051	260	13.65	19149	318	16.61

*With known birthweight and gestation.
†Based on less than 20 cases.

Table 12-60. Cardiac Conditions — Newborn

Birthweight (gm)	WHITE			BLACK		
	Livebirths with Newborn Exam (number)	With Condition		Livebirths with Newborn Exam (number)	With Condition	
		(number)	(percent)		(number)	(percent)
Under 2501	1287	4	0.31	2570	4	0.16
Over 2500	16742	11	0.07	16689	12	0.07
Total	18029	15	0.08	19259	16	0.08

Neonatal Deaths

	Livebirths with Newborn Exam (number)	Neonatal Deaths		Livebirths with Newborn Exam (number)	Neonatal Deaths	
		(number)	(rate)		(number)	(rate)
With condition						
Under 2501	4	1	250.00†	4	3	750.00†
Over 2500	11	5	454.55†	12	8	666.67†
Total	15	6	400.00†	16	11	687.50†
Without condition						
Under 2501	857*	9	10.50	1854*	5	2.70
Over 2500	15338*	25	1.63	15504*	23	1.48
Total	16195*	34	2.10	17358*	28	1.61

Neurologically Abnormal at One Year

	One-Year Exam (number)	Neurologically Abnormal		One-Year Exam (number)	Neurologically Abnormal	
		(number)	(rate)		(number)	(rate)
With condition						
Under 2501	2	0	0 †	0	0	–
Over 2500	3	0	0 †	4	0	0 †
Total	5	0	0 †	4	0	0 †
Without condition						
Under 2501	675	25	37.04	1656	56	33.82
Over 2500	12501	167	13.36	13892	166	11.95
Total	13176	192	14.57	15548	222	14.28

Mean birthweight (gm): White — with condition: 2954   Without condition: 3304
Black — with condition: 2892   Without condition: 3085

*Excludes cases with other abnormalities within the system.
†Based on less than 20 cases.

Table 12–61. Respiratory Abnormality
with Central Nervous System Abnormality — Newborn

	WHITE			BLACK		
Birthweight (gm)	Livebirths with Newborn Exam (number)	With Condition		Livebirths with Newborn Exam (number)	With Condition	
		(number)	(percent)		(number)	(percent)
Under 2501	1287	10	0.78	2570	19	0.74
Over 2500	16742	13	0.08	16689	15	0.09
Total	18029	23	0.13	19259	34	0.18

Neonatal Deaths

	Livebirths with Newborn Exam (number)	Neonatal Deaths		Livebirths with Newborn Exam (number)	Neonatal Deaths	
		(number)	(rate)		(number)	(rate)
With condition						
Under 2501	10	8	800.00†	19	14	736.84†
Over 2500	13	6	461.54†	15	7	466.67†
Total	23	14	608.70	34	21	617.65
Without condition						
Under 2501	857*	9	10.50	1854*	5	2.70
Over 2500	15338*	25	1.63	15504*	23	1.48
Total	16195*	34	2.10	17358*	28	1.61

Neurologically Abnormal at One Year

	One-Year Exam (number)	Neurologically Abnormal		One-Year Exam (number)	Neurologically Abnormal	
		(number)	(rate)		(number)	(rate)
With condition						
Under 2501	1	1	1000.00†	4	3	750.00†
Over 2500	3	0	0 †	7	0	0 †
Total	4	1	250.00†	11	3	272.73†
Without condition						
Under 2501	675	25	37.04	1656	56	33.82
Over 2500	12501	167	13.36	13892	166	11.95
Total	13176	192	14.57	15548	222	14.28

Mean birthweight (gm): White — with condition: 2346   Without condition: 3304
Black — with condition: 2126   Without condition: 3085

*Excludes cases with other abnormalities within the system.
†Based on less than 20 cases.

In infants of both birthweight groups (above 2500 grams and 2500 grams and below), when respiratory abnormalities were reported, the mortality rate was greatly increased. The neonatal death rate was only 2.1 per 1000 live births for white infants, and 1.6 for blacks, when *no* respiratory problems were noted, as compared with rates of 13.6 for whites and 19.7 for blacks, when *all* infants were considered.

The newborn diagnoses reported covered a wide range of pathological conditions; however, when those associated with immaturity resulting from early delivery and low birthweight for gestational age were excluded, life-threatening conditions were indeed rare. For example, a definite diagnosis of congenital heart disease was made during the neonatal period in only 40 white (0.2 percent), and 21 black (0.1 percent). Surgical procedures (excluding such minor and routine procedures as circumcisions, the tying of supernumerary digits, and the removal of skin tags) were carried out in only 64 white, and 100 black neonates. General anesthesia was administered to 38 white, and 33 black babies during the nursery stay. Tracheo-esophageal fistula occurred once in 18,029 white and three times in the 19,259 black neonates, while duodenal atresia occurred in one white and two black babies.

A number of points must be considered in evaluating the implications of the low frequencies of specific conditions reported in this chapter.

1. The organization and design of the study minimized underreporting and the low frequencies are valid.

2. The specific diagnostic categories did not include the majority of infants in trouble, as "low birthweight" was not itself considered a diagnostic category. However, in terms of risk of mortality and its continuum of adversity in survivors, low birthweight was the single most important condition. Overall, approximately 8 percent of white, and 14 percent of the black babies weighed under 2501 grams at birth and were, by definition, of low birthweight. The low-birthweight infants experienced a higher mortality and poorer long-range outcome in almost every diagnostic category than larger infants. However, the risks of low-birthweight infants are being significantly reduced and the prognosis for normal growth and development enhanced by meticulous attention to all aspects of perinatal care. The publications of Usher and McLean (20) in Canada, of McDonald (21) and of Stewart and Reynolds (22) of England, and of Stahlman et al. (23) in the United States attest to this.

3. The increasing availability of facilities for prenatal diagnosis of genetic and other fetal abnormalities, coupled with the broadening of indications for abortion, should result in the delivery of fewer abnormal babies. A trend in this direction has already been documented by Lanman et al. (24). Also, family planning and population control measures have significantly reduced all births.

The data presented in this chapter are unique in their completeness and comprehensiveness, and the follow-up of the children provides an unusual dimension. The information from the NCPP has implications for the comprehensive planning of health care for pregnant women and their newborn infants. While optimal care must be provided, the low frequency and diversity of life-threatening conditions in the

(Continued on page 212)

Table 12-62. Newborn Summary Data
Neurologic Abnormalities — White

Condition, Abnormality or Procedure	Livebirths Total No.	%	Under 2501 gm No.	%	Over 2500 gm No.	%	Neonatal Deaths Total No.	Rate	Under 2501 gm No.	Rate	Over 2500 gm No.	Rate	Neuro. Abn. 1 Year Total No.	Rate	Under 2501 gm No.	Rate	Over 2500 gm No.	Rate	Mean Bwt.
Brain abnormality	137	0.8	52	4.0	85	0.5	56	408.8	31	596.2	25	294.1	24	363.6	3	214.3	21	403.9	2638
Seizures	46	0.3	12	0.9	34	0.2	11	239.1	2	166.7	9	264.7	4	148.2	0	0	4	190.5	3003
Myoclonus	29	0.2	2	0.2	27	0.2	1	34.5	0		1	37.0	2	80.0	0		2	87.0	3317
Hypertonia	92	0.5	10	0.8	82	0.5	6	65.2	1	100.0	5	61.0	9	126.8	1	125.0	8	127.0	3151
Jitteriness or tremulousness	237	1.3	31	2.4	206	1.2	4	16.9	0	0	4	19.4	11	53.9	4	148.2	7	39.6	3172
Hyperactivity	9	0.1	1	0.1	8	0.1	0	0	0	0	0	0	0	0	0	0	0	0	3015
Hypotonia	324	1.8	116	9.0	208	1.2	70	216.1	48	413.8	22	105.8	37	175.4	12	235.3	25	156.3	2747
Hypoactivity	151	0.8	66	5.1	85	0.5	54	357.6	37	560.6	17	200.0	15	185.2	6	250.0	9	157.9	2546
Lethargy	129	0.7	50	3.9	79	0.5	40	310.1	27	540.0	13	164.6	7	92.1	1	52.6	6	105.3	2614
Asym. of reflexes, activity, or tone	31	0.2	2	0.2	29	0.2	0	0	0		0	0	4	153.9	0	0	4	160.0	3350
Symmetrical, but abnormal reflexes	113	0.6	34	2.6	79	0.5	18	159.3	10	294.1	8	101.3	14	177.2	4	235.3	10	161.3	2880
Abnormal moro	150	0.8	56	4.4	94	0.6	38	253.3	23	410.7	15	159.6	17	186.8	6	250.0	11	164.2	2749
Abnormal cry	153	0.9	43	3.3	110	0.7	32	209.2	17	395.4	15	136.4	13	132.7	3	136.4	10	131.6	2799
Abnormal suck	91	0.5	34	2.6	57	0.3	24	263.7	12	352.9	12	210.5	11	211.5	3	200.0	8	216.2	2694
Other manifestations	77	0.4	18	1.4	59	0.4	15	194.8	12	666.7	3	50.9	6	125.0	0	0	6	136.4	2848
Brachial plexus abnormality	15	0.1	1	0.1	14	0.1	0	0	0		0	0	2	166.7	0	0	2	166.7	3719
Facial nerve abnormality	62	0.3	7	0.5	55	0.3	0	0	0		0	0	7	132.1	0	0	7	148.9	3338
Ocular nerve abnormality	21	0.1	2	0.2	19	0.1	0	0	0		0	0	3	176.5	0	0	3	187.5	3237
Other peripheral cranial abnormality	5	0.0	0	0	5	0.0	0	0	0		0	0	2	500.0	–		2	500.0	3459
Fractured skull	7	0.0	0	0	7	0.0	0	0	0		0	0	0	0	–		0	0	3495
Cephalhematoma	251	1.4	10	0.8	241	1.4	4	15.9	2	200.0	2	8.3	1	4.9	0	0	1	5.0	3378
Intracranial hemorrhage	39	0.2	27	2.1	12	0.1	35	897.4	27	*	8	666.7	2	666.7	0	0	2	666.7	1828
Spinal cord abnormality	5	0.0	4	0.3	1	0.0	3	600.0	3	750.0	0	0	0	0	0	0	0	0	1786
Other neurologic abnormality	8	0.0	2	0.2	6	0.0	5	625.0	2	*	3	500.0	0	0	0	0	0	0	3041
None †	15760		915		14845		90	5.7	58	63.4	32	2.2	158	12.3	24	34.6	134	11.1	3293
Total	18029		1287		16742														

*Rate is 1000.0.
† No abnormalities within the system.

Table 12-63. Newborn Summary Data
Neurologic Abnormalities — Black

Condition, Abnormality or Procedure	Livebirths						Neonatal Deaths						Neuro. Abn. 1 Year						Mean Bwt.
	Total		Under 2501 gm		Over 2500 gm		Total		Under 2501 gm		Over 2500 gm		Total		Under 2501 gm		Over 2500 gm		
	No.	%	No.	%	No.	%	No.	Rate	No.	Rate	No.	Rate	No.	Rate	No.	Rate	No.	Rate	
Brain abnormality	192	1.0	89	3.5	103	0.6	91	474.0	60	674.2	31	301.0	16	200.0	6	300.0	10	166.7	2354
Seizures	62	0.3	20	0.8	42	0.3	25	403.2	10	500.0	15	357.1	6	193.6	1	142.9	5	208.3	2736
Myoclonus	47	0.2	14	0.5	33	0.2	2	42.6	2	142.9	0	0	3	83.3	1	125.0	2	71.4	2837
Hypertonia	156	0.8	35	1.4	121	0.7	11	70.5	1	28.6	10	82.6	6	45.8	1	35.7	5	48.5	2915
Jitteriness or tremulousness	398	2.1	91	3.5	307	1.8	9	22.6	6	65.9	3	9.8	17	48.7	7	93.3	10	36.5	2906
Hyperactivity	23	0.1	7	0.3	16	0.1	0	0	0	0	0	0	0	0	0	0	0	0	2957
Hypotonia	415	2.2	189	7.4	226	1.4	103	248.2	75	396.8	28	123.9	38	138.2	17	175.3	21	118.0	2468
Hypoactivity	287	1.5	129	5.0	158	1.0	82	285.7	59	457.4	23	145.6	16	87.9	6	96.8	10	83.3	2490
Lethargy	153	0.8	62	2.4	91	0.6	37	241.8	27	435.5	10	109.9	7	67.3	4	129.0	3	41.1	2508
Asym. of reflexes, activity, or tone	73	0.4	16	0.6	57	0.3	7	95.9	4	250.0	3	52.6	9	152.5	2	200.0	7	142.9	2949
Symmetrical, but abnormal reflexes	189	1.0	63	2.5	126	0.8	27	142.9	14	222.2	13	103.2	14	96.6	5	119.1	9	87.4	2727
Abnormal moro	343	1.8	126	4.9	217	1.3	70	204.1	48	381.0	22	101.4	26	105.3	14	205.9	12	67.0	2619
Abnormal cry	250	1.3	124	4.8	126	0.8	76	304.0	54	435.5	22	174.6	21	138.2	10	166.7	11	119.6	2407
Abnormal suck	144	0.8	85	3.3	59	0.4	51	354.2	36	423.5	15	254.2	11	135.8	5	116.3	6	157.9	2238
Other manifestations	143	0.7	53	2.1	90	0.5	32	223.8	24	452.8	8	88.9	8	82.5	3	136.4	5	66.7	2687
Brachial plexus abnormality	32	0.2	2	0.1	30	0.2	0	0	0	0	0	0	2	69.0	0	0	2	74.1	3638
Facial nerve abnormality	45	0.2	1	0.0	44	0.3	0	0	0	0	0	0	6	142.9	0	0	6	146.3	3328
Ocular nerve abnormality	26	0.1	2	0.1	24	0.1	1	38.5	1	500.0	0	0	1	41.7	1	*	0	0	3128
Other peripheral cranial abnormality	6	0.0	1	0.0	5	0.0	0	0	0	0	0	0	1	166.7	0	0	1	200.0	3369
Fractured skull	5	0.0	0	0	5	0.0	0	0	0	–	0	0	0	0	0	–	0	0	3583
Cephalhematoma	127	0.7	16	0.6	111	0.7	10	78.7	8	500.0	2	18.0	3	26.8	0	0	3	28.9	3024
Intracranial hemorrhage	61	0.3	43	1.7	18	0.1	61	*	43	*	18	*	0	–	0	–	0	–	1843
Spinal cord abnormality	6	0.0	3	0.1	3	0.0	4	666.7	2	666.7	2	666.7	2	*	1	*	1	*	2244
Other neurologic abnormality	11	0.1	3	0.1	8	0.1	9	818.2	3	*	6	750.0	0	0	0	–	0	0	2809
None †	16974		1998		14976		142	8.4	97	48.6	45	3.0	182	12.1	50	29.5	132	9.9	3064
Total	19259		2570		16689														

*Rate is 1000.0.
† No abnormalities within the system.

Table 12-64. Newborn Summary Data
Central Nervous System Malformations and Related Conditions — White

Condition, Abnormality or Procedure	Livebirths Total		Livebirths Under 2501 gm		Livebirths Over 2500 gm		Neonatal Deaths Total		Neonatal Deaths Under 2501 gm		Neonatal Deaths Over 2500 gm		Neuro. Abn. 1 Year Total		Neuro. Abn. 1 Year Under 2501 gm		Neuro. Abn. 1 Year Over 2500 gm		Mean Bwt.
	No.	%	No.	%	No.	%	No.	Rate	No.	Rate	No.	Rate	No.	Rate	No.	Rate	No.	Rate	
Anencephaly	8	0.0	4	0.3	4	0.0	8	*	4	*	4	*	0	–	0	–	0	–	2452
Microcephaly	6	0.0	2	0.2	4	0.0	1	166.7	1	500.0	0	0	2	500.0	0	0	2	666.7	2868
Hydranencephaly	1	0.0	0	0	1	0.0	0	0	0	–	0	0	1	*	0	0	1	*	2948
Hydrocephaly	7	0.0	1	0.1	6	0.0	3	428.6	1	*	2	333.3	3	750.0	0	–	3	750.0	3244
Craniosynostosis	5	0.0	2	0.2	3	0.0	0	0	0	0	0	0	1	250.0	1	500.0	0	0	2846
Abn. sep. of sutures	19	0.1	4	0.3	15	0.1	1	52.6	0	0	1	66.7	1	71.4	0	0	1	100.0	3085
Abn. shape of skull	27	0.2	1	0.1	26	0.2	3	111.1	1	*	2	76.9	4	200.0	0	–	4	200.0	3243
Encephalocele	3	0.0	1	0.1	2	0.0	1	333.3	1	*	0	0	2	*	0	–	2	*	2693
Meningomyelocele/ meningocele	8	0.0	4	0.3	4	0.0	3	375.0	2	500.0	1	250.0	1	500.0	0	0	1	*	2438
Pilonidal sinus	18	0.1	0	0	18	0.1	0	0	0	–	0	0	0	0	0	–	0	0	3512
Cong. dermal sinus	2	0.0	0	0	2	0.0	1	500.0	0	–	1	500.0	0	0	0	–	0	0	3317
Rare CNS malformations	32	0.2	9	0.7	23	0.1	6	187.5	4	444.4	2	87.0	7	350.0	4	*	3	187.5	2906
None†	17917		1266		16651		199	11.1	135	106.6	64	3.8	227	15.7	41	45.6	186	13.7	
Total	18029		1287		16742														3272

*Rate is 1000.0.
†No abnormalities within the system.

Table 12-65. Newborn Summary Data
Central Nervous System Malformations and Related Conditions — Black

Condition, Abnormality or Procedure	Livebirths						Neonatal Deaths						Neuro. Abn. 1 Year						Mean Bwt.
	Total		Under 2501 gm		Over 2500 gm		Total		Under 2501 gm		Over 2500 gm		Total		Under 2501 gm		Over 2500 gm		
	No.	%	No.	%	No.	%	No.	Rate	No.	Rate	No.	Rate	No.	Rate	No.	Rate	No.	Rate	
Anencephaly	1	0.0	0	0.0	1	0.0	1	*	0	–	1	*	0	–	0	–	0	–	3090
Microcephaly	5	0.0	3	0.1	2	0.0	0	0	0	0	0	0	1	333.3	0	0	1	500.0	2495
Hydranencephaly	2	0.0	1	0.0	1	0.0	0	0	0	0	0	0	1	*	1	*	0	0	2325
Hydrocephaly	9	0.1	2	0.1	7	0.0	2	222.2	0	0	2	285.7	4	666.7	1	500.0	3	750.0	2873
Craniosynostosis	1	0.0	0	0	1	0.0	0	0	0	–	0	0	0	0	0	–	0	0	3487
Abn. sep. of sutures	49	0.3	7	0.3	42	0.3	2	40.8	0	0	2	47.6	2	46.5	0	0	2	55.6	3056
Abn. shape of skull	21	0.1	5	0.2	16	0.1	1	47.6	0	0	1	62.5	3	166.7	2	400.0	1	76.9	2785
Encephalocele	1	0.0	0	0	1	0.0	1	*	0	–	1	*	0	–	0	–	0	–	2608
Meningomyelocele/ meningocele	9	0.1	3	0.1	6	0.0	0	0	0	0	0	0	5	714.3	1	500.0	4	800.0	2892
Pilonidal sinus	18	0.1	4	0.2	14	0.1	0	0	0	0	0	0	1	62.5	1	250.0	0	0	2799
Cong. dermal sinus	1	0.0	0	0	1	0.0	0	0	0	–	0	0	0	0	0	–	0	0	3317
Rare CNS malformations	32	0.2	10	0.4	22	0.1	3	93.8	1	100.0	2	90.9	4	148.2	1	142.9	3	150.0	2705
None†	19129		2539		16590		323	16.9	233	91.8	90	5.4	257	15.3	80	39.1	177	12.0	3042
Total	19259		2570		16689														

*Rate is 1000.0.
†No abnormalities within the system.

Table 12-66. Newborn Summary Data
Musculoskeletal Abnormalities — White

Condition, Abnormality or Procedure	Livebirths						Neonatal Deaths						Neuro. Abn. 1 Year						Mean Bwt.
	Total		Under 2501 gm		Over 2500 gm		Total		Under 2501 gm		Over 2500 gm		Total		Under 2501 gm		Over 2500 gm		
	No.	%	No.	%	No.	%	No.	Rate	No.	Rate	No.	Rate	No.	Rate	No.	Rate	No.	Rate	
Vertebral abnormality	9	0.1	2	0.2	7	0.0	3	333.3	2	*	1	142.9	2	500.0	0	0	2	500.0	2910
Talipes equinovarus	31	0.2	6	0.5	25	0.2	7	225.8	5	833.3	2	80.0	2	111.1	0	0	2	111.1	2969
Metatarsus adductus	25	0.1	2	0.2	23	0.1	1	40.0	1	500.0	0	0	0	0	0	0	0	0	3209
Calcaneo valgus	14	0.1	1	0.1	13	0.1	1	71.4	0	0	1	76.9	1	100.0	0	0	1	111.1	3120
Congenital dislocation or dysplasia of the hip	20	0.1	4	0.3	16	0.1	2	100.0	2	500.0	0	0	1	71.4	1	500.0	0	0	3333
Absence or hypoplasia of extremity or part	15	0.1	5	0.4	10	0.1	2	133.3	1	200.0	1	100.0	5	416.7	2	666.7	3	333.3	2672
Polydactyly	27	0.2	3	0.2	24	0.1	3	111.1	1	333.3	2	83.3	2	100.0	0	0	2	111.1	3095
Syndactyly	34	0.2	7	0.5	27	0.2	0	0	0	0	0	0	4	153.9	1	250.0	3	136.4	3071
Torticollis	3	0.0	0	0	3	0.0	0	0	0	–	0	0	0	0	0	–	0	0	3317
Arthrogryposis multiplex	1	0.0	1	0.1	0	0	1	*	1	*	0	–	0	–	0	–	0	–	1361
Achondroplasia	0	0	0	0	0	0	0	–	0	–	0	–	0	–	0	–	0	–	–
Fractured clavicle	24	0.1	0	0	24	0.1	0	0	0	0	0	0	0	0	0	–	0	0	–
Other fractures	10	0.1	3	0.2	7	0.0	1	100.0	1	333.3	0	0	2	333.3	1	500.0	1	250.0	3796
Other abn. non-neuro.	60	0.3	14	1.1	46	0.3	7	116.7	6	428.6	1	21.7	11	314.3	4	666.7	7	241.4	3056
None†	17791		1255		16536		196	11.0	130	103.6	66	4.0	224	15.6	41	45.8	183	13.6	2996
Total	18029		1287		16742														3273

*Rate is 1000.0.
†No abnormalities within the system.

Table 12-67. Newborn Summary Data
Musculoskeletal Abnormalities — Black

Condition, Abnormality or Procedure	Livebirths						Neonatal Deaths						Neuro. Abn. 1 Year						Mean Bwt.
	Total		Under 2501 gm		Over 2500 gm		Total		Under 2501 gm		Over 2500 gm		Total		Under 2501 gm		Over 2500 gm		
	No.	%	No.	%	No.	%	No.	Rate	No.	Rate	No.	Rate	No.	Rate	No.	Rate	No.	Rate	
Vertebral abnormality	5	0.0	4	0.2	1	0.0	0	0	0	0	0	0	2	500.0	1	333.3	1	*	2421
Talipes equinovarus	24	0.1	5	0.2	19	0.1	3	125.0	3	600.0	0	0	4	210.5	1	*	3	166.7	2840
Metatarsus adductus	33	0.2	1	0.0	32	0.2	0	0	0	0	0	0	0	0	0	0	0	0	3392
Calcaneo valgus	4	0.0	0	0	4	0.0	0	0	0	-	0	0	0	0	0	-	0	0	3778
Congenital dislocation or dysplasia of the hip	4	0.0	1	0.0	3	0.0	1	250.0	1	*	0	0	0	0	0	-	0	0	2417
Absence or hypoplasia of extremity or part	13	0.1	3	0.1	10	0.1	2	153.9	2	666.7	0	0	0	0	0	0	0	0	2902
Polydactyly	265	1.4	27	1.1	238	1.4	4	15.1	4	148.2	0	0	4	16.8	1	52.6	3	13.7	3083
Syndactyly	19	0.1	1	0.0	18	0.1	0	0	0	0	0	0	1	58.8	0	0	1	62.5	3304
Torticollis	1	0.0	1	0.0	0	0.0	0	0	0	0	0	-	0	0	0	0	0	-	2240
Arthrogryposis multiplex	1	0.0	1	0.0	0	0.0	1	*	1	*	0	-	0	-	0	-	0	-	1956
Achondroplasia	1	0.0	0	0.0	1	0.0	0	0	0	-	0	0	0	0	0	-	0	0	3203
Fractured clavicle	28	0.2	1	0.0	27	0.2	0	0	0	0	0	0	2	74.1	0	0	2	76.9	3123
Other fractures	7	0.0	2	0.1	5	0.0	2	285.7	1	500.0	1	200.0	0	0	0	0	0	0	2649
Other abn. non-neuro.	58	0.3	7	0.3	51	0.3	5	86.2	2	285.7	3	58.8	4	83.3	0	0	4	90.9	3084
None†	18815		2520		16295		316	16.8	223	88.5	93	5.7	254	15.3	82	40.2	172	11.8	
Total	19259		2570		16689														3039

*Rate is 1000.0.
†No abnormalities within the system.

Table 12-68. Newborn Summary Data
Eye Conditions — White

Condition, Abnormality or Procedure	Livebirths						Neonatal Deaths						Neuro. Abn. 1 Year						Mean Bwt.
	Total		Under 2501 gm		Over 2500 gm		Total		Under 2501 gm		Over 2500 gm		Total		Under 2501 gm		Over 2500 gm		
	No.	%	No.	%	No.	%	No.	Rate	No.	Rate	No.	Rate	No.	Rate	No.	Rate	No.	Rate	
Chorio-retinitis	0	0	0	0	0	0	0	–	0	–	0	–	0	–	0	–	0	–	–
Retrolental fibroplasia	0	0.0	0	0.0	0	0.0	0	–	0	–	0	0	0	–	0	–	0	–	–
Cataract	7	0.0	2	0.2	5	0.0	0	0	0	0	0	0	2	333.3	1	500.0	1	250.0	2851
Corneal opacity	2	0.0	1	0.1	1	0.0	2	*	1	*	1	*	0	–	0	–	0	–	2396
Microphthalmia	3	0.0	1	0.1	2	0.0	2	666.7	1	*	1	500.0	0	0	0	–	0	0	2731
Blindness	0	0	0	0	0	0	0	–	0	–	0	–	0	–	0	–	0	–	–
Nystagmus	10	0.1	0	0	10	0.1	0	0	0	–	0	0	2	200.0	0	–	2	200.0	3547
Other eye conditions	33	0.2	9	0.7	24	0.1	4	121.2	3	333.3	1	41.7	8	470.6	3	*	5	357.1	2948
None†	17978		1275		16703		209	11.6	138	108.2	71	4.3	233	16.1	42	46.4	191	14.1	3272
Total	18029		1287		16742														

*Rate is 1000.0.
†No abnormalities within the system.

Table 12-69. Newborn Summary Data
Eye Conditions — Black

Condition, Abnormality or Procedure	Livebirths						Neonatal Deaths						Neuro. Abn. 1 Year						Mean Bwt.
	Total		Under 2501 gm		Over 2500 gm		Total		Under 2501 gm		Over 2500 gm		Total		Under 2501 gm		Over 2500 gm		
	No.	%	No.	%	No.	%	No.	Rate	No.	Rate	No.	Rate	No.	Rate	No.	Rate	No.	Rate	
Chorio-retinitis	1	0.0	1	0.0	0	0	0	0	0	0	0	–	0	0	0	0	0	–	2381
Retrolental fibroplasia	1	0.0	1	0.0	0	0	0	0	0	0	0	–	1	*	1	*	0	–	1191
Cataract	11	0.1	5	0.2	6	0.0	0	0	0	0	0	0	4	400.0	1	250.0	3	500.0	2629
Corneal opacity	3	0.0	1	0.0	2	0.0	1	333.3	1	*	0	0	1	500.0	0	–	1	500.0	2863
Microphthalmia	3	0.0	3	0.1	0	0	1	333.3	1	333.3	0	–	0	0	0	0	0	–	1795
Blindness	1	0.0	1	0.0	0	0	0	0	0	0	0	–	0	0	0	0	0	–	2296
Nystagmus	22	0.1	1	0.0	21	0.1	0	0	0	0	0	0	2	105.3	0	0	2	105.3	3274
Other eye conditions	26	0.1	7	0.3	19	0.1	2	76.9	1	142.9	1	52.6	2	100.0	0	0	2	125.0	2782
None†	19195		2554		16641														
Total	19259		2570		16689		328	17.1	232	90.8	96	5.8	260	15.4	83	40.3	177	11.9	3041

*Rate is 1000.0.
†No abnormalities within the system

Table 12-70. Newborn Summary Data
Ear Conditions — White

Condition, Abnormality or Procedure	Livebirths						Neonatal Deaths						Neuro. Abn. 1 Year						Mean Bwt.
	Total		Under 2501 gm		Over 2500 gm		Total		Under 2501 gm		Over 2500 gm		Total		Under 2501 gm		Over 2500 gm		
	No.	%	No.	%	No.	%	No.	Rate	No.	Rate	No.	Rate	No.	Rate	No.	Rate	No.	Rate	
Low-set ears	23	0.1	9	0.7	14	0.1	8	347.8	4	444.4	4	285.7	4	363.6	2	666.7	2	250.0	2771
Deformed ear pinna	31	0.2	3	0.2	28	0.2	1	32.3	1	333.3	0	0	4	181.8	1	*	3	142.9	3159
Branchial cleft anomaly	28	0.2	2	0.2	26	0.2	0	0	0	0	0	0	1	47.6	0	–	1	52.6	3283
Deafness	1	0.0	0	0.0	1	0.0	0	0	0	–	0	0	0	0	0	0	0	0	3118
Other ear conditions	23	0.1	2	0.2	21	0.1	1	43.5	0	0	1	47.6	1	52.6	0	0	1	55.6	3345
None†	17930		1272		16658		206	11.5	137	107.7	69	4.1	236	16.3	43	47.6	193	14.3	
Total	18029		1287		16742														3272

*Rate is 1000.0.
†No abnormalities within the system.

Table 12-71. Newborn Summary Data
Ear Conditions — Black

Condition, Abnormality or Procedure	Livebirths						Neonatal Deaths						Neuro. Abn. 1 Year						Mean Bwt.
	Total		Under 2501 gm		Over 2500 gm		Total		Under 2501 gm		Over 2500 gm		Total		Under 2501 gm		Over 2500 gm		
	No.	%	No.	%	No.	%	No.	Rate	No.	Rate	No.	Rate	No.	Rate	No.	Rate	No.	Rate	
Low-set ears	47	0.2	9	0.4	38	0.2	3	63.8	2	222.2	1	26.3	3	75.0	1	142.9	2	60.6	2997
Deformed ear pinna	50	0.3	8	0.3	42	0.3	2	40.0	2	250.0	0	0	2	43.5	0	0	2	48.8	2999
Branchial cleft anomaly	249	1.3	34	1.3	215	1.3	1	4.0	0	0	1	4.7	5	21.8	1	32.3	4	20.2	3024
Deafness	1	0.0	1	0.0	0	0	0	0	0	0	0	–	0	0	0	0	0	–	2296
Other ear conditions	33	0.2	6	0.2	27	0.2	0	0	0	0	0	0	0	0	0	0	0	0	3000
None†	18892		2518		16374		326	17.3	231	91.7	95	5.8	260	15.7	83	41.0	177	12.1	
Total	19259		2570		16689														3041

†No abnormalities within the system.

Table 12-72. Newborn Summary Data
Upper Respiratory Tract and Mouth Conditions — White

Condition, Abnormality or Procedure	Livebirths						Neonatal Deaths						Neuro. Abn. 1 Year						Mean Bwt.
	Total		Under 2501 gm		Over 2500 gm		Total		Under 2501 gm		Over 2500 gm		Total		Under 2501 gm		Over 2500 gm		
	No.	%	No.	%	No.	%	No.	Rate	No.	Rate	No.	Rate	No.	Rate	No.	Rate	No.	Rate	
Choanal atresia	1	0.0	0	0	1	0.0	0	0	0	–	0	0	0	0	0	–	0	0	2948
Cleft palate	19	0.1	4	0.3	15	0.1	2	105.3	1	250.0	1	66.7	3	214.3	2	666.7	1	90.9	3141
Cleft uvula (bifid)	6	0.0	3	0.2	3	0.0	0	0	0	0	0	0	1	200.0	1	333.3	0	0	2788
Cleft lip	24	0.1	2	0.2	22	0.1	2	83.3	0	0	2	90.9	2	125.0	1	500.0	1	71.4	3228
Cleft gum	16	0.1	1	0.1	15	0.1	0	0	0	0	0	0	2	133.3	0	0	2	142.9	3492
Micrognathia	11	0.1	1	0.1	10	0.1	0	0	0	0	0	0	0	0	0	0	0	0	2995
Malformation of epiglottis and larynx	0	0	0	0	0	0	0	–	0	–	0	–	0	–	0	–	0	–	–
Other respiratory tract and mouth conditions	49	0.3	11	0.9	38	0.2	3	61.2	2	181.8	1	26.3	11	289.5	4	666.7	7	218.8	3132
None†	17929		1268		16661														
Total	18029		1287		16742		209	11.7	139	109.6	70	4.2	231	16.0	41	45.6	190	14.0	3272

†No abnormalities within the system.

Table 12-73. Newborn Summary Data
Upper Respiratory Tract and Mouth Conditions — Black

Condition, Abnormality or Procedure	Livebirths						Neonatal Deaths						Neuro. Abn. 1 Year						Mean Bwt.
	Total		Under 2501 gm		Over 2500 gm		Total		Under 2501 gm		Over 2500 gm		Total		Under 2501 gm		Over 2500 gm		
	No.	%	No.	%	No.	%	No.	Rate	No.	Rate	No.	Rate	No.	Rate	No.	Rate	No.	Rate	
Choanal atresia	1	0.0	1	0.0	0	0	1	*	1	*	0	–	0	–	0	–	0	–	2126
Cleft palate	15	0.1	6	0.2	9	0.1	1	66.7	1	166.7	0	0	0	0	0	0	0	0	2519
Cleft uvula (bifid)	4	0.0	0	0	4	0.0	0	0	0	–	0	0	0	0	0	0	0	0	3360
Cleft lip	11	0.1	4	0.2	7	0.0	1	90.9	1	250.0	0	0	0	0	0	0	0	0	2603
Cleft gum	83	0.4	15	0.6	68	0.4	2	24.1	0	0	2	29.4	1	13.7	1	100.0	0	0	2979
Micrognathia	3	0.0	0	0	3	0.0	0	0	0	–	0	0	0	0	0	–	0	0	2825
Malformation of epiglottis and larynx	0	0	0	0	0	0	0	–	0	–	0	–	0	–	0	–	0	–	–
Other respiratory tract and mouth conditions	78	0.4	12	0.5	66	0.4	4	51.3	1	83.3	3	45.5	0	0	0	0	0	0	3035
None†	19082		2537		16545														–
Total	19259		2570		16689		323	16.9	231	91.1	92	5.6	269	16.0	84	41.0	185	12.5	3041

*Rate is 1000.0.
†No abnormalities within the system.

Table 12-74. Newborn Summary Data
Thoracic Abnormalities — White

Condition, Abnormality or Procedure	Livebirths						Neonatal Deaths						Neuro. Abn. 1 Year						Mean Bwt.
	Total		Under 2501 gm		Over 2500 gm		Total		Under 2501 gm		Over 2500 gm		Total		Under 2501 gm		Over 2500 gm		
	No.	%	No.	%	No.	%	No.	Rate	No.	Rate	No.	Rate	No.	Rate	No.	Rate	No.	Rate	
Anomaly of diaphragm	9	0.1	3	0.2	6	0.0	5	555.6	3	*	2	333.3	0	0	0	–	0	0	2659
Anomaly of lung	9	0.1	4	0.3	5	0.0	9	*	4	*	5	*	0	–	0	–	0	–	2482
Anomaly of chest wall	6	0.0	2	0.2	4	0.0	1	166.7	1	500.0	0	0	1	200.0	0	0	1	250.0	2915
Pectus excavatum	4	0.0	2	0.2	2	0.0	0	0	0	0	0	0	0	0	0	0	0	0	2353
Other thoracic abn.	9	0.1	5	0.4	4	0.0	6	666.7	4	800.0	2	500.0	0	0	0	0	0	0	2258
None†	17999		1274		16725														
Total	18029		1287		16742		200	11.1	133	104.4	67	4.0	244	16.8	46	50.7	198	14.6	3272

*Rate is 1000.0.
†No abnormalities within the system.

Table 12-75. Newborn Summary Data
Thoracic Abnormalities — Black

Condition, Abnormality or Procedure	Livebirths						Neonatal Deaths						Neuro. Abn. 1 Year						Mean Bwt.
	Total		Under 2501 gm		Over 2500 gm		Total		Under 2501 gm		Over 2500 gm		Total		Under 2501 gm		Over 2500 gm		
	No.	%	No.	%	No.	%	No.	Rate	No.	Rate	No.	Rate	No.	Rate	No.	Rate	No.	Rate	
Anomaly of diaphragm	6	0.0	1	0.0	5	0.0	3	500.0	1	*	2	400.0	0	0	0	–	0	0	3132
Anomaly of lung	10	0.1	7	0.3	3	0.0	10	*	7	*	3	*	0	–	0	–	0	–	2200
Anomaly of chest wall	2	0.0	0	0.0	2	0.0	0	0	0	–	0	0	1	*	0	–	1	*	3558
Pectus excavatum	6	0.0	4	0.2	2	0.0	2	333.3	2	500.0	0	0	0	0	0	0	0	0	2183
Other thoracic abn.	14	0.1	8	0.3	6	0.0	10	714.3	7	875.0	3	500.0	0	0	0	0	0	0	2260
None†	19226		2552		16674														
Total	19259		2570		16689		311	16.2	219	85.8	92	5.5	269	15.9	85	41.1	184	12.4	3042

*Rate is 1000.0.
†No abnormalities within the system.

Table 12-76. Newborn Summary Data
Respiratory Abnormalities — White

Condition, Abnormality or Procedure	Livebirths						Neonatal Deaths						Neuro. Abn. 1 Year						Mean Bwt.
	Total		Under 2501 gm		Over 2500 gm		Total		Under 2501 gm		Over 2500 gm		Total		Under 2501 gm		Over 2500 gm		
	No.	%	No.	%	No.	%	No.	Rate	No.	Rate	No.	Rate	No.	Rate	No.	Rate	No.	Rate	
Respiratory abnormality associated with:																			
Hyaline membrane disease	81	0.5	60	4.7	21	0.1	49	604.9	39	650.0	10	476.2	1	40.0	0	0	1	100.0	2042
Primary atelectasis	74	0.4	48	3.7	26	0.2	49	662.2	40	833.3	9	346.2	0	0	0	0	0	0	2066
Pneumonia	75	0.4	35	2.7	40	0.2	24	320.0	15	428.6	9	225.0	3	76.9	2	117.7	1	45.5	2537
Aspiration before or during delivery	44	0.2	17	1.3	27	0.2	18	409.1	13	764.7	5	185.2	2	90.9	0	0	2	111.1	2536
Aspiration after del.	10	0.1	4	0.3	6	0.0	1	100.0	0	0	1	166.7	1	142.9	1	333.3	0	0	2444
Pulmonary hemorrhage	16	0.1	9	0.7	7	0.0	15	937.5	9	*	6	857.1	0	0	0	0	0	0	2240
Cardiac conditions	15	0.1	4	0.3	11	0.1	6	400.0	1	250.0	5	454.6	0	0	0	0	0	0	2954
C.N.S. abnormality	23	0.1	10	0.8	13	0.1	14	608.7	8	800.0	6	461.5	1	250.0	1	*	0	0	2345
Metabolic imbalance	6	0.0	3	0.2	3	0.0	1	166.7	1	333.3	0	0	0	0	0	0	0	0	1918
Other specified	90	0.5	28	2.2	62	0.4	28	311.1	21	750.0	7	112.9	2	39.2	2	285.7	0	0	2729
Unknown resp. cond.	62	0.3	11	0.9	51	0.3	1	16.1	1	90.9	0	0	2	40.0	1	111.1	1	24.4	3157
Signif. respiratory events:																			
Primary apnea	158	0.9	43	3.3	115	0.7	31	196.2	27	627.9	4	34.8	4	38.1	1	71.4	3	33.0	2856
Resuscitation-during first 5 min. of life	1089	6.0	185	14.4	904	5.4	76	69.8	56	302.7	20	22.1	34	40.2	12	114.3	22	29.7	3074
Resuscitation-after first 5 min. of life	484	2.7	141	11.0	343	2.1	101	208.7	75	531.9	26	75.8	9	29.3	4	74.1	5	19.8	2854
None†	16195		857		15338		34	2.1	9	10.5	25	1.6	192	14.6	25	37.0	167	13.4	3304
Total	18029		1287		16742														

*Rate is 1000.0.
† No abnormalities within the system.

Table 12-77. Newborn Summary Data
Respiratory Abnormalities — Black

Condition, Abnormality or Procedure	Livebirths						Neonatal Deaths						Neuro. Abn. 1 Year						Mean Bwt.
	Total		Under 2501 gm		Over 2500 gm		Total		Under 2501 gm		Over 2500 gm		Total		Under 2501 gm		Over 2500 gm		
	No.	%	No.	%	No.	%	No.	Rate	No.	Rate	No.	Rate	No.	Rate	No.	Rate	No.	Rate	
Respiratory abnormality associated with:																			
Hyaline membrane disease	86	0.5	74	2.9	12	0.1	55	639.5	48	648.7	7	583.3	9	333.3	7	318.2	2	400.0	1695
Primary atelectasis	111	0.6	90	3.5	21	0.1	98	882.9	85	944.4	13	619.1	0	0	0	0	0	0	1561
Pneumonia	101	0.5	61	2.4	40	0.2	61	604.0	41	672.1	20	500.0	1	27.0	1	55.6	0	0	2212
Aspiration before or during delivery	59	0.3	29	1.1	30	0.2	41	694.9	27	931.0	14	466.7	1	62.5	0	0	1	71.4	2237
Aspiration after del.	17	0.1	7	0.3	10	0.1	6	352.9	4	571.4	2	200.0	0	0	0	0	0	0	2628
Pulmonary hemorrhage	45	0.2	34	1.3	11	0.1	44	977.8	33	970.6	11	*	0	0	0	0	0	–	1797
Cardiac conditions	16	0.1	4	0.2	12	0.1	11	687.5	3	750.0	8	666.7	0	0	0	0	0	0	2892
C.N.S. abnormality	34	0.2	19	0.7	15	0.1	21	617.7	14	736.8	7	466.7	3	272.7	3	750.0	0	0	2126
Metabolic imbalance	6	0.0	2	0.1	4	0.0	4	666.7	1	500.0	3	750.0	0	0	0	0	0	0	2840
Other specified	152	0.8	84	3.3	68	0.4	73	480.3	57	678.6	16	235.3	3	42.9	2	80.0	1	22.2	2129
Unknown resp. cond.	133	0.7	42	1.6	91	0.6	2	15.0	2	47.6	0	0	3	25.0	3	85.7	0	0	2741
Signif. respiratory events:																			
Primary apnea	376	2.0	137	5.3	239	1.4	89	236.7	67	489.1	22	92.1	8	31.1	3	48.4	5	25.6	2582
Resuscitation-during first 5 min. of life	1146	6.0	358	13.9	788	4.7	149	130.0	109	304.5	40	50.8	25	28.8	12	57.1	13	19.8	2771
Resuscitation-after first 5 min. of life	626	3.3	269	10.5	357	2.1	178	284.4	134	498.1	44	123.3	16	40.4	9	76.9	7	25.1	2486
None †	17358		1854		15504		28	1.6	5	2.7	23	1.5	222	14.3	56	33.8	166	12.0	3085
Total	19259		2570		16689														

*Rate is 1000.0.
† No abnormalities within the system.

Table 12-78. Newborn Summary Data
Cardiovascular Conditions — White

Condition, Abnormality or Procedure	Livebirths						Neonatal Deaths						Neuro. Abn. 1 Year						Mean Bwt.
	Total		Under 2501 gm		Over 2500 gm		Total		Under 2501 gm		Over 2500 gm		Total		Under 2501 gm		Over 2500 gm		
	No.	%	No.	%	No.	%	No.	Rate	No.	Rate	No.	Rate	No.	Rate	No.	Rate	No.	Rate	
Acyanotic CHD	22	0.1	10	0.8	12	0.1	9	409.1	5	500.0	4	333.3	3	333.3	2	666.7	1	166.7	2589
Cyanotic CHD	18	0.1	3	0.2	15	0.1	9	500.0	2	666.7	7	466.7	0	0	0	0	0	0	2870
Fibroelastosis	0	0	0	0	0	0	0	–	0	–	0	–	0	–	0	–	0	–	–
Cardiac arrythmia	22	0.1	6	0.5	16	0.1	9	409.1	4	666.7	5	312.5	0	0	0	0	0	0	2782
Abn. heart rate	43	0.2	18	1.4	25	0.2	19	441.9	13	722.2	6	240.0	1	62.5	1	333.3	0	0	2592
Cardiac enlargement	19	0.1	7	0.5	12	0.1	9	473.7	3	428.6	6	500.0	1	200.0	1	500.0	0	0	2608
Cardiac decompensation	18	0.1	6	0.5	12	0.1	11	611.1	4	666.7	7	583.3	0	0	0	0	0	0	2712
Specific C-V diagnosis	37	0.2	16	1.2	21	0.1	24	648.7	12	750.0	12	571.4	1	142.9	1	333.3	0	0	2666
Other cardiovascular conditions	13	0.1	5	0.4	8	0.1	6	461.5	4	800.0	2	250.0	0	0	0	0	0	0	2558
None†	17916		1246		16670														
Total	18029		1287		16742		168	9.4	115	92.3	53	3.2	242	16.2	44	48.8	198	14.6	3275

†No abnormalities within the system.

Table 12-79. Newborn Summary Data
Cardiovascular Conditions — Black

Condition, Abnormality or Procedure	Livebirths Total No.	%	Under 2501 gm No.	%	Over 2500 gm No.	%	Neonatal Deaths Total No.	Rate	Under 2501 gm No.	Rate	Over 2500 gm No.	Rate	Neuro. Abn. 1 Year Total No.	Rate	Under 2501 gm No.	Rate	Over 2500 gm No.	Rate	Mean Bwt.
Acyanotic CHD	16	0.1	9	0.4	7	0.0	3	187.5	2	222.2	1	142.9	2	222.2	1	200.0	1	250.0	2445
Cyanotic CHD	5	0.0	1	0.0	4	0.0	4	800.0	1	*	3	750.0	0	0	0	–	0	0	2580
Fibroelastosis	0		0		0		0	–	0	–	0	–	0	–	0	–	0	–	–
Cardiac arrythmia	18	0.1	6	0.2	12	0.1	4	222.2	1	166.7	3	250.0	0	0	0	0	0	0	2814
Abn. heart rate	49	0.3	21	0.8	28	0.2	19	387.8	11	523.8	8	285.7	2	76.9	1	125.0	1	55.6	2462
Cardiac enlargement	15	0.1	6	0.2	9	0.1	10	666.7	3	500.0	7	777.8	0	0	0	0	0	0	2723
Cardiac decompensation	18	0.1	5	0.2	13	0.1	11	611.1	3	600.0	8	615.4	1	250.0	0	0	1	250.0	2906
Specific C-V diagnosis	32	0.2	12	0.5	20	0.1	20	625.0	9	750.0	11	550.0	1	100.0	1	333.3	0	0	2500
Other cardiovascular conditions	28	0.2	16	0.6	12	0.1	21	750.0	15	937.5	6	500.0	0	0	0	0	0	0	2273
None†	19136		2514		16622		274	14.3	202	80.4	72	4.3	266	15.7	83	40.4	183	12.3	3044
Total	19259		2570		16689														

*Rate is 1000.0.
†No abnormalities within the system.

Table 12-80. Newborn Summary Data
Alimentary Tract Malformations and Other Conditions — White

Condition, Abnormality or Procedure	Livebirths Total No.	Livebirths Total %	Livebirths Under 2501 gm No.	Livebirths Under 2501 gm %	Livebirths Over 2500 gm No.	Livebirths Over 2500 gm %	Neonatal Deaths Total No.	Neonatal Deaths Total Rate	Neonatal Deaths Under 2501 gm No.	Neonatal Deaths Under 2501 gm Rate	Neonatal Deaths Over 2500 gm No.	Neonatal Deaths Over 2500 gm Rate	Neuro. Abn. 1 Year Total No.	Neuro. Abn. 1 Year Total Rate	Neuro. Abn. 1 Year Under 2501 gm No.	Neuro. Abn. 1 Year Under 2501 gm Rate	Neuro. Abn. 1 Year Over 2500 gm No.	Neuro. Abn. 1 Year Over 2500 gm Rate	Mean Bwt.
Tracheo-esophageal fistula	1	0.0	0	0	1	0.0	0	0	0	–	0	0	0	0	0	–	0	0	2551
Duodenal atresia	1	0.0	0	0	1	0.0	0	0	0	–	0	0	1	*	0	–	1	*	2693
Malrotation	3	0.0	2	0.2	1	0.0	2	666.7	2	*	0	0	0	0	0	–	0	0	2722
Omphalocele	1	0.0	1	0.1	0	0.0	1	*	1	*	0	–	0	–	0	–	0	–	2353
Visceral perforation	3	0.0	1	0.1	2	0.0	1	333.3	1	*	0	–	0	0	0	–	0	0	2807
Imperforate anus	5	0.0	1	0.1	4	0.0	2	400.0	1	*	1	250.0	0	0	0	–	0	0	2909
Inguinal hernia	10	0.1	8	0.6	2	0.0	1	100.0	1	125.0	0	0	1	125.0	1	166.7	0	0	1993
Femoral hernia	0	0.0	0	0	0	0.0	0	–	0	–	0	–	0	–	0	–	0	–	–
Other hernia	2	0.0	0	0	2	0.0	1	500.0	0	–	1	500.0	0	0	0	–	0	0	2793
Other non-infectious G.I.	44	0.2	17	1.3	27	0.2	16	363.6	9	529.4	7	259.3	4	200.0	2	333.3	2	142.9	2585
Nonet	17969		1263		16706		197	11.0	133	105.3	64	3.8	239	16.5	43	47.8	196	14.4	3274
Total	18029		1287		16742														

*Rate is 1000.0.
†No abnormalities within the system.

Table 12-81. Newborn Summary Data
Alimentary Tract Malformations and Other Conditions — Black

Condition, Abnormality or Procedure	Livebirths						Neonatal Deaths						Neuro. Abn. 1 Year						Mean Bwt.
	Total		Under 2501 gm		Over 2500 gm		Total		Under 2501 gm		Over 2500 gm		Total		Under 2501 gm		Over 2500 gm	
	No.	%	No.	%	No.	%	No.	Rate	No.	Rate	No.	Rate	No.	Rate	No.	Rate	No.	Rate	
Tracheo-esophageal fistula	3	0.0	2	0.1	1	0.0	1	333.3	1	500.0	0	0	0	0	0	0	0	0	2580
Duodenal atresia	2	0.0	2	0.1	0	0.0	1	500.0	1	500.0	0	—	0	0	0	0	0	—	1999
Malrotation	4	0.0	1	0.0	3	0.0	3	750.0	1	*	2	666.7	0	0	0	0	0	0	2970
Omphalocele	7	0.0	1	0.0	6	0.0	2	285.7	0	0	2	333.3	0	0	0	0	0	0	2972
Visceral perforation	7	0.0	3	0.1	4	0.0	5	714.3	3	*	2	500.0	0	0	0	0	0	0	2450
Imperforate anus	4	0.0	3	0.1	1	0.0	0	0	0	0	0	0	1	250.0	1	333.3	0	0	2353
Inguinal hernia	19	0.1	12	0.5	7	0.0	0	0	0	0	0	0	3	176.5	3	272.7	0	—	2059
Femoral hernia	0	0.0	0	0.0	0	0.0	0	—	0	—	0	—	0	—	0	—	0	—	—
Other hernia	3	0.0	1	0.0	2	0.0	0	0	0	0	0	0	0	0	0	0	0	0	3052
Other non-infectious G.I.	61	0.3	18	0.7	43	0.3	23	377.1	10	555.6	13	302.3	1	32.3	1	142.9	0	0	2756
None†	19161		2533		16628														
Total	19259		2570		16689		302	15.8	220	86.9	82	4.9	266	15.8	81	39.5	185	12.5	3043

*Rate is 1000.0.
†No abnormalities within the system.

Table 12-82. Newborn Summary Data
Liver, Bile Ducts, and/or Spleen Abnormalities — White

Condition, Abnormality or Procedure	Livebirths						Neonatal Deaths						Neuro. Abn. 1 Year						Mean Bwt.
	Total		Under 2501 gm		Over 2500 gm		Total		Under 2501 gm		Over 2500 gm		Total		Under 2501 gm		Over 2500 gm		
	No.	%	No.	%	No.	%	No.	Rate	No.	Rate	No.	Rate	No.	Rate	No.	Rate	No.	Rate	
Abn. of liver, bile ducts, and/or spleen	42	0.2	21	1.6	21	0.1	24	571.4	14	666.7	10	476.2	1	66.7	0	0	1	111.1	2547
None†	17987		1266		16721		191	10.6	128	101.1	63	3.8	244	16.8	46	50.8	198	14.6	3273
Total	18029		1287		16742														

†No abnormalities within the system.

Table 12-83. Newborn Summary Data
Liver, Bile Ducts, and/or Spleen Abnormalities — Black

Condition, Abnormality or Procedure	Livebirths						Neonatal Deaths						Neuro. Abn. 1 Year						Mean Bwt.
	Total		Under 2501 gm		Over 2500 gm		Total		Under 2501 gm		Over 2500 gm		Total		Under 2501 gm		Over 2500 gm		
	No.	%	No.	%	No.	%	No.	Rate	No.	Rate	No.	Rate	No.	Rate	No.	Rate	No.	Rate	
Abn. of liver, bile ducts, and/or spleen	50	0.3	27	1.1	23	0.1	34	680.0	22	814.8	12	521.7	2	181.8	1	250.0	1	142.9	2282
None†	19209		2543		16666		297	15.5	212	83.4	85	5.1	268	15.8	84	40.7	184	12.4	3043
Total	19259		2570		16689														

†No abnormalities within the system.

Table 12-84. Newborn Summary Data
Genitourinary Conditions — White

Condition, Abnormality or Procedure	Livebirths Total No.	%	Under 2501 gm No.	%	Over 2500 gm No.	%	Neonatal Deaths Total No.	Rate	Under 2501 gm No.	Rate	Over 2500 gm No.	Rate	Neuro. Abn. 1 Year Total No.	Rate	Under 2501 gm No.	Rate	Over 2500 gm No.	Rate	Mean Bwt.
Hypospadias‡	68	0.7	12	2.1	56	0.6	1	14.7	1	83.3	0	0	2	36.4	0	0	2	44.4	3193
Chordee‡	7	0.1	0	0	7	0.1	0	0	0	–	0	0	1	200.0	0	–	1	200.0	3086
None†	9243		580		8773														3330
Total‡	9353																		
Other abn. of external genitalia	20	0.1	5	0.4	15	0.1	1	50.0	1	200.0	0	0	4	250.0	1	333.3	3	230.8	3001
Bladder outflow or urethral obstruction	1	0.0	0	0	1	0.0	0	0	0	–	0	0	0	0	0	–	0	0	5046
Hydronephrosis or hydro–ureter obstruction	9	0.1	2	0.2	7	0.0	4	444.4	2	*	2	285.7	0	0	0	–	0	0	3131
Cystic kidney	7	0.0	5	0.4	2	0.0	5	714.3	4	800.0	1	500.0	0	0	0	0	0	0	2179
Other non–infectious genitourinary cond.	28	0.2	9	0.7	19	0.1	11	392.9	7	777.8	4	210.5	2	142.9	1	500.0	1	83.3	2891
None†	17908		1258		16650		199	11.1	131	104.1	68	4.1	238	16.5	44	49.2	194	14.3	3273
Total	18029		1287		16742														

*Rate is 1000.0.
†No abnormalities within the system.
‡Males only.

Table 12-85. Newborn Summary Data
Genitourinary Conditions — Black

Condition, Abnormality or Procedure	Livebirths Total		Under 2501 gm		Over 2500 gm		Neonatal Deaths Total		Under 2501 gm		Over 2500 gm		Neuro. Abn. 1 Year Total		Under 2501 gm		Over 2500 gm		Mean Bwt.
	No.	%	No.	%	No.	%	No.	Rate	No.	Rate	No.	Rate	No.	Rate	No.	Rate	No.	Rate	
Hypospadias‡	46	0.5	14	1.2	32	0.4	1	21.7	0	–	1	31.3	0	0	0	0	0	0	2859
Chordee‡	1	0.0	0	0	1	0.0	0	0	0	–	0	0	0	0	0	–	0	0	2637
None†	9562																		
Total‡	9643		1161		8482														3098
Other abn. of external genitalia	13	0.1	4	0.2	9	0.1	2	153.9	2	500.0	0	0	1	100.0	0	0	1	125.0	2800
Bladder outflow or urethral obstruction	6	0.0	1	0.0	5	0.0	3	500.0	1	*	2	400.0	1	333.3	0	–	1	333.3	3095
Hydronephrosis or hydro-ureter obstruction	12	0.1	5	0.2	7	0.0	6	500.0	3	600.0	3	428.6	0	0	0	0	0	0	2414
Cystic kidney	11	0.1	6	0.2	5	0.0	9	818.2	6	*	3	600.0	0	0	0	–	0	0	2245
Other non-infectious genitourinary cond.	19	0.1	6	0.2	13	0.1	9	473.7	3	500.0	6	461.5	3	333.3	2	666.7	1	166.7	2845
None†	19166		2541		16625														
Total	19259		2570		16689		311	16.2	225	88.6	86	5.2	265	15.7	83	40.4	182	12.3	3042

*Rate is 1000.0.
†No abnormalities within the system.
‡Males only.

Table 12-86. Newborn Summary Data
Neoplastic Disease and/or Other Tumors — White

Condition, Abnormality or Procedure	Livebirths						Neonatal Deaths						Neuro. Abn. 1 Year						Mean Bwt.
	Total		Under 2501 gm		Over 2500 gm		Total		Under 2501 gm		Over 2500 gm		Total		Under 2501 gm		Over 2500 gm		
	No.	%	No.	%	No.	%	No.	Rate	No.	Rate	No.	Rate	No.	Rate	No.	Rate	No.	Rate	
Neoplastic disease and/or other tumors	5	0.0	0	0	5	0.0	0	0	0	–	0	0	0	0	0	–	0	0	3340
Nonet	18024		1286		16737		215	11.9	142	110.4	73	4.4	245	16.9	46	50.5	199	14.6	3271
Total	18029		1287		16742														

†No abnormalities within the system.

Table 12-87. Newborn Summary Data
Neoplastic Disease and/or Other Tumors — Black

Condition, Abnormality or Procedure	Livebirths						Neonatal Deaths						Neuro. Abn. 1 Year						Mean Bwt.
	Total		Under 2501 gm		Over 2500 gm		Total		Under 2501 gm		Over 2500 gm		Total		Under 2501 gm		Over 2500 gm		
	No.	%	No.	%	No.	%	No.	Rate	No.	Rate	No.	Rate	No.	Rate	No.	Rate	No.	Rate	
Neoplastic disease and/or other tumors	10	0.1	2	0.1	8	0.1	1	100.0	1	500.0	0	0	0	0	0	0	0	0	3155
Nonet	19249		2568		16681		330	17.1	233	90.7	97	5.8	270	15.9	85	41.1	185	12.4	3040
Total	19259		2570		16689														

†No abnormalities within the system.

Table 12-88. Newborn Summary Data
Hematologic Conditions — White

Condition, Abnormality or Procedure	Livebirths						Neonatal Deaths						Neuro. Abn. 1 Year						Mean Bwt.
	Total		Under 2501 gm		Over 2500 gm		Total		Under 2501 gm		Over 2500 gm		Total		Under 2501 gm		Over 2500 gm		
	No.	%	No.	%	No.	%	No.	Rate	No.	Rate	No.	Rate	No.	Rate	No.	Rate	No.	Rate	
Erythroblastosis	167	0.9	34	2.6	133	0.8	12	71.9	7	105.9	5	37.6	3	22.6	1	40.0	2	18.5	2965
Rh	113	0.6	26	2.0	87	0.5	10	88.5	6	230.8	4	46.0	0	0	0	0	0	0	2888
ABO	43	0.2	6	0.5	37	0.2	1	25.3	0	0	1	27.0	3	85.7	1	200.0	2	66.7	3132
Other	1	0.0	1	0.1	0	0	1	*	1	*	0	–	0	–	0	–	0	–	1644
Other hemolytic dis.	2	0.0	1	0.1	1	0.0	0	0	0	0	0	0	1	500.0	1	*	0	0	2367
Coagulation defect	10	0.1	2	0.2	8	0.1	1	100.0	0	0	1	125.0	2	285.7	0	0	2	400.0	3221
Intra–uterine blood loss	3	0.0	1	0.1	2	0.0	1	333.3	1	*	0	0	1	500.0	0	–	1	500.0	2825
Other major hemorrhage	19	0.1	7	0.5	12	0.1	7	368.4	6	857.1	1	83.3	2	250.0	0	0	2	250.0	2811
Other hematologic conditions	30	0.2	17	1.3	13	0.1	5	166.7	3	176.5	2	153.9	2	83.3	1	71.4	1	100.0	2373
None†	17804		1226		16578		191	10.7	126	102.8	65	3.9	236	16.5	43	49.4	193	14.3	3276
Total	18029		1287		16742														

*Rate is 1000.0.
†No abnormalities within the system.

Table 12-89. Newborn Summary Data
Hematologic Conditions — Black

Condition, Abnormality or Procedure	Livebirths						Neonatal Deaths						Neuro. Abn. 1 Year						Mean Bwt.
	Total		Under 2501 gm		Over 2500 gm		Total		Under 2501 gm		Over 2500 gm		Total		Under 2501 gm		Over 2500 gm		
	No.	%	No.	%	No.	%	No.	Rate	No.	Rate	No.	Rate	No.	Rate	No.	Rate	No.	Rate	
Erythroblastosis	105	0.6	22	0.9	83	0.5	3	28.6	2	90.9	1	12.1	1	10.8	0	0	1	12.8	2901
Rh	32	0.2	8	0.3	24	0.1	1	31.3	1	125.0	0	0	1	34.5	0	0	1	43.5	2840
ABO	63	0.3	11	0.4	52	0.3	1	15.9	0	0	1	19.2	0	0	0	0	0	0	2940
Other	2	0.0	1	0.0	1	0.0	0	0	0	0	0	0	0	0	0	0	0	0	2665
Other hemolytic dis.	3	0.0	2	0.1	1	0.0	0	0	0	0	0	0	0	0	0	0	0	0	2816
Coagulation defect	11	0.1	3	0.1	8	0.1	3	272.7	1	333.3	2	250.0	1	142.9	1	*	0	0	2956
Intra-uterine blood loss	3	0.0	1	0.0	2	0.0	0	0	0	0	0	0	0	0	0	0	0	0	2731
Other major hemorrhage	29	0.2	13	0.5	16	0.1	15	517.2	12	923.1	3	187.5	0	0	0	0	0	0	2355
Other hematologic conditions	67	0.4	51	2.0	16	0.1	5	74.6	3	58.8	2	125.0	7	129.6	6	139.5	1	90.9	1867
Nonet	19044		2480		16564														
Total	19259		2570		16689		307	16.1	217	87.5	90	5.4	261	15.6	78	38.9	183	12.4	3046

*Rate is 1000.0.
†No abnormalities within the system.

Table 12-90. Newborn Summary Data
Skin Conditions and Malformations — White

Condition, Abnormality or Procedure	Livebirths						Neonatal Deaths						Neuro. Abn. 1 Year						Mean Bwt.
	Total		Under 2501 gm		Over 2500 gm		Total		Under 2501 gm		Over 2500 gm		Total		Under 2501 gm		Over 2500 gm		
	No.	%	No.	%	No.	%	No.	Rate	No.	Rate	No.	Rate	No.	Rate	No.	Rate	No.	Rate	
Strawberry/portwine hemangioma	106	0.6	11	0.9	95	0.6	1	9.4	0	0	1	10.5	1	11.0	0	0	1	12.2	3270
Cavernous hemangioma	20	0.1	3	0.2	17	0.1	0	0	0	0	0	0	0	0	0	0	0	0	3118
Hairy nevus	7	0.0	0	0	7	0.0	0	0	0	–	0	0	0	0	0	–	0	0	3280
Lymphangioma	2	0.0	0	0	2	0.0	0	0	0	–	0	0	0	0	0	–	0	0	3600
Sclerema	8	0.0	6	0.5	2	0.0	4	500.0	4	666.7	0	0	0	0	0	0	0	0	2024
Severe ecchymosis	51	0.3	22	1.7	29	0.2	10	196.1	10	454.6	0	0	3	103.5	1	125.0	2	95.2	2581
Significant petechiae	73	0.4	11	0.9	62	0.4	2	27.4	1	90.9	1	16.1	4	67.8	3	333.3	1	20.0	3359
Supernumerary nipples	14	0.1	0	0	14	0.1	0	0	0	–	0	0	1	76.9	0	–	1	76.9	3210
Café au lait spots	0	0	0	0	0	0	0	–	0	–	0	–	0	–	0	–	0	–	–
Other skin cond. and malformations	76	0.4	12	0.9	64	0.4	8	105.3	4	333.3	4	62.5	5	94.3	2	285.7	3	65.2	3152
None†	17695		1229		16466														
Total	18029		1287		16742		193	10.9	125	101.7	68	4.1	232	16.3	41	46.8	191	14.3	3274

†No abnormalities within the system.

Table 12-91. Newborn Summary Data
Skin Conditions and Malformations — Black

Condition, Abnormality or Procedure	Livebirths						Neonatal Deaths						Neuro. Abn. 1 Year						Mean Bwt.
	Total		Under 2501 gm		Over 2500 gm		Total		Under 2501 gm		Over 2500 gm		Total		Under 2501 gm		Over 2500 gm		
	No.	%	No.	%	No.	%	No.	Rate	No.	Rate	No.	Rate	No.	Rate	No.	Rate	No.	Rate	
Strawberry/portwine hemangioma	62	0.3	8	0.3	54	0.3	0	0	0	0	0	0	0	0	0	0	0	0	3151
Cavernous hemangioma	14	0.1	6	0.2	8	0.1	1	71.4	1	166.7	0	0	0	0	0	0	0	0	2499
Hairy nevus	4	0.0	0	0	4	0.0	0	0	0	–	0	0	0	0	0	–	0	0	3154
Lymphangioma	4	0.0	0	0	4	0.0	0	0	0	–	0	0	0	0	0	–	0	0	3048
Sclerema	5	0.0	4	0.2	1	0.0	4	800.0	3	750.0	1	*	1	*	1	*	0	–	1871
Severe ecchymosis	56	0.3	36	1.4	20	0.1	21	375.0	20	555.6	1	50.0	3	90.9	3	200.0	0	0	2066
Significant petechiae	50	0.3	16	0.6	34	0.2	9	180.0	8	500.0	1	29.4	1	25.6	1	142.9	0	0	2731
Supernumerary nipples	238	1.2	19	0.7	219	1.3	0	0	0	0	0	0	4	19.0	1	55.6	3	15.5	3155
Café au lait spots	37	0.2	1	0.0	36	0.2	0	0	0	0	0	0	2	60.6	0	0	2	62.5	3364
Other skin cond. and malformations	149	0.8	31	1.2	118	0.7	11	73.8	7	225.8	4	33.9	5	40.7	3	142.9	2	19.6	2963
None†	18668		2457		16211		288	15.4	198	80.6	90	5.6	256	15.6	78	39.0	178	12.3	
Total	19259		2570		16689														3043

*Rate is 1000.0.
†No abnormalities within the system.

Table 12-92. Newborn Summary Data Infections — White

Condition, Abnormality or Procedure	Livebirths						Neonatal Deaths						Neuro. Abn. 1 Year						Mean Bwt.
	Total		Under 2501 gm		Over 2500 gm		Total		Under 2501 gm		Over 2500 gm		Total		Under 2501 gm		Over 2500 gm		
	No.	%	No.	%	No.	%	No.	Rate	No.	Rate	No.	Rate	No.	Rate	No.	Rate	No.	Rate	
Septicemia	17	0.1	6	0.5	11	0.1	6	352.9	2	333.3	4	363.6	1	100.0	1	250.0	0	0	2758
Infection of CNS	5	0.0	0	0	5	0.0	2	400.0	0	–	2	400.0	1	333.3	0	–	1	333.3	3311
Infection of resp. system	74	0.4	26	2.0	48	0.3	14	189.2	9	346.2	5	104.2	3	61.2	2	142.9	1	28.6	2731
Infection of urinary tract	24	0.1	9	0.7	15	0.1	2	83.3	1	111.1	1	66.7	1	55.6	1	142.9	0	0	2836
Infect. of bone and joint	0	0	0	0	0	0	0	–	0	–	0	–	0	–	0	–	0	–	–
Infection of heart	0	0	0	0	0	0	0	–	0	–	0	–	0	–	0	–	0	–	–
Infect. of G.I. system	32	0.2	11	0.9	21	0.1	2	62.5	2	181.8	0	0	2	87.0	0	0	2	111.1	2891
Infection of eye	22	0.1	6	0.5	16	0.1	0	0	0	0	0	0	0	–	0	–	0	0	3108
Infection of ear	1	0.0	1	0.1	0	0	1	*	1	*	0	–	0	–	0	–	0	–	2353
Infection of skin	63	0.4	17	1.3	46	0.3	3	47.6	3	176.5	0	0	2	39.2	1	90.9	1	25.0	2987
Infect. of mucous membrane	18	0.1	9	0.7	9	0.1	0	0	0	0	0	0	0	0	0	0	0	0	2493
Other infection	4	0.0	2	0.2	2	0.0	1	250.0	1	500.0	0	0	0	0	0	0	0	0	2218
None†	17806		1212		16594		188	10.6	125	103.1	63	3.8	237	16.5	42	48.3	195	14.5	3277
Total	18029		1287		16742														

*Rate is 1000.0.
†No abnormalities within the system.

Table 12-93. Newborn Summary Data
Infections — Black

Condition, Abnormality or Procedure	Livebirths						Neonatal Deaths						Neuro. Abn. 1 Year						Mean Bwt.
	Total		Under 2501 gm		Over 2500 gm		Total		Under 2501 gm		Over 2500 gm		Total		Under 2501 gm		Over 2500 gm		
	No.	%	No.	%	No.	%	No.	Rate	No.	Rate	No.	Rate	No.	Rate	No.	Rate	No.	Rate	
Septicemia	31	0.2	27	1.1	4	0.0	19	612.9	16	592.6	3	750.0	1	100.0	1	111.1	0	0	1700
Infection of CNS	11	0.1	7	0.3	4	0.0	7	636.4	6	857.1	1	250.0	1	333.3	0	0	1	333.3	2209
Infection of resp. system	108	0.6	62	2.4	46	0.3	40	370.4	25	403.2	15	326.1	3	48.4	3	85.7	0	0	2342
Infection of urinary tract	12	0.1	8	0.3	4	0.0	0	0	0	0	0	0	0	0	0	0	0	0	2320
Infect. of bone and joint	0	0	0	0	0	–	0	–	0	–	0	–	0	–	0	–	0	–	–
Infection of heart	1	0.0	0	0	1	0.0	1	*	0	–	1	*	0	–	0	–	0	–	3374
Infect. of G.I. system	61	0.3	37	1.4	24	0.1	5	82.0	4	108.1	1	41.7	5	106.4	5	172.4	0	0	2304
Infection of eye	93	0.5	42	1.6	51	0.3	0	0	0	0	0	0	3	38.0	1	28.6	2	45.5	2608
Infection of ear	4	0.0	2	0.1	2	0.0	2	500.0	2	*	0	0	0	0	0	–	0	0	2374
Infection of skin	90	0.5	43	1.7	47	0.3	14	155.6	11	255.6	3	63.8	5	74.6	4	142.9	1	25.6	2497
Infect. of mucous membrane	16	0.1	9	0.4	7	0.0	1	62.5	1	111.1	0	0	3	214.3	2	250.0	1	166.7	2512
Other infection	22	0.1	12	0.5	10	0.1	7	318.2	4	333.3	3	300.0	0	0	0	0	0	0	2430
None†	18898		2387		16511		274	14.5	197	82.5	77	4.7	253	15.2	73	37.6	180	12.2	3051
Total	19259		2570		16689														

*Rate is 1000.0.
†No abnormalities within the system.

Table 12-94. Newborn Summary Data
Syndromes — White

Condition, Abnormality or Procedure	Livebirths						Neonatal Deaths						Neuro. Abn. 1 Year						Mean Bwt.
	Total		Under 2501 gm		Over 2500 gm		Total		Under 2501 gm		Over 2500 gm		Total		Under 2501 gm		Over 2500 gm		
	No.	%	No.	%	No.	%	No.	Rate	No.	Rate	No.	Rate	No.	Rate	No.	Rate	No.	Rate	
Mongolism	18	0.1	6	0.5	12	0.1	2	111.1	1	166.7	1	83.3	11	*	3	*	8	*	2783
Gonadal dysgenesis	3	0.0	3	0.2	0	0	2	666.7	2	666.7	0	–	1	*	1	*	0	–	2306
Adrenogenital	0	0	0	0	0	0	0	–	0	–	0	–	0	–	0	–	0	–	–
Marfan's	0	0	0	0	0	0	0	–	0	–	0	–	0	–	0	–	0	–	–
Pierre robin	2	0.0	0	0	2	0.0	0	0	0	0	0	0	0	0	0	–	0	0	3105
Other syndromes	14	0.1	3	0.2	11	0.1	2	142.9	0	0	2	181.8	5	555.6	3	*	2	333.3	2995
None†	17992		1275		16717														
Total	18029		1287		16742		209	11.6	139	109.0	70	4.2	228	15.7	39	43.1	189	13.9	3272

*Rate is 1000.0.
†No abnormalities within the system.

Table 12-95. Newborn Summary Data
Syndromes — Black

Condition, Abnormality or Procedure	Livebirths						Neonatal Deaths						Neuro. Abn. 1 Year						Mean Bwt.
	Total		Under 2501 gm		Over 2500 gm		Total		Under 2501 gm		Over 2500 gm		Total		Under 2501 gm		Over 2500 gm		
	No.	%	No.	%	No.	%	No.	Rate	No.	Rate	No.	Rate	No.	Rate	No.	Rate	No.	Rate	
Mongolism	15	0.1	1	0.0	14	0.1	0	0	0	0	0	0	7	875.0	1	*	6	857.1	3206
Gonadal dysgenesis	0	0	0	0	0	0	0	–	0	–	0	–	0	–	0	–	0	–	–
Adrenogenital	0	0	0	0	0	0	0	–	0	–	0	–	0	–	0	–	0	–	–
Marfan's	0	0	0	0	0	0	0	–	0	–	0	–	0	–	0	–	0	–	–
Pierre robin	1	0.0	0	0	1	0.0	0	0	0	0	0	0	0	0	0	–	0	0	2608
Other syndromes	5	0.0	3	0.1	2	0.0	3	600.0	2	666.7	1	500.0	1	500.0	1	*	0	0	1899
None†	19238		2566		16672		328	17.1	232	90.4	96	5.8	262	15.5	83	40.1	179	12.0	3041
Total	19259		2570		16689														

*Rate is 1000.0.
†No abnormalities within the system.

Table 12-96. Newborn Summary Data
Other Endocrine or Metabolic Diseases — White

Condition, Abnormality or Procedure	Livebirths						Neonatal Deaths						Neuro. Abn. 1 Year						Mean Bwt.
	Total		Under 2501 gm		Over 2500 gm		Total		Under 2501 gm		Over 2500 gm		Total		Under 2501 gm		Over 2500 gm		
	No.	%	No.	%	No.	%	No.	Rate	No.	Rate	No.	Rate	No.	Rate	No.	Rate	No.	Rate	
Cretinism	0	0	0	0	0	0	0	–	0	–	0	–	0	–	0	–	0	–	–
Fibrocystic disease of pancreas	2	0.0	0	0	2	0.0	0	0	0	–	0	–	0	0	0	–	0	0	3232
Presumed symptomatic hypocalcemia	18	0.1	6	0.5	12	0.1	1	55.6	1	166.7	0	0	0	0	0	0	0	0	2901
Presumed symptomatic hypoglycemia	8	0.0	4	0.3	4	0.0	1	125.0	0	0	1	250.0	0	0	0	0	0	0	2846
Inborn errors of metabolism	2	0.0	1	0.1	1	0.0	0	0	0	0	0	0	2	*	1	*	1	*	2552
Other endocrine or metabolic diseases	26	0.1	12	0.9	14	0.1	16	615.4	8	666.7	8	571.4	0	0	0	0	0	0	2482
None†	17974		1265		16709		197	11.0	133	105.1	64	3.8	243	16.8	45	49.9	198	14.6	3273
Total	18029		1287		16742														

*Rate is 1000.0.
†No abnormalities within the system.

Table 12-97. Newborn Summary Data
Other Endocrine or Metabolic Diseases — Black

Condition, Abnormality or Procedure	Livebirths Total		Livebirths Under 2501 gm		Livebirths Over 2500 gm		Neonatal Deaths Total		Neonatal Deaths Under 2501 gm		Neonatal Deaths Over 2500 gm		Neuro. Abn. 1 Year Total		Neuro. Abn. 1 Year Under 2501 gm		Neuro. Abn. 1 Year Over 2500 gm		Mean Bwt.
	No.	%	No.	%	No.	%	No.	Rate	No.	Rate	No.	Rate	No.	Rate	No.	Rate	No.	Rate	
Cretinism	0	0	0	0	0	0	0	–	0	–	0	–	0	–	0	–	0	–	–
Fibrocystic disease of pancreas	0	0	0	0	0	0	0	–	0	–	0	–	0	–	0	–	0	–	–
Presumed symptomatic hypocalcemia	4	0.0	1	0.0	3	0.0	0	0	0	0	0	0	0	0	0	0	0	0	3055
Presumed symptomatic hypoglycemia	9	0.1	4	0.2	5	0.0	0	0	0	0	0	0	1	142.9	0	0	1	250.0	2932
Inborn errors of metabolism	5	0.0	0	0	5	0.0	1	200.0	0	–	1	200.0	0	0	0	–	0	0	3011
Other endocrine or metabolic diseases	13	0.1	4	0.2	9	0.1	6	461.5	3	750.0	3	333.3	0	0	0	0	0	0	2704
None†	19229		2561		16668		324	16.9	231	90.2	93	5.6	269	15.9	85	41.2	184	12.4	3041
Total	19259		2570		16689														

†No abnormalities within the system.

Table 12-98. Newborn Summary Data Procedures — White

Condition, Abnormality or Procedure	Livebirths Total No.	%	Livebirths Under 2501 gm No.	%	Livebirths Over 2500 gm No.	%	Neonatal Deaths Total No.	Rate	Under 2501 gm No.	Rate	Over 2500 gm No.	Rate	Neuro. Abn. 1 Year Total No.	Rate	Under 2501 gm No.	Rate	Over 2500 gm No.	Rate	Mean Bwt.
Blood transfusions	57	0.3	24	1.9	33	0.2	12	210.5	7	291.7	5	151.5	4	117.7	1	100.0	3	125.0	2660
Exchange transfusions	172	1.0	63	4.9	109	0.7	13	75.6	8	127.0	5	45.9	4	29.6	3	66.7	1	11.1	2743
Parenteral fluids	157	0.9	82	6.4	75	0.5	41	261.2	29	353.7	12	160.0	8	93.0	3	83.3	5	100.0	2392
Spinal puncture	262	1.5	67	5.2	195	1.2	22	84.0	12	179.1	10	51.3	25	132.3	5	116.3	20	137.0	3019
Subdural puncture	44	0.2	11	0.9	33	0.2	6	136.4	1	90.9	5	151.5	7	218.8	3	428.6	4	160.0	3040
Ventricular puncture	10	0.1	3	0.2	7	0.0	4	400.0	1	333.3	3	428.6	3	600.0	0	0	3	750.0	2897
General anesthesia	38	0.2	5	0.4	33	0.2	3	79.0	0	0	3	90.9	4	148.2	0	0	4	166.7	3262
Surgery performed	64	0.4	14	1.1	50	0.3	9	140.6	3	214.3	6	120.0	5	122.0	1	125.0	4	121.2	3040
Chromosome studies	13	0.1	5	0.4	8	0.1	4	307.7	2	400.0	2	250.0	6	857.1	3	*	3	750.0	2636
X-ray and/or fluoroscopy	1069	5.9	273	21.2	796	4.8	84	78.6	45	164.8	39	49.0	65	82.2	22	123.6	43	70.2	3016
Antibiotics — internal	916	5.1	290	22.5	626	3.7	81	88.4	54	186.2	27	43.1	41	58.6	17	90.9	24	46.8	2846
EEG record	669	3.7	99	7.7	570	3.4	5	7.5	1	10.1	4	7.0	22	39.6	6	79.0	16	33.3	3193
Other procedures administered	286	1.6	125	9.7	161	1.0	74	258.7	47	376.0	27	167.7	13	77.8	5	83.3	8	74.8	2664
None†	15929		818		15111		79	5.0	58	70.9	21	1.4	156	12.1	16	26.5	140	11.4	3302
Total	18029		1287		16742														

*Rate is 1000.0.
†No abnormalities within the system.

Table 12-99. Newborn Summary Data Procedures — Black

Condition, Abnormality or Procedure	Livebirths						Neonatal Deaths						Neuro. Abn. 1 Year						Mean Bwt.
	Total		Under 2501 gm		Over 2500 gm		Total		Under 2501 gm		Over 2500 gm		Total		Under 2501 gm		Over 2500 gm		
	No.	%	No.	%	No.	%	No.	Rate	No.	Rate	No.	Rate	No.	Rate	No.	Rate	No.	Rate	
Blood transfusions	82	0.4	50	2.0	32	0.2	9	109.8	3	60.0	6	187.5	14	212.1	8	190.5	6	250.0	2220
Exchange transfusions	136	0.7	57	2.2	79	0.5	5	36.8	2	35.1	3	38.0	8	67.8	5	106.4	3	42.3	2644
Parenteral fluids	193	1.0	112	4.4	81	0.5	47	243.5	26	232.1	21	259.3	23	182.5	16	213.3	7	137.3	2314
Spinal puncture	215	1.1	78	3.0	137	0.8	25	116.3	6	76.9	19	138.7	16	93.0	6	96.8	10	90.9	2707
Subdural puncture	38	0.2	9	0.4	29	0.2	2	52.6	0	0	2	69.0	5	172.4	1	166.7	4	173.9	2948
Ventricular puncture	14	0.1	4	0.2	10	0.1	3	214.3	0	0	3	300.0	4	500.0	2	666.7	2	400.0	2940
General anesthesia	33	0.2	9	0.4	24	0.1	7	212.1	2	222.2	5	208.3	4	181.8	2	333.3	2	125.0	2856
Surgery performed	100	0.5	31	1.2	69	0.4	14	140.0	6	193.6	8	115.9	13	173.3	6	272.7	7	132.1	2761
Chromosome studies	7	0.0	3	0.1	4	0.0	1	142.9	1	333.3	0	0	1	333.3	1	500.0	0	0	2721
X-ray and/or fluoroscopy	879	4.6	324	12.6	555	3.3	106	120.6	59	182.1	47	84.7	53	75.8	26	111.1	27	58.1	2718
Antibiotics — internal	1070	5.6	513	20.0	557	3.3	129	120.6	90	175.4	39	70.0	55	67.6	30	83.1	25	55.2	2526
EEG record	629	3.3	116	4.5	513	3.1	5	8.0	3	25.9	2	3.9	13	22.5	6	58.8	7	14.7	2993
Other procedures administered	515	2.7	245	9.5	270	1.6	121	235.0	82	334.7	39	144.4	29	83.8	18	134.3	11	51.9	2478
None†	17017		1800		15217														
Total	19259		2570		16689		121	7.1	91	50.6	30	2.0	185	12.2	44	28.8	141	10.4	3081

†No abnormalities within the system.

neonatal period indicate the need for thoughtful planning to provide the highly sophisticated care required, without the proliferation of duplicate, underutilized, and expensive facilities. An appropriate number of well-equipped and specially staffed regional centers may be a solution. Such centers, however, in no way preclude the need, in every hospital where babies are born, for experienced personnel and appropriate equipment for the management of resuscitation problems in the delivery room, and for emergency situations which may arise unexpectedly in the newborn nursery.

REFERENCES

(1) N. C. Myrianthopoulos and C. S. Chung. 1974. Congenital malformations in singletons: Epidemiologic survey. *Birth Defects: Original Article Series. The National Foundation-March of Dimes.* Vol. X, No. 11: 1–58.

(2) M. Gordon, H. Rich, J. Deutschberger, and M. Green. 1973. The immediate and long-term outcome of obstetric birth trauma. I. Brachial plexus paralysis. *American Journal of Obstetrics and Gynecology* 117: 51–56.

(3) V. Chernick. 1974. Modern therapy of hyaline membrane disease by stabilization of alveoli. In L. Gluck (ed.), *Modern Perinatal Medicine,* p. 409. Chicago: Medical Year Book Publishing Co.

(4) M. E. Avery and J. Mead. 1959. Surface properties in relation to atelectasis and hyaline membrane disease. *American Journal of Diseases of Children* 97: 517–23.

(5) A. J. Schaffer and M. E. Avery. 1971. Atelectasis and hyaline membrane disease. In *Diseases of the Newborn,* 3rd ed., pp. 76–77, 90–91. Philadelphia: W. B. Saunders Co.

(6) C. W. Brumley, W. A. Hodson, and M. E. Avery. 1967. Lung phospholipids and surface tension correlations in infants with and without hyaline membrane disease and in adults. *Pediatrics* 40: 13–19.

(7) R. O. Fisch, H. J. Gravem, and R. R. Engel. 1968. Neurological status of survivors of neonatal respiratory distress syndrome. *Journal of Pediatrics* 73: 395–403.

(8) R. O. Fisch, M. K. Bilek, L. D. Miller, and R. R. Engel. 1975. Physical and mental status at 4 years of age of survivors of the respiratory distress syndrome. *Journal of Pediatrics* 86: 497–503.

(9) M. T. Stahlman, E. J. Battersby, F. M. Shepard, and W. J. Blankenship. 1967. Prognosis in hyaline membrane disease. *New England Journal of Medicine* 276: 303–309.

(10) N. R. Butler and E. D. Alberman (eds.). 1969. *Perinatal Problems. The Second Report of the 1958 British Perinatal Mortality Survey.* Edinburgh and London: Livingstone.

(11) P. Gruenwald. 1969. In N. R. Butler and E. D. Alberman (eds.), *Perinatal Problems. The Second Report of the 1958 British Perinatal Mortality Survey,* p. 188. Edinburgh and London: Livingstone.

(12) R. V. Kotas. 1972. The estimation of perinatal pulmonary maturity: A commentary. *Journal of Pediatrics* 81: 378–83.

(13) J. B. Hardy, G. H. McCracken, Jr., M. R. Gilkeson, and J. L. Sever. 1969. Adverse fetal outcome following maternal rubella after the first trimester of pregnancy. *Journal of the American Medical Association* 207: 2414–20.

(14) J. E. Kurent and J. L. Sever. 1973. Perinatal infections and epidemiology of anencephaly and spina bifida. *Teratology* 8: 359–62.

(15) J. L. Sever, K. B. Nelson, and M. R. Gilkeson. 1965. Rubella epidemic, 1964: Effect on 6,000 pregnancies. *American Journal of Diseases of Children* 110: 395–407.

(16) J. L. Sever, J. B. Hardy, K. B. Nelson, and M. R. Gilkeson. 1969. Rubella in the Collaborative Perinatal Research Study. II. Clinical and laboratory findings in children through 3 years of age. *American Journal of Diseases of Children* 118: 123–32.

(17) J. L. Sever. 1970. Viral teratogens: A status report. *Hospital Practice* 5: 75–83.

(18) J. L. Sever, M. R. Gilkeson, T. C. Chen, A. C. Ley, and D. Edmonds. 1970. Epidemiology of mongolism in the Collaborative Project. *Annals of the New York Academy of Sciences* 171: 328–40.

(19) J. L. Sever, D. A. Fuccillo, J. Ellenberg, and M. R. Gilkeson. 1975. Infection and low birth weight in an industrialized society. *American Journal of Diseases of Children.* 129: 557–58.

(20) R. Usher and F. McLean. 1969. Intrauterine growth of liveborn Caucasian infants. *Journal of Pediatrics* 74: 901–10.

(21) A. D. McDonald. 1967. Children of very low birthweight. In *MEIU Research Monograph, No. 1.* London: Heineman.

(22) A. L. Stewart and E. O. R. Reynolds. 1974. Improved prognosis for infants of very low birthweight. *Pediatrics* 54: 724–34.

(23) M. T. Stahlman. 1968. What evidence exists that intensive care has changed the incidence of intact survival? In *Problems of Neonatal Intensive Care Units,* presented at the 59th Ross Conference on Pediatric Research, University of Vermont College of Medicine, Stowe, Vermont, Aug. 4–6.

(24) J. T. Lanman, S. G. Kohl, and J. H. Bedell. 1974. Changes in pregnancy outcome after liberalization of the New York State abortion law. *American Journal of Obstetrics and Gynecology* 118:485.

13

DEVELOPMENTAL STATUS
AT EIGHT MONTHS

INTRODUCTION

During intrauterine life, fetal development normally proceeds in sequential fashion according to a rigorous timetable. Deviations from this schedule reflect abnormalities in the genetic material received from the parents, the impact of an abnormal fetal environment, or interactions between unfavorable genetic and environmental influences. Normal growth and development after birth also proceed within well defined limits. Growth implies multiplication of physical mass resulting from increased numbers and/or size of cells forming tissues and organs. Development, on the other hand, reflects increasing maturation, with the orderly acquisition of an increased complexity of function. As this study is concerned with the identification of causes of neurological abnormality, the function of the central nervous system, as measured by neurosensory, neuromotor, and intellectual aspects of development, is of particular importance. In infancy, where the relationship between maturity level and neurological integrity is particularly strong, the attainment of specific skills at the expected age levels represents milestones or markers that can be used to assess neurological integrity and to screen out children with deviant patterns of development. Over the years, the developmental assessment of infant behavior has become a major tool in pediatric neurology and a part of the health maintenance armamentarium.

Intellectual performance, as measured later in childhood, depends upon complex interactions between genetic endowment and environmental influences, both intrauterine and postnatal, with the effects of the postnatal environment becoming increasingly important as the child grows through the preschool years. It is well recognized (1) that "global" developmental scores or quotients derived from the examination of infants cannot generally be considered to be predictive of IQ scores obtained in early school age, except in a gross way. However, the failure of an infant to develop specific skills by the expected age may be a sensitive indicator of neurological impairment (2). The Bayley Mental and Motor Scores were found by Boggs, Hardy, and Frazier (3), using NINCDS Collaborative Perinatal Project data, to be sensitive endpoints in the evaluation of possible adverse effects of neonatal hyperbilirubinemia.

Developmental tests during infancy and intelligence tests later in life measure different aspects of central nervous system function. Infant tests depend primarily on the evaluation of skills involving fine and gross motor function. Correlations that exist between developmental scores during infancy and later intelligence test scores may, therefore, reflect the effect of underlying factors basic to the development of both motor and intellectual function.

On the premise that developmental failure may reflect neurological impairment, an objective evaluation of the developmental status of each infant became a part of the protocol of the NCPP. The Bayley Scales of Mental and Motor Development were chosen as the best instrument available at that time. They were modified and standardized for use in the NCPP.

A developmental evaluation early in life was included in the protocol for several reasons. First, it was believed that it would serve to identify children with deviant neurological function at an early age. Second, the validity of early developmental findings as predictors of later neurological and intellectual development could be tested and if these predictions were useful they might compensate in part in those instances where later follow-up was not possible. Finally, it was hoped to identify items that could be incorporated into a screening test to enable practicing physicians to identify more accurately those children with deviant and less than optimal patterns of development. Data analysis presently under way will relate outcome variables at the seven-year level to developmental findings at eight months, as well as to prenatal factors, perinatal stress, birthweight, race, sex, and to postnatal influences, both biological and environmental.

The descriptive analyses presented in this chapter provide a general overview of the developmental status of the study children, based on the use of "motor" and "mental" test scores. The wealth of data available pertaining to the acquisition of individual skills and their value in predicting later outcome (for example, fine motor skills as measured by the maturity of prehensile grasp) strongly indicates the need for specific in-depth analyses. Preliminary studies along these lines indicate that such research might prove rewarding (4,5).

METHOD OF EXAMINATION

The Bayley Scales of Infant Mental and Motor Development (6) were the primary instruments chosen for the early developmental evaluation at eight months. They were selected because a global development score could be derived for each scale, and because each item could also be examined and recorded individually. The scales were extensively pretested and standardized at each of the collaborating institutions before becoming a part of the NCPP protocol, in January 1961. The background and standardization of the scales are described in the revised (1969) manual for the Bayley Scales of Infant Development (7).

The age of eight months was chosen, because a number of clear developmental milestones are normally achieved between seven and eight months of age. It was required that the baby be examined as close as possible to his eight-month birthday, within a two-week period, before or afterward, and the data presented here are restricted to cases tested within these time limits.

After a suitable "warm-up" period, the tests of mental development were administered in a quiet test room, at a table with the infant seated, comfortably supported, on the mother's lap, on one side, and the examiner, facing the baby, on the other. The tests of motor development were, for the most part, administered in a playpen or crib, or on the floor, where gross motor activity could be evaluated. Every effort was made to maintain a warm, friendly, relaxed, and nonclinical atmosphere.

For the most part, the mother's role in the test situation was that of a passive observer. However, for some items, such as "frolic play" or "responds selectively to name or nickname," the mother was asked to participate.

Each test item was scored *Pass* or *Fail* on the basis of the performance actually observed by the examiner. Several exceptions were permitted; they pertained to the vocalization items on the Mental Scale and to a few gross motor items where it was sometimes necessary to depend on the mother's report of the child's performance at home. When this information was dependent upon reported rather than observed performance, the fact was recorded. Space was also provided on the record for comments about unusual behavior. On the Mental Scale, possible scores range from 0 to 106, covering age levels of 0 to 14.9 months. The Motor Scale contained fewer test items, with a possible range of scores from 0 to 43.

In addition to the Bayley Scales, the developmental test battery administered at eight months included: (1) An Infant Behavior Profile; (2) Additional Observations; and (3) A Maternal Rating Scale. The Infant Behavior Profile was included to evaluate the qualitative aspects of the child's behavior as observed in the course of the psychological examination, both during testing and in free play. Five-point scales were developed to represent degrees of manifestations of specified behavior for those major dimensions considered to be of diagnostic value. Included were items such as speed, duration and intensity of response, persistence in pursuit, orientation to persons, social responses, activity level, and the like. This material is available in the data file, but is not included in this report.

The additional observations made by the examiner provided for the recording of supplemental information on hearing, vision and motor responses, which were not obtained on the Scales of Mental and Motor Development, and for the notation of physical abnormalities and/or unusual behavior.

The Maternal Rating Scales completed by the examiner were designed to bring to light certain variables in the mother-child relationships that might have had an effect on eight-month test performance.

The examiner, on the basis of observations during the 45 minutes, or more, spent with the mother and child, was required to record a clinical impression of the child's development. In addition, the data pertaining to each item was reviewed, a narrative summary written, and the objective scores for mental and motor performance computed.

Quality control measures included careful training and supervision of examiners, interinstitutional workshops, and the use of standardized forms and manuals. The records were carefully edited and checked by staff at the local institutions and in the Perinatal Research Branch prior to data processing.

OBSERVATIONS

The observations reported here are intended to provide an overview of some of the factors that influence the developmental status of children at eight months of age.

As indicated above, the protocol specified that children should be tested using the modified Bayley Scales of Infant Mental and Motor Development as close to the eight-month birthday as possible. Among the whites 0.8 percent and among blacks 1.2 percent were tested prior to 7.5 months of age, and 19.4 percent of the whites and 14.2 percent of the blacks were over 8.5 months at the time of testing. As this report deals with the absolute scores rather than developmental quotients, and because of the correlation of scores with chronological age, test results from children less than 7.5 or greater than 8.5 months of age have been excluded from further consideration here. Babies born prior to April 1, 1960 were examined using a pretest form and on this basis have also been excluded from these tabulations.

The material presented in this chapter includes the findings from 11,534 white and 13,516 black babies examined between 7.5 and 8.5 months of age. As the data were found to be consistent by institution, this report is confined to the presentation of analyses carried out on the pooled data from all institutions.

The descriptive analyses that follow consider the effect of a number of variables on developmental status as measured by: (1) the distributions of the Bayley Mental and Motor Scores obtained by the children, by race; (2) the distributions of "low" mental and motor scores, i.e., below 75 on the Mental Scale and below 27 on the Motor Scale (these being the cut-off points that define approximately the lowest 8 percent of the children); and (3) the distributions of mean or average scores obtained by children in various groupings.

Race: Association with Developmental Status

The distributions of Bayley Mental and Motor Scores are displayed for the 11,534 whites and the 13,516 black infants tested within the 7.5- to 8.5-month time limits. The general distribution curves presented in Tables 13–1 and 13–2 and Figures 13–1 and 13–2 are essentially similar by race. When considered by birthweight and gestational age, some differences that became apparent are discussed in the section that follows.

The lack of overall difference between the developmental test scores of white

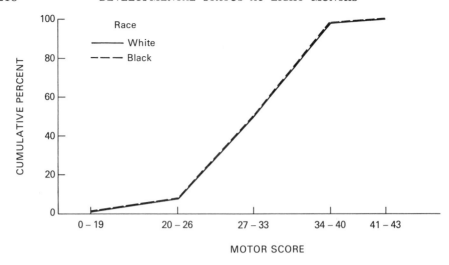

Figure 13-1. 8-Month Motor Score by Race

Table 13-1. 8-Month Motor Score by Race

	WHITE			BLACK		
Score	Number Tested	Percent	Cumulative Percent	Number Tested	Percent	Cumulative Percent
0–19	81	0.70	0.70	138	1.02	1.02
20–26	811	7.04	7.74	829	6.14	7.16
27–33	4869	42.25	49.99	5763	42.67	49.83
34–40	5505	47.77	97.75	6541	48.43	98.25
41–43	259	2.25	100.00	236	1.75	100.00
Total	11525	100.00		13507	100.00	
Unknown	9	0.08		9	0.07	
Grand total	11534	100.00		13516	100.00	

and black infants is in accord with the findings of others, particularly those of Knobloch and Pasamanick (2). It is of particular interest because the distributions of Binet IQ scores at age four years in this same population of children were found to be greatly different for whites and blacks. As discussed earlier, it is recognized that the tests at eight months and four years evaluate different aspects of function. Knobloch and Pasamanick, whose studies showed similar divergencies in later test scores, have suggested that the measures of intelligence in later life appeared to be greatly influenced by environmental factors relating to life experiences that tend to limit opportunities for learning. The possible effects of environmental influences will be discussed in more detail later in this chapter, after data pertaining to the effects of birthweight and gestational age have been presented.

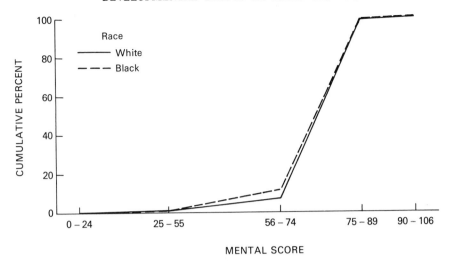

Figure 13-2. 8-Month Mental Score by Race

Table 13-2. 8-Month Mental Score by Race

	WHITE			BLACK		
Score	Number Tested	Percent	Cumulative Percent	Number Tested	Percent	Cumulative Percent
0–24	8	0.07	0.07	17	0.13	0.13
25–55	59	0.51	0.58	143	1.06	1.18
56–74	732	6.35	6.93	1386	10.26	11.45
75–89	10621	92.13	99.06	11841	87.66	99.10
90–106	108	0.94	100.00	121	0.90	100.00
Total	11528	100.00		13508	100.00	
Unknown	6	0.05		8	0.06	
Grand total	11534	100.00		13516	100.00	

Relationships between Motor and Mental Scores

Figures 13–3 and 13–4 and Tables 13–3 and 13–4 show the slightly curvilinear relationships that exist between the mental and motor scores for white and black children. When the mean motor score is examined by groupings of mental scores, it is clear that there is a progressive increase in motor scores with increases in the mental score. There is little difference between the races, except for the lowest group of mental scores. Here, small sample size may be exerting an effect, and the significance of the finding is questionable. When the relationship between scores is examined along the other axis (i.e., in terms of the mean mental score for each grouping of motor scores), the same relationship is observed but there is a slight, but consistent difference between the two racial groups, with the white children having a slightly higher average mental score for each motor score grouping. How-

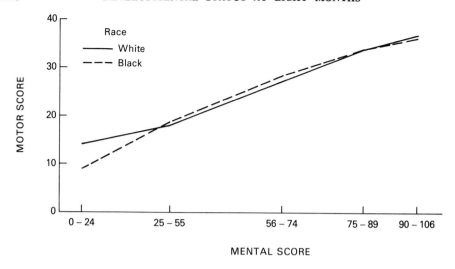

Figure 13-3. Mean 8-Month Motor Score by Mental Score by Race

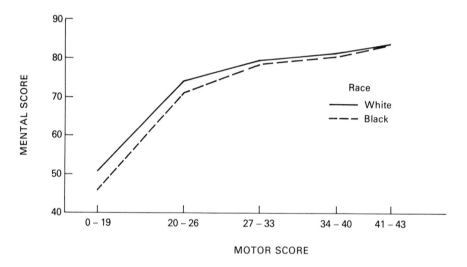

Figure 13-4. Mean 8-Month Mental Score by Motor Score by Race

ever, it must be remembered that in excess of 90 percent of the children attained scores above 27 on the Motor Scale, and at this higher end of the curve the differences between blacks and whites are very small.

Relationships with Birthweight

The possible relationships between birthweight and developmental performance at eight months were examined in a number of ways (Figs. 13–5 to 13–12 and Tables 13–5 to 13–8):

Table 13-3. 8-Month Motor Score by 8-Month Mental Score — White

	Number Tested								
	Motor Score								
Mental Score	0-19	20-26	27-33	34-40	41-43	Total	Unknown	Grand total	Mean
0-24	6	1	1	0	0	8	0	8	14.13
25-55	38	18	3	0	0	59	0	59	18.07
56-74	32	307	307	86	0	732	0	732	27.28
75-89	5	483	4537	5344	248	10617	4	10621	33.66
90-106	0	0	21	75	11	107	1	108	36.52
Total	81	809	4869	5505	259	11523	5	11528	33.19
Unknown	0	2	0	0	0	2	4	6	25.00*
Grand total	81	811	4869	5505	259	11525	9	11534	33.18
Mean	50.72	74.09	79.38	81.21	83.40	79.77	82.50	79.77	

*Based on less than 5 cases.

Table 13-4. 8-Month Motor Score by 8-Month Mental Score — Black

	Number Tested								
	Motor Score								
Mental Score	0-19	20-26	27-33	34-40	41-43	Total	Unknown	Grand total	Mean
0-24	16	1	0	0	0	17	0	17	8.94
25-55	84	52	6	0	0	142	1	143	18.81
56-74	34	419	752	178	2	1385	1	1386	28.48
75-89	2	354	4983	6287	211	11837	4	11841	33.86
90-106	1	1	20	76	23	121	0	121	36.00
Total	137	827	5761	6541	236	13502	6	13508	33.15
Unknown	1	2	2	0	0	5	3	8	26.00
Grand total	138	829	5763	6541	236	13507	9	13516	33.14
Mean	45.74	71.06	78.36	80.40	83.47	78.90	73.50	78.90	

1. *The mean mental and motor scores, within each birthweight category*, for black and white children, are presented in the accompanying graphs and tables. For children of both races there is a progressive increase in scores accompanying increasing birthweight. In the group weighing less than 1001 grams, where sample size was smallest, black infants performed somewhat better than the whites. There is a particularly large increase in average score with each weight increment under 2500 grams. The babies of 1001 to 1500 grams had average mental scores of 64 for the blacks and 67 for the whites, while babies of 3500 grams (7 lbs. and 11½ oz.) or above, of both races, had mental scores which averaged 80 points, an increase of 13 points in the white babies and 16 points in the blacks. The relationship between birthweight and average motor score followed a similar pattern, except that the black babies within each birthweight group had, on the average, consistently, but very slightly, higher scores (about one point) than the white.

2. *The percentage distribution of low mental and motor scores, in each birthweight category*, is displayed in the accompanying graphs and tables. The important

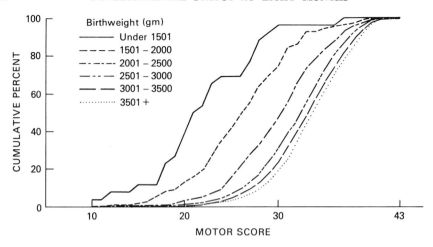

Figure 13-5. 8-Month Motor Score by Birthweight — White

Table 13-5. 8-Month Motor Score by Birthweight — White

Number Tested

Motor Score	Birthweight (gm)							Total	Mean
	Under 1001	1001– 1500	1501– 2000	2001– 2500	2501– 3000	3001– 3500	3501+		
0–19	2	5	10	10	25	16	13	81	2683
20–26	1	10	43	109	184	288	176	811	3038
27–33	0	7	48	291	1011	1969	1543	4869	3269
34–40	0	1	8	144	968	2321	2063	5505	3365
41–43	0	0	0	5	30	104	120	259	3463
Total	3	23	109	559	2218	4698	3915	11525	3299
Unknown	0	0	1	0	2	2	4	9	3509
Grand total	3	23	110	559	2220	4770	3919	11534	3299
Mean	16.00*	23.22	26.68	30.52	32.50	33.40	33.94	33.18	

Percent

Motor Score	Under 1001	1001– 1500	1501– 2000	2001– 2500	2501– 3000	3001– 3500	3501+	Total
0–19	66.67†	21.74	9.17	1.79	1.13	0.34	0.33	0.70
20–26	33.33†	43.48	39.45	19.50	8.30	6.13	4.50	7.04
27–33	0 †	30.43	44.04	52.06	45.58	41.91	39.41	42.25
34–40	0 †	4.35	7.34	25.76	43.64	49.40	52.69	47.77
41–43	0 †	0	0	0.89	1.35	2.21	3.07	2.25
Total	100.00	100.00	100.00	100.00	100.00	100.00	100.00	100.00
Unknown	0	0	0.91	0	0.09	0.04	0.10	0.08
Grand total	100.00	100.00	100.00	100.00	100.00	100.00	100.00	100.00

*Based on less than 5 cases.
†Based on less than 20 cases.

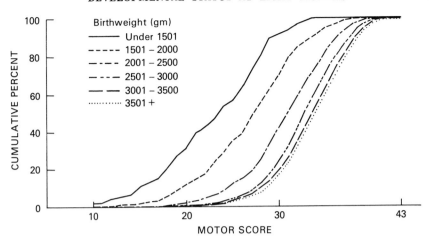

Figure 13-6. 8-Month Motor Score by Birthweight — Black

Table 13-6. 8–Month Motor Score by Birthweight — Black

Number Tested

Motor Score	Under 1001	1001–1500	1501–2000	2001–2500	2501–3000	3001–3500	3501+	Total	Mean
0–19	4	21	25	21	23	32	12	138	2418
20–26	3	30	83	164	234	230	85	829	2735
27–33	3	30	139	655	1876	2153	907	5763	3014
34–40	0	1	33	410	1867	2887	1343	6541	3157
41–43	0	0	0	4	46	106	80	236	3334
Total	10	82	280	1254	4046	5408	2427	13507	3066
Unknown	0	0	0	1	4	3	1	9	2892
Grand total	10	82	280	1255	4050	5411	2428	13516	3066
Mean	21.50	23.44	27.37	31.14	33.03	33.73	34.09	33.14	

Percent

Motor Score	Under 1001	1001–1500	1501–2000	2001–2500	2501–3000	3001–3500	3501+	Total
0–19	40.00*	25.61	8.93	1.67	0.57	0.59	0.49	1.02
20–26	30.00*	36.59	29.64	13.08	5.78	4.25	3.50	6.14
27–33	30.00*	36.59	49.64	52.03	46.37	39.81	37.37	42.67
34–40	0 *	1.22	11.79	32.70	46.14	53.38	55.34	48.43
41–43	0 *	0	0	0.32	1.14	1.96	3.30	1.75
Total	100.00	100.00	100.00	100.00	100.00	100.00	100.00	100.00
Unknown	0 *	0	0	0.08	0.10	0.06	0.04	0.07
Grand total	100.00	100.00	100.00	100.00	100.00	100.00	100.00	100.00

*Based on less than 20 cases.

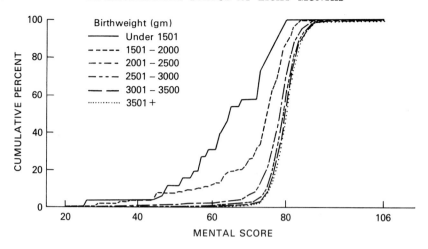

Figure 13-7. 8-Month Mental Score by Birthweight — White

Table 13-7. 8-Month Mental Score by Birthweight — White

Number Tested

Mental Score	Under 1001	1001–1500	1501–2000	2001–2500	2501–3000	3001–3500	3501+	Total	Mean
0–24	0	0	1	2	1	2	2	8	2902
25–55	2	3	9	8	16	15	6	59	2633
56–74	1	14	36	87	164	253	177	732	3049
75–89	0	6	63	457	2024	4384	3687	10621	3320
90–106	0	0	0	3	14	44	47	108	3414
Total	3	23	109	557	2219	4698	3919	11528	3299
Unknown	0	0	1	2	1	2	0	6	2698
Grand total	3	23	110	559	2220	4700	3919	11534	3299
Mean	43.67*	67.30	71.73	77.54	79.26	80.01	80.42	79.77	

Percent

Mental Score	Under 1001	1001–1500	1501–2000	2001–2500	2501–3000	3001–3500	3501+	Total	
0–24	0 †	0	0.92	0.36	0.05	0.04	0.05	0.07	
25–55	66.67†	13.04	8.26	1.44	0.72	0.32	0.15	0.51	
56–74	33.33†	60.87	33.03	15.62	7.39	5.39	4.52	6.35	
75–89	0 †	26.09	57.80	82.05	91.21	93.32	94.08	92.13	
90–106	0 †	0	0	0.54	0.63	0.94	1.20	0.94	
Total	100.00	100.00	100.00	100.00	100.00	100.00	100.00	100.00	
Unknown	0	0	0.91	0.36	0.05	0.04	0	0.05	
Grand total	100.00	100.00	100.00	100.00	100.00	100.00	100.00	100.00	

*Based on less than 5 cases.
†Based on less than 20 cases.

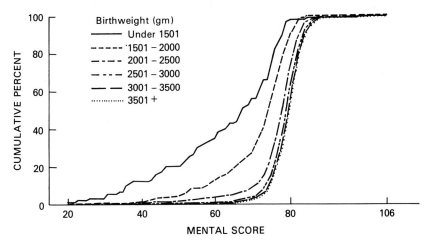

Figure 13-8. 8-Month Mental Score by Birthweight — Black

Table 13-8. 8-Month Mental Score by Birthweight — Black

	Number Tested								
	Birthweight (gm)								
Mental Score	Under 1001	1001–1500	1501–2000	2001–2500	2501–3000	3001–3500	3501+	Total	Mean
0–24	0	2	0	4	3	5	3	17	2786
25–55	5	20	23	26	30	29	10	143	2394
56–74	4	29	113	214	436	424	166	1386	2830
75–89	1	29	144	1004	3552	4903	2208	11841	3100
90–106	0	1	0	7	27	46	40	121	3286
Total	10	81	280	1255	4048	5407	2427	13508	3066
Unknown	0	1	0	0	2	4	1	8	2906
Grand total	10	82	280	1255	4050	5411	2428	13516	3066
Mean	55.20	64.00	71.84	76.94	78.89	79.53	79.93	78.90	

	Percent								
0–24	0 *	2.47	0	0.32	0.07	0.09	0.12	0.13	
25–55	50.00*	24.69	8.21	2.07	0.74	0.54	0.41	1.06	
56–74	40.00*	35.80	40.36	17.05	10.77	7.84	6.84	10.26	
75–89	10.00*	35.80	51.43	80.00	87.75	90.68	90.98	87.66	
90–106	0 *	1.23	0	0.56	0.67	0.85	1.65	0.90	
Total	100.00	100.00	100.00	100.00	100.00	100.00	100.00	100.00	
Unknown	0	1.22	0	0	0.05	0.07	0.04	0.06	
Grand total	100.00	100.00	100.00	100.00	100.00	100.00	100.00	100.00	

*Based on less than 20 cases.

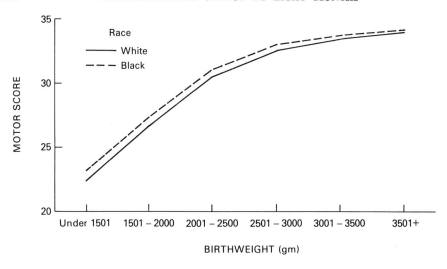

Figure 13-9. Mean 8-Month Motor Score by Birthweight by Race

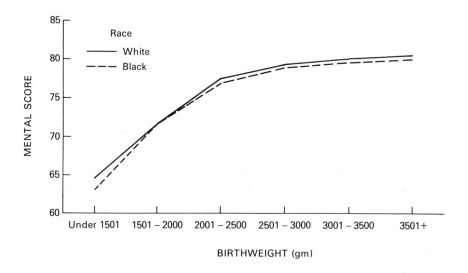

Figure 13-10. Mean 8-Month Mental Score by Birthweight by Race

relationship between low birthweight and low developmental scores, i.e., the risk of falling below 75 on the Mental and 27 on the Motor Scale, is clearly seen. An extremely high percentage of low-weight babies obtained low scores, almost 100 percent of those weighing less than 1001 grams (2.2 lbs.) and over 35 percent of those who weighed between 1501 and 2000 grams. There is a progressive decrease in the risk of low scores with each 500-gram increment increase in birthweight, with only 2 to 3 percent of the babies who weighed 3501 grams and above falling into the low-scoring group.

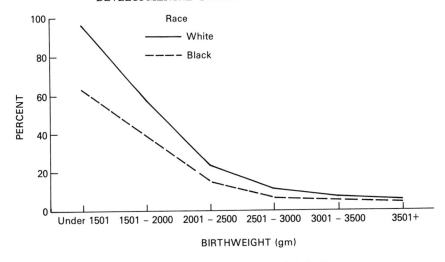

Figure 13-11. 8-Month Motor Scores Under 27 by Birthweight by Race

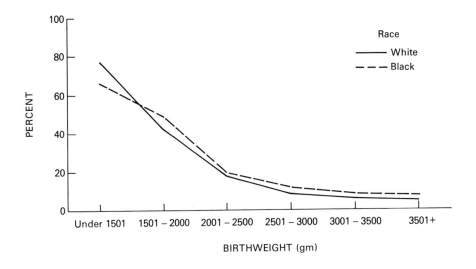

Figure 13-12. 8-Month Mental Scores Under 75 by Birthweight by Race

It will be noted, again, that the distributions are not greatly different by race. However, in infants weighing below 1501 grams, slightly fewer black infants than white obtained low scores; and in each category above 1501 grams, the reverse was true with whites having, on the average, fewer low scores. The distributions of low motor scores, like the general distribution of motor scores by birthweight, show a slight but consistent difference between children in the two racial groups. Again, the black babies show consistently lower percentages of low scores in each birthweight category. The difference, however, is very small.

A progressive increase in mean score is noted with each increase in birthweight.

Because of relatively small numbers, the lowest two birthweight categories have been combined in the accompanying graph. Only small differences by birthweight are seen in the scores of babies who weighed in excess of 2500 grams at birth. However, even small differences may be important, as more than 90 percent of the white babies and more than 85 percent of the black infants were above this weight.

3. *Birthweight by Sex of Child.* Because of the recognized effect of birthweight upon developmental scores at eight months, and because female infants were, on the average, about 100 grams less than males, the possible relationship of sex to developmental level attained at eight months was examined within the 500-gram birthweight categories. The sex of the child appeared to have no meaningful effect on development at this age.

Birthweight and Gestational Age

As the gestational age* of a fetus at birth is a major determinant of the degree of maturity attained in utero, it is reasonable to suppose that this parameter may be strongly related to developmental status at eight months of age. Thus, the developmental level of a child at eight months, reflects both gestational age and chronological age from birth. Some workers, notably Knobloch, Harper, and their colleagues (8), when examining infants, made allowance for premature delivery by using conceptional rather than chronological age. However, as it is not known whether development proceeds at the same rate within and outside the uterus, the date of birth was chosen as the starting point and chronological age was used for this report. As the Bayley Development tests are scaled and can be adjusted for age, further explorations of the NCPP data may clarify the problem of adjustment for shortened gestational age.

Consideration of the possible effects upon developmental status at eight months of the duration of intrauterine life is complicated. A strong relationship exists between gestational age and birthweight and, under normal circumstances, the duration of gestation at the time of delivery of the fetus is a powerful determinant of its birthweight. Babies of short gestation and low birthweight and, in addition, those whose birthweight falls outside the normal ranges for gestational age have increased risks of perinatal mortality and of neurological abnormality if they survive. While this is particularly true for the "small for dates" baby, there is evidence that it also pertains, to a lesser extent, for the baby who is excessively large for his gestational age. For further discussion, please see Chapter 7.

Perusal of Figures 13–13 through 13–20 and Tables 13–9 through 13–12 shows a clear relationship between gestational age at birth and developmental status at eight months; as gestational age increases, so do the motor and mental scores obtained on the Bayley Developmental Scales.

The mean mental and motor scores were evaluated for groups of babies classified by gestational age within the various 500-gram birthweight categories (extending from 1501 grams, and below, to 3501 grams and above). The gestational age groupings included three-week intervals from those under 34 weeks to 40 weeks

* See Chapter 7 for discussion of gestational age.

and above. The graphs and tables that accompany this section show the effect of gestational age on developmental status at eight months within birthweight groups.

Within each birthweight grouping with longer gestational age, there was, in general, an increase in average motor and mental scores obtained by babies of each race. While the average differences in scores between low-weight infants of short and long gestations tended to be relatively substantial, the differences between large babies of short gestation and those of longer gestation were very small. When one examines the proportion of children in each birthweight-gestational age category obtaining low mental and motor scores, the same general trends are evident. However, the consistent trend for small babies of 43 weeks gestation and above to have a higher risk of low scores with birthweight below 2501 grams than babies of 40 to 42 weeks gestation is of interest. It points up the increased risk of adverse outcome for low-birthweight babies of long gestations (small for dates).

In summary, it is quite clear that both gestational age and birthweight are associated with developmental status at eight months. Gestational age has an effect, and above and beyond it there is a strong effect of birthweight. However, the relative contribution of each variable cannot be precisely determined from this analysis.

The most favored babies in terms of development were those of normal birthweight (3001 grams or above) and normal gestational age (40 weeks or more). Lower scores were obtained by babies who were of low birthweight and correspondingly low gestation and by those whose birthweight was inappropriately low or high for relatively normal gestational age.

MATERNAL FACTORS AND DEVELOPMENTAL STATUS

The maternal parameters of age, race, and parity have demonstrable associations with perinatal mortality and birthweight (9). It seemed possible, therefore, that their interactions might also influence the developmental status of the children. These variables were examined singly, in combination, and finally with appropriate controls on birthweight. When one examines the motor scores, the increasing frequency of low scores with increasing maternal age over 20 is seen, and the crossing over of the distribution curves for the infants of white and black women is again apparent. The babies of white women over 20 years of age had higher percentages of low motor scores than the blacks.

Maternal Age and Birthweight

When the relationships between maternal age and mean motor and mental developmental scores were examined by maternal age, within birthweight subgroups, no striking relationships were identified beyond the clear association between birthweight and developmental status at eight months, which existed at every maternal age, with the larger babies greatly favored over those in the lowest weight group. With increasing maternal age, excepting for the babies of 2000 grams and below, there is, overall, a gradual and slight decline in scores for both races. (Figs. 13–21 through 13–24 and Tables 13–13 through 13–16.)

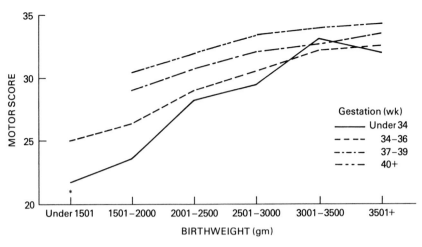

*Based on less than 5 cases.

Figure 13-13. Mean 8-Month Motor Score by Birthweight by Gestation at Delivery — White

Table 13-9. 8-Month Motor Score by Birthweight by Gestation at Delivery — White

Number Tested with Known Score

Gestation (wk)	Under 1001	1001– 1500	1501– 2000	2001– 2500	2501– 3000	3001– 3500	3501+	Total	Mean Birthweight
Under 34	3	16	35	32	36	31	24	177	2534
34–36	0	5	32	133	155	114	69	508	2807
37–39	0	0	27	210	861	1282	564	2944	3127
40–42	0	1	12	156	987	2776	2599	6531	3397
43+	0	1	3	26	173	472	633	1308	3486

The header spanning the birthweight columns reads: Birthweight (gm)

Mean Motor Score

Gestation (wk)	Under 1001	1001– 1500	1501– 2000	2001– 2500	2501– 3000	3001– 3500	3501+	Total
Under 34	16.00*	22.75	23.60	28.22	29.42	32.97	31.83	28.17
34–36	–	25.00	26.34	28.97	30.45	32.07	32.41	30.38
37–39	–	–	29.00	30.68	31.99	32.54	33.37	32.37
40–42	–	18.00*	28.92	31.85	33.28	33.80	34.04	33.76
43+	–	27.00*	36.33*	32.12	33.00	33.73	34.36	33.90

Percent with Scores under 27

Gestation (wk)	Under 1001	1001– 1500	1501– 2000	2001– 2500	2501– 3000	3001– 3500	3501+	Total
Under 34	100.00†	68.75†	68.57	34.38	30.56	12.91	20.83	38.98
34–36	–	60.00†	53.13	30.08	17.42	13.16	11.59	21.65
37–39	–	–	33.33	18.09	11.27	8.89	7.62	10.23
40–42	–	100.00†	25.00†	14.74	5.78	5.08	3.92	5.01
43+	–	0 †	0 †	23.08	9.82	5.93	4.74	6.20

*Based on less than 5 cases.
†Based on less than 20 cases.

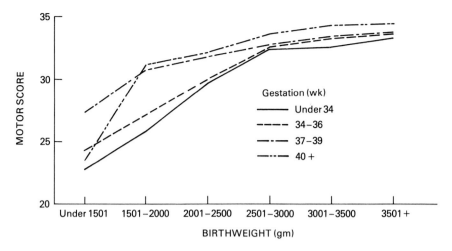

Figure 13-14. Mean 8-Month Motor Score by Birthweight by Gestation at Delivery — Black

Table 13-10. 8-Month Motor Score by Birthweight by Gestation at Delivery — Black

Number Tested with Known Score

Gestation (wk)	Under 1001	1001– 1500	1501– 2000	2001– 2500	2501– 3000	3001– 3500	3501+	Total	Mean Birthweight
Under 34	8	58	127	136	174	197	67	767	2577
34–36	0	17	87	328	454	393	115	1394	2782
37–39	1	2	42	479	1662	1747	566	4499	3012
40–42	1	4	17	234	1425	2509	1326	5516	3214
43+	0	1	5	64	295	524	333	1222	3231

Mean Motor Score

Gestation (wk)	Under 1001	1001– 1500	1501– 2000	2001– 2500	2501– 3000	3001– 3500	3501+	Total
Under 34	20.00	23.14	25.84	29.65	32.34	32.48	33.19	30.07
34–36	–	24.24	27.15	29.94	32.52	33.17	33.50	31.74
37–39	24.00*	29.00*	30.69	31.75	32.72	33.22	33.71	32.91
40–42	31.00*	23.00*	32.00	32.14	33.61	34.17	34.28	33.95
43+	–	18.00*	28.00	32.00	33.28	34.32	34.49	33.95

Percent with Scores under 27

Gestation (wk)	Under 1001	1001– 1500	1501– 2000	2001– 2500	2501– 3000	3001– 3500	3501+	Total
Under 34	75.00†	67.24	49.61	19.85	8.05	8.63	8.95	22.43
34–36	–	52.94†	40.23	19.20	8.59	7.64	6.09	13.13
37–39	100.00†	50.00†	14.28	11.48	6.98	6.41	4.06	6.97
40–42	0 †	25.00†	5.88†	12.82	4.98	3.39	3.70	4.29
43+	–	100.00†	40.00†	14.07	4.75	2.86	3.00	4.17

*Based on less than 5 cases.
†Based on less than 20 cases.

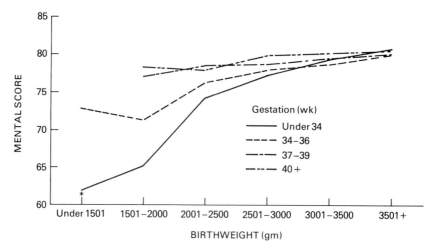

*Based on less than 5 cases.

Figure 13-15. Mean 8-Month Mental Score by Birthweight by Gestation at Delivery — White

Table 13-11. 8-Month Mental Score by Birthweight by Gestation at Delivery — White

Number Tested with Known Score

Gestation (wk)	Under 1001	1001– 1500	1501– 2000	2001– 2500	2501– 3000	3001– 3500	3501+	Total	Mean Birthweight
Under 34	3	16	35	32	36	31	24	177	2534
34–36	0	5	32	133	155	114	69	508	2807
37–39	0	0	27	209	861	1282	564	2943	3127
40–42	0	1	12	155	988	2777	2602	6535	3397
43+	0	1	3	26	173	471	634	1308	3487

Mean Mental Score

Gestation (wk)	Under 1001	1001– 1500	1501– 2000	2001– 2500	2501– 3000	3001– 3500	3501+	Total	
Under 34	43.67*	65.31	65.20	74.25	77.25	79.39	80.67	73.51	
34–36	–	72.80	71.31	76.35	78.02	78.75	79.77	77.51	
37–39	–	–	77.07	78.51	78.69	79.57	80.07	79.31	
40–42	–	62.00*	77.58	77.79	79.95	80.24	80.51	80.24	
43+	–	77.00*	81.00*	78.62	79.61	80.27	80.41	80.22	

Percent with Scores under 75

Gestation (wk)	Under 1001	1001– 1500	1501– 2000	2001– 2500	2501– 3000	3001– 3500	3501+	Total	
Under 34	100.00†	75.00†	65.71	31.26	19.44	9.68	0	32.76	
34–36	–	80.00†	46.88	21.81	10.33	10.53	4.35	15.55	
37–39	–	–	18.51	14.36	11.15	7.02	5.50	8.57	
40–42	–	100.00†	25.00†	14.84	4.85	5.11	4.34	5.05	
43+	–	0 †	0 †	15.38	8.09	4.23	5.68	5.68	

*Based on less than 5 cases.
†Based on less than 20 cases.

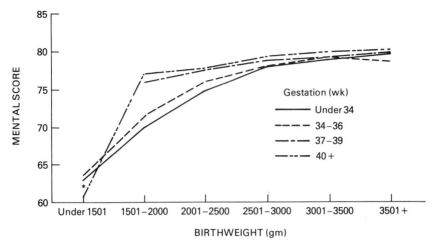

*Based on less than 5 cases.

Figure 13-16. Mean 8-Month Mental Score by Birthweight by Gestation at Delivery — Black

Table 13-12. 8-Month Mental Score by Birthweight by Gestation at Delivery — Black

				Number Tested with Known Score				
				Birthweight (gm)				
Gestation (wk)	Under 1001	1001– 1500	1501– 2000	2001– 2500	2501– 3000	3001– 3500	3501+	Total	Mean Birthweight
Under 34	8	57	127	136	174	197	67	766	2579
34–36	0	17	87	328	454	392	115	1393	2781
37–39	1	2	42	479	1665	1747	566	4502	3012
40–42	1	4	17	235	1424	2508	1326	5515	3214
43+	0	1	5	64	295	525	333	1223	3231
				Mean Mental Score				
Under 34	49.63	64.70	69.96	74.82	77.89	78.81	79.58	75.14	
34–36	–	63.59	71.57	76.06	78.02	79.15	78.48	77.33	
37–39	70.00*	68.00*	75.90	77.50	78.80	79.12	79.76	78.87	
40–42	85.00*	58.75*	77.88	78.27	79.26	79.84	80.00	79.64	
43+	–	44.00*	74.20	75.95	79.75	79.92	80.56	79.80	
				Percent with Scores under 75				
Under 34	100.00†	64.91	57.48	27.94	14.94	12.19	8.95	27.67	
34–36	–	64.70†	48.28	25.92	14.76	9.19	12.17	18.31	
37–39	100.00†	50.00†	33.33	16.08	11.77	9.90	6.90	11.12	
40–42	0 †	25.00†	17.65†	14.47	10.25	7.46	7.02	8.41	
43+	–	100.00†	60.00†	15.63	9.83	6.47	7.21	8.26	

*Based on less than 5 cases.
†Based on less than 20 cases.

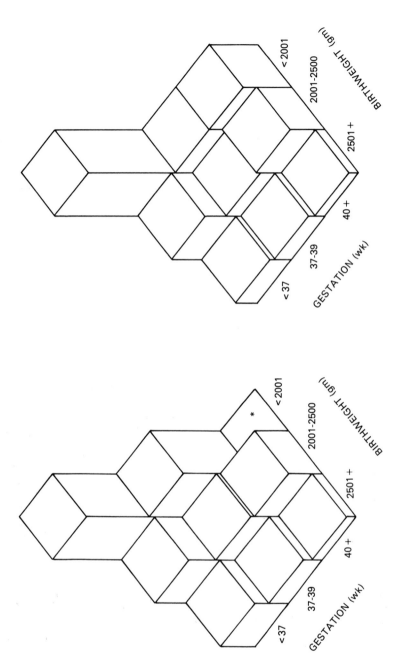

Figure 13-18. Percent With 8-Month Motor Scores Below 27 by Birthweight by Gestation at Delivery-Black

* Not shown for less than 20 cases.

Figure13-17. Percent With 8-Month Motor Scores Below 27 by Birthweight by Gestation at Delivery-White

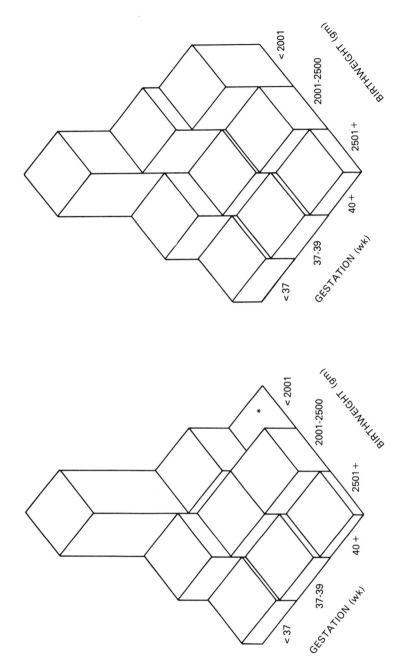

Figure 13-20. Percent With 8-Month Mental Scores Below 75 by Birthweight by Gestation at Delivery-Black

* Not shown for less than 20 cases.

Figure 13-19. Percent With 8-Month Mental Scores Below 75 by Birthweight by Gestation at Delivery-White

Table 13-13. 8-Month Motor Score by Age of Gravida by Birthweight — White

Number Tested with Known Score

| Age of Gravida | Birthweight (gm) | | | | |
	Under 2001	2001– 2500	2501– 3000	3001+	Total
10-15	1	5	17	57	80
16-17	6	28	131	402	567
18-19	21	66	328	1146	1561
20-24	40	206	863	3396	4505
25-29	32	122	459	1885	2498
30-34	21	76	245	999	1341
35-39	10	41	137	568	756
40+	4	15	38	160	217

Mean Motor Score

Age of Gravida	Under 2001	2001– 2500	2501– 3000	3001+	Total
10-15	19.00*	31.80	33.35	34.16	33.65
16-17	28.50	31.68	33.87	34.57	34.20
18-19	25.62	31.08	33.00	34.43	33.87
20-24	27.70	31.02	32.40	33.91	33.44
25-29	23.72	29.48	32.47	33.17	32.74
30-34	25.29	30.86	31.96	32.68	32.33
35-39	26.10	29.95	31.85	33.23	32.71
40+	25.75*	27.27	31.45	33.01	32.21

Percent with Scores under 27

Age of Gravida	Under 2001	2001– 2500	2501– 3000	3001+	Total
10-15	100.00†	0 †	0 †	3.50	3.75
16-17	16.67†	25.00	6.87	2.99	5.12
18-19	47.62	21.21	7.31	3.66	5.76
20-24	35.00	16.02	8.92	4.71	6.30
25-29	78.13	29.51	10.24	6.74	9.41
30-34	57.15	21.06	12.24	9.11	11.11
35-39	60.00†	19.51	12.41	7.74	9.92
40+	50.00†	33.33†	13.16	9.38	12.44

*Based on less than 5 cases.
†Based on less than 20 cases.

Maternal Age and Parity

When the relationships between maternal age and mean scores were reexamined, controlling on parity rather than birthweight, the trends were not so clear. There was, however, a very slight but consistent difference between the mean scores of the infants of nulliparous women, which were slightly higher, and those of infants of women with prior pregnancies. The difference was greatest when the mother was less than twenty years old; the average developmental scores being lowest for the infants of multiparous women in the youngest age brackets. (Tables 13–17 through 13–20.)

When maternal age and parity were examined individually, within race, only trivial effects were noted. However, when the variables were examined simultaneously, even these minor effects tended to disappear.

Table 13-14. 8-Month Motor Score by Age of Gravida by Birthweight — Black

| | Number Tested with Known Score | | | | |
| | Birthweight (gm) | | | | |
Age of Gravida	Under 2001	2001–2500	2501–3000	3001+	Total
10-15	28	92	253	379	752
16-17	58	150	534	745	1487
18-19	62	218	675	1136	2091
20-24	108	385	1281	2459	4233
25-29	47	202	680	1518	2447
30-34	35	116	390	947	1488
35-39	24	75	187	520	806
40+	10	16	46	131	203
	Mean Motor Score				
10-15	27.18	31.30	33.77	34.22	33.45
16-17	27.91	31.18	33.57	34.19	33.42
18-19	25.90	31.07	33.20	33.97	33.18
20-24	26.19	31.03	32.95	33.77	33.08
25-29	25.62	31.06	32.70	33.80	33.11
30-34	25.49	31.87	32.86	33.65	33.11
35-39	26.42	30.52	32.28	33.69	32.85
40+	25.70	32.00	31.93	33.65	32.74
	Percent with Scores under 27				
10-15	42.86	10.87	3.56	2.90	5.58
16-17	36.21	11.33	3.56	2.95	5.31
18-19	50.00	15.13	6.37	3.61	7.08
20-24	39.81	14.55	6.48	5.00	7.21
25-29	51.06	16.42	7.94	4.32	7.23
30-34	54.29	15.52	6.67	6.13	8.13
35-39	41.67	21.33	9.62	6.15	9.43
40+	60.00*	12.50*	10.87	4.58	9.36

*Based on less than 20 cases.

Education of Gravida and Birthweight

In order to obtain some insight into possible relationships between the education of the mother and the developmental status of the child at eight months, the developmental scores were examined by the years of schooling completed by the mother. Tables 13–21 through 13–24 and Figures 13–25 through 13–32 show the results of an examination of mean mental and motor scores and percentages of low scores, within birthweight groups, for mothers who had completed varying years of schooling. A very slight relationship between increasing scores and increased schooling was noted for babies of either race. Again the strong and strikingly consistent effect of birthweight was noted. Within each birthweight category, increased education of the mother had relatively little effect on the mean developmental scores.

Table 13-15. 8-Month Mental Score by Age of Gravida by Birthweight — White

	Number Tested with Known Score				
	Birthweight (gm)				
Age of Gravida	Under 2001	2001–2500	2501–3000	3001+	Total
10–15	1	5	17	57	80
16–17	6	28	131	403	568
18–19	21	66	328	1146	1561
20–24	40	206	864	3397	4507
25–29	32	121	459	1886	2498
30–34	21	76	245	999	1341
35–39	10	40	137	569	756
40+	4	15	38	160	217
	Mean Mental Score				
10–15	53.00*	79.40	80.53	81.19	80.59
16–17	72.17	78.04	79.70	80.54	80.13
18–19	72.52	77.44	79.47	80.32	79.92
20–24	74.20	78.18	79.33	80.11	79.82
25–29	67.50	77.11	79.30	80.07	79.62
30–34	67.19	77.30	78.74	80.19	79.56
35–39	64.20	77.35	78.67	80.58	79.85
40+	77.00*	73.00	78.71	80.04	79.26
	Percent with Scores under 75				
10–15	100.00†	0 †	0 †	1.75	2.50
16–17	50.00†	21.43	5.34	2.73	4.76
18–19	42.85	15.16	5.78	4.54	5.76
20–24	30.00	16.99	8.10	5.33	6.60
25–29	68.76	18.19	7.62	6.36	7.97
30–34	61.91	15.79	12.24	6.11	8.64
35–39	50.00†	17.50	10.22	3.17	5.82
40+	25.00†	33.34†	15.79	6.88	10.60

*Based on less than 5 cases.
†Based on less than 20 cases.

Summary and Discussion

On the basis of the descriptive analyses performed, a number of relationships between developmental status at eight months, as measured by motor and mental scores, and antecedent factors emerge.

The birthweight and gestational age of the infant, when considered singly, have relationships with developmental status at eight months that were similar; i.e., mean developmental scores, in general, increase progressively with both increasing birthweight and gestational age. When the variables were examined together, the babies with the highest average scores were those weighing over 3000 grams, born at term. The low-birthweight infants of short gestational age and those infants whose birthweight was inappropriate for their gestational age (small for dates) had lower mean scores and higher frequencies of low developmental scores.

Table 13-16. 8-Month Mental Score by Age of Gravida by Birthweight — Black

	Birthweight (gm)				
Age of Gravida	Under 2001	2001– 2500	2501– 3000	3001+	Total

Number Tested with Known Score

Age of Gravida	Under 2001	2001–2500	2501–3000	3001+	Total
10-15	28	92	253	379	752
16-17	58	150	534	745	1487
18-19	62	218	676	1134	2090
20-24	107	386	1281	2458	4232
25-29	47	202	680	1519	2448
30-34	35	116	390	948	1489
35-39	24	75	188	520	807
40+	10	16	46	131	203

Mean Mental Score

Age of Gravida	Under 2001	2001–2500	2501–3000	3001+	Total
10-15	70.07	77.47	79.64	79.87	79.13
16-17	72.57	76.64	79.34	79.70	78.98
18-19	69.90	76.56	78.41	79.59	78.60
20-24	69.52	76.99	78.97	79.54	78.88
25-29	68.81	77.32	78.74	79.65	79.00
30-34	67.71	77.68	79.00	79.60	79.01
35-39	67.42	75.92	78.43	80.20	79.01
40+	68.40	75.13	77.74	79.74	78.36

Percent with Scores under 75

Age of Gravida	Under 2001	2001–2500	2501–3000	3001+	Total
10-15	50.00	15.22	11.86	7.39	11.43
16-17	44.83	19.33	6.93	6.44	9.42
18-19	53.22	21.56	12.14	7.85	12.01
20-24	55.14	20.26	11.71	8.21	11.56
25-29	53.20	17.82	12.50	8.43	11.19
30-34	62.85	16.38	13.59	8.65	11.83
35-39	54.17	25.33	13.30	8.65	12.63
40+	40.00*	12.50*	15.21	11.45	13.79

*Based on less than 20 cases.

The birthweight associations with later developmental status are quite striking and appear of greater magnitude than the effects of the other antecedent variables considered.

Race was observed to have little association with developmental motor and mental scores at this age. A slight tendency for white infants to show minimally greater mental scores and black infants minimally higher motor scores was noted in low-weight infants.

Relationships between parity and developmental level, particularly when controlled by the related variables of maternal age and race, were in general unclear. The infants of multiparous women had slightly lower scores than first-born infants. The difference between the first-born and later-born infants was greatest where the mother was less than twenty years old at registration for prenatal care. This observation is in accord with the increased risk of adverse pregnancy outcome of young multiparous women.

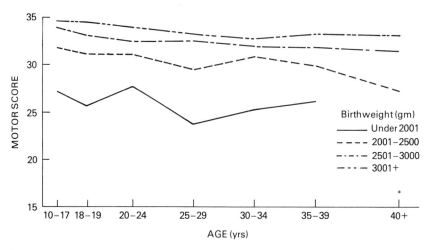

*Based on less than 5 cases.

Figure 13-21. Mean 8-Month Motor Score by Age of Gravida by Birthweight — White

Table 13-17. 8-Month Motor Score by Age of Gravida by Parity — White

				Number Tested					
				Motor Score					
Age (yrs)	0–19	20–26	27–33	34–40	41–43	Total	Unknown	Grand Total	Mean
				Parity 0					
10–15	2	1	33	36	5	77	1	78	33.74
16–17	1	20	180	291	22	514	1	515	34.36
18–19	1	45	411	675	36	1168	1	1169	34.42
20–24	6	76	857	1286	71	2296	2	2298	34.17
25–29	3	20	228	277	19	547	0	547	33.75
30–34	1	9	66	65	1	142	0	142	33.16
35–39	0	2	21	21	2	46	0	46	33.43
40+	0	0	7	5	0	12	0	12	32.25
Total	14	173	1803	2656	156	4802	5	4807	34.16
Unknown	0	0	0	0	0	0	0	0	–
Grand Total	14	173	1803	2656	156	4802	5	4807	34.16
				Parity 1+					
10–15	0	0	2	1	0	3	0	3	31.33*
16–17	0	8	17	26	2	53	0	53	32.66
18–19	7	37	173	169	5	391	0	391	32.25
20–24	13	189	1000	974	21	2197	2	2199	32.66
25–29	20	191	886	810	38	1945	1	1946	32.46
30–34	16	123	573	469	17	1198	0	1198	32.23
35–39	8	65	306	318	12	709	1	710	32.66
40+	3	24	97	72	8	204	0	204	32.22
Total	67	637	3054	2839	103	6700	4	6704	32.49
Unknown	0	0	0	0	0	0	0	0	–
Grand Total	67	637	3054	2839	103	6700	4	6704	32.49

*Based on less than 5 cases.

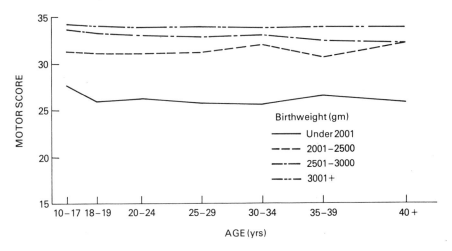

Figure 13-22. Mean 8-Month Motor Score by Age of Gravida by Birthweight — Black

Table 13-18. 8-Month Motor Score by Age of Gravida by Parity — Black

Number Tested

Age (yrs)	0–19	20–26	27–33	34–40	41–43	Total	Unknown	Grand Total	Mean
			Motor Score						
Parity 0									
10–15	7	32	294	374	8	715	0	715	33.51
16–17	7	47	503	636	21	1214	2	1216	33.71
18–19	9	51	483	704	17	1264	0	1264	33.84
20–24	2	41	514	684	21	1262	0	1262	33.90
25–29	1	7	101	124	8	241	0	241	33.89
30–34	1	5	29	45	0	80	0	80	33.40
35–39	0	4	15	18	2	39	0	39	33.44
40+	0	1	6	4	0	11	0	11	32.55
Total	27	188	1945	2589	77	4826	2	4828	33.76
Unknown	0	0	0	0	0	0	0	0	–
Grand Total	27	188	1945	2589	77	4826	2	4828	33.76
Parity 1+									
10–15	1	2	16	17	0	36	0	36	32.25
16–17	6	18	141	104	3	272	0	272	34.14
18–19	15	73	383	347	6	824	1	825	32.15
20–24	41	221	1301	1352	54	2969	2	2971	32.73
25–29	16	153	979	1001	51	2200	1	2201	33.03
30–34	18	97	582	682	28	1407	1	1408	33.10
35–39	10	62	325	358	12	767	1	768	32.82
40+	4	14	86	83	5	192	0	192	32.75
Total	111	640	3813	3944	159	8667	6	8673	32.80
Unknown	0	0	0	0	0	0	0	0	–
Grand Total	111	640	3813	3944	159	8667	6	8673	32.80

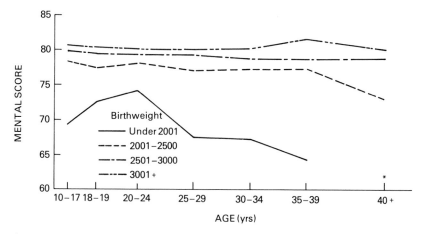

*Based on less than 5 cases.

Figure 13-23. Mean 8-Month Mental Score by Age of Gravida by Birthweight — White

Table 13-19. 8-Month Mental Score by Age of Gravida by Parity — White

					Number Tested				
			Mental Score						
Age (yrs)	0–24	25–55	56–74	75–89	90–106	Total	Unknown	Grand Total	Mean
Parity 0									
10–15	0	1	1	74	1	77	1	78	80.57
16–17	0	1	23	484	7	515	0	515	80.23
18–19	1	2	48	1109	8	1168	1	1169	80.25
20–24	2	3	102	2165	25	2297	1	2298	80.18
25–29	0	2	27	512	6	547	0	547	80.20
30–34	0	0	7	134	1	142	0	142	80.21
35–39	0	0	2	44	0	46	0	46	79.78
40+	0	0	0	12	0	12	0	12	79.42
Total	3	9	210	4534	48	4804	3	4807	80.21
Unknown	0	0	0	0	0	0	0	0	—
Grand Total	3	9	210	4534	48	4804	3	4807	80.21
Parity 1+									
10–15	0	0	0	3	0	3	0	3	81.00*
16–17	0	0	3	50	0	53	0	53	79.21
18–19	2	3	34	350	2	391	0	391	78.92
20–24	0	11	180	1993	14	2198	1	2199	79.45
25–29	2	15	151	1767	10	1945	1	1946	79.47
30–34	1	9	99	1075	14	1198	0	1198	79.48
35–39	0	10	32	650	17	709	1	710	79.85
40+	0	2	21	178	3	204	0	204	79.26
Total	5	50	520	6066	60	6701	3	6704	79.47
Unknown	0	0	0	0	0	0	0	0	—
Grand Total	5	50	520	6066	60	6701	3	6704	79.47

*Based on less than 5 cases

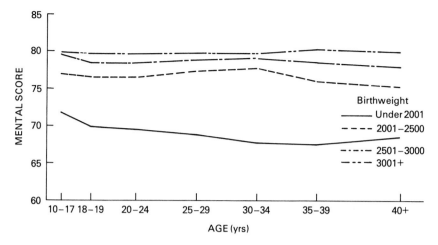

Figure 13-24. Mean 8-Month Mental Score by Age of Gravida by Birthweight — Black

Table 13-20. 8-Month Mental Score by Age of Gravida by Parity — Black

				Number Tested					
				Mental Score					
Age (yrs)	0-24	25-55	56-74	75-89	90-106	Total	Unknown	Grand Total	Mean
Parity 0									
10-15	0	7	76	625	7	715	0	715	79.16
16-17	3	4	87	1115	5	1214	2	1216	79.32
18-19	4	6	104	1137	12	1263	1	1264	79.31
20-24	0	2	92	1152	15	1261	1	1262	79.79
25-29	0	0	12	222	7	241	0	241	80.58
30-34	0	1	6	71	2	80	0	80	79.34
35-39	0	0	6	33	0	39	0	39	79.10
40+	0	0	2	9	0	11	0	11	78.64
Total	7	20	385	4364	48	4824	4	4828	79.48
Unknown	0	0	0	0	0	0	0	0	–
Grand Total	7	20	385	4364	48	4824	4	4828	79.48
Parity 1+									
10-15	0	1	2	33	0	36	0	36	78.58
16-17	1	5	40	226	0	272	0	272	77.50
18-19	0	16	121	679	8	824	1	825	77.50
20-24	5	41	349	2556	18	2969	2	2971	78.49
25-29	2	21	239	1924	15	2201	0	2201	78.82
30-34	1	20	146	1223	17	1407	1	1408	79.02
35-39	1	14	81	658	14	768	0	768	79.01
40+	0	4	22	165	1	192	0	192	78.35
Total	10	122	1000	7464	73	8669	4	8673	78.58
Unknown	0	0	0	0	0	0	0	0	–
Grand Total	10	122	1000	7464	73	8669	4	8673	78.58

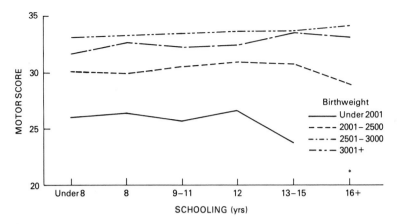

*Based on less than 5 cases.

Figure 13-25. Mean 8-Month Motor Score by Years of Schooling Completed by Gravida by Birthweight — White

Table 13-21. 8-Month Motor Score
by Years of Schooling Completed by Gravida by Birthweight — White

Number Tested with Known Score

Years	Birthweight (gm)				
	Under 2001	2001–2500	2501–3000	3001+	Total
0–4	1	12	17	90	120
5–7	7	35	96	343	481
8	12	48	147	501	708
9–11	61	184	719	2396	3360
12	39	185	775	3124	4123
13–15	9	50	257	1170	1486
16	1	22	130	631	784
17+	1	10	42	208	261
Total	131	546	2183	8463	11323

Mean Motor Score

Years	Under 2001	2001–2500	2501–3000	3001+	Total
0–4	21.00*	29.08	29.82	32.71	31.84
5–7	26.71	30.43	32.01	33.16	32.64
8	26.42	29.96	32.67	33.27	32.80
9–11	25.66	30.57	32.23	33.43	32.88
12	26.62	30.94	32.40	33.61	33.20
13–15	23.78	30.74	33.49	34.30	33.98
16	28.00*	27.86	33.49	34.00	33.74
17+	25.00*	31.50	31.79	34.45	33.87
Total	25.92	30.52	32.51	33.66	33.19

Percent with Score under 27

Years	Under 2001	2001–2500	2501–3000	3001+	Total
0–4	100.00†	33.33†	23.52†	7.78	13.33
5–7	57.15†	20.00	12.50	9.33	11.43
8	50.00†	18.75	10.20	7.98	9.89
9–11	49.18	23.37	10.01	6.76	9.14
12	48.72	19.46	10.71	5.32	7.37
13–15	77.78†	18.00	5.06	3.59	4.78
16	0 †	27.28	2.31	3.81	4.21
17+	100.00†	10.00†	7.14	3.85	4.98
Total	51.91	21.06	9.39	5.68	7.67

*Based on less than 5 cases.
†Based on less than 20 cases.

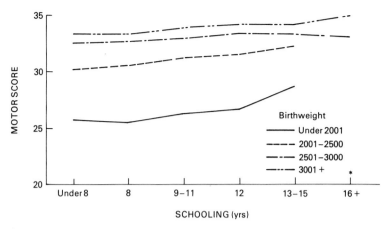

* Based on less than 5 cases.

Figure 13-26. Mean 8-Month Motor Score by Years of Schooling Completed by Gravida by Birthweight — Black

Table 13-22. 8-Month Motor Score
by Years of Schooling Completed by Gravida by Birthweight — Black

	Number Tested with Known Score				
		Birthweight (gm)			
Years	Under 2001	2001– 2500	2501– 3000	3001+	Total
0–4	6	27	62	103	198
5–7	35	99	329	659	1122
8	40	144	363	677	1224
9–11	162	574	1859	3494	6089
12	104	346	1192	2392	4034
13–15	15	45	161	372	593
16	2	4	26	54	86
17+	0	0	6	8	14
Total	364	1239	3998	7759	13360
	Mean Motor Score				
0–4	26.50	31.04	32.39	32.97	32.33
5–7	25.60	30.05	32.56	33.42	32.63
8	25.47	30.56	32.72	33.35	32.58
9–11	26.24	31.21	32.95	33.80	33.09
12	26.66	31.50	33.38	34.14	33.50
13–15	28.67	32.20	33.30	34.08	33.59
16	27.00*	31.00*	33.54	34.80	34.06
17+	–	–	30.83	35.75	33.64
Total	26.32	31.15	33.03	33.84	33.15
	Percent with Score under 27				
0–4	50.00†	7.41	11.29	8.74	10.61
5–7	48.57	23.23	7.59	6.68	9.71
8	60.00	16.67	6.62	5.91	9.15
9–11	45.68	14.11	7.00	4.63	7.34
12	39.42	13.30	4.78	3.51	5.65
13–15	33.33†	8.89	5.59	4.03	5.57
16	0 †	25.00†	3.85	3.70	4.65
17+	–	–	16.67†	0 †	7.14†
Total	45.06	14.60	6.35	4.59	7.15

*Based on less than 5 cases.
†Based on less than 20 cases.

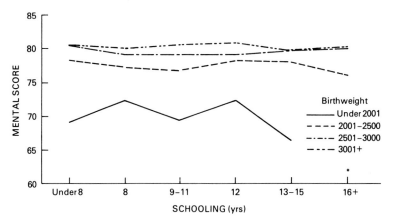

* Based on less than 5 cases.

Figure 13-27. Mean 8-Month Mental Score by Years of Schooling Completed by Gravida by Birthweight — White

Table 13-23. 8-Month Mental Score
by Years of Schooling Completed by Gravida by Birthweight — White

	Number Tested with Known Score				
	Birthweight (gm)				
Years	Under 2001	2001– 2500	2501– 3000	3001+	Total
0–4	1	12	17	90	120
5–7	7	35	96	343	481
8	12	48	147	502	709
9–11	61	182	719	2397	3359
12	39	185	776	3126	4126
13–15	9	50	257	1170	1486
16	1	22	130	631	784
17+	1	10	42	208	261
Total	131	544	2184	8467	11326
	Mean Mental Score				
0–4	64.06*	74.08	78.47	80.40	79.36
5–7	69.86	79.69	80.79	80.26	80.17
8	72.42	77.35	79.16	80.05	79.55
9–11	69.44	76.84	79.14	80.17	79.57
12	72.38	78.18	79.04	80.30	79.89
13–15	66.33	78.00	79.61	80.20	79.94
16	74.00*	74.59	79.87	79.89	79.73
17+	70.00*	79.10	78.71	80.07	79.78
Total	70.40	77.52	79.27	80.20	79.78
	Percent with Score under 75				
0–4	100.00†	50.00†	11.76†	2.22	9.17
5–7	42.86†	8.57	6.25	8.16	8.32
8	41.66†	20.83	10.20	4.78	7.62
9–11	50.82	19.78	8.90	5.59	7.89
12	38.46	11.89	8.63	4.83	6.17
13–15	77.78†	16.00	5.06	4.53	5.45
16	100.00†	31.82	3.85	6.03	6.50
17+	100.00†	20.00†	9.52	7.21	8.43
Total	48.85	17.28	8.07	5.26	6.88

*Based on less than 5 cases.
†Based on less than 20 cases.

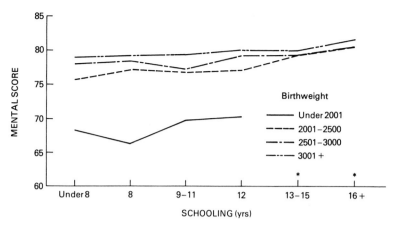

* Based on less than 5 cases.

Figure 13-28. Mean 8-Month Mental Score by Years of Schooling Completed by Gravida by Birthweight — Black

Table 13-24. 8-Month Mental Score by Years of Schooling Completed by Gravida by Birthweight — Black

Number Tested with Known Score

Years	Birthweight (gm)				
	Under 2001	2001– 2500	2501– 3000	3001+	Total
0–4	6	27	62	104	199
5–7	35	99	330	659	1123
8	40	144	363	677	1224
9–11	161	575	1861	3493	6090
12	104	346	1191	2391	4032
13–15	15	45	161	372	593
16	2	4	26	54	86
17+	0	0	6	8	14
Total	363	1240	4000	7758	13361

Mean Mental Score

Years	Under 2001	2001– 2500	2501– 3000	3001+	Total
0–4	71.83	77.04	77.97	78.64	78.01
5–7	67.54	75.37	78.03	78.94	78.00
8	66.25	77.20	78.44	79.27	78.35
9–11	69.68	76.80	78.83	79.49	78.77
12	70.33	77.29	79.32	80.10	79.37
13–15	74.20	79.40	79.35	80.03	79.65
16	76.00*	79.25*	80.42	81.44	80.91
17+	–	–	81.17	82.88	82.14
Total	69.54	76.97	78.89	79.64	78.90

Percent with Score under 75

Years	Under 2001	2001– 2500	2501– 3000	3001+	Total
0–4	66.67†	14.81	16.13	13.46	16.08
5–7	57.15	28.28	16.97	12.29	16.48
8	62.50	20.13	15.43	8.28	13.56
9–11	54.65	18.78	11.88	8.59	11.78
12	48.07	19.07	8.47	6.20	9.05
13–15	33.34†	11.11	8.07	7.80	8.77
16	50.00†	0 †	7.69	5.56	6.98
17+	–	–	16.67†	0 †	7.14†
Total	53.16	19.36	11.49	8.13	11.41

*Based on less than 5 cases.
†Based on less than 20 cases.

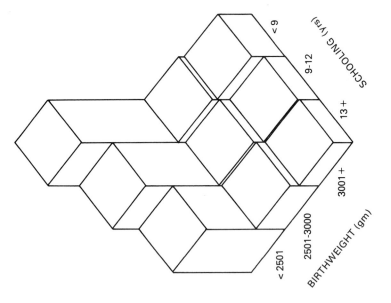

Figure 13-30. Percent With 8-Month Motor Scores Below 27 by Birthweight by Years of Schooling Completed by Gravida-Black

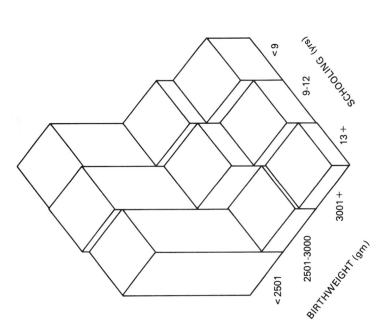

Figure 13-29. Percent With 8-Month Motor Scores Below 27 by Birthweight by Years of Schooling Completed by Gravida-White

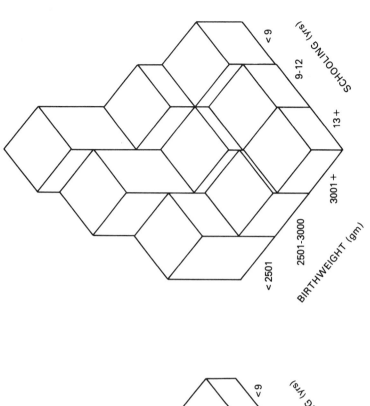

Figure 13-32. Percent With 8-Month Mental Scores Below 75 by Birthweight by Years of Schooling Completed by Gravida-Black

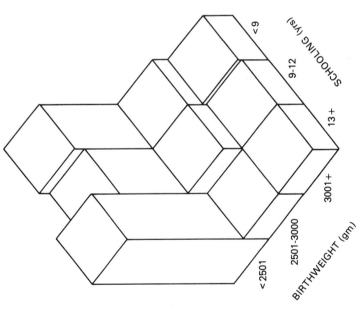

Figure 13-31. Percent With 8-Month Mental Scores Below 75 by Birthweight by Years of Schooling Completed by Gravida-White

The finding of little association between maternal educational level and the developmental scores of their children at eight months, when birthweight was controlled, is intriguing. This appears in sharp contrast to findings in later childhood; Binet IQ at age four years is strongly associated with the level of maternal education in this study (5). At four years, within each racial group, there was a steady increase in average IQ score as maternal education increased. Also, a substantial difference in average IQ score between white and black children was noted at each level of maternal education.

The factors underlying the observation that the developmental level of white and black children appeared little different at eight months but substantially different at four years are not entirely clear. One must bear in mind that the normal intellectual repertoire that can be tested at eight months is very limited, as compared with the more extensive array that can be tested at four years. The central nervous system functions tested at the two ages are perforce somewhat different, with heavy dependence on evaluations of motor skills at the younger age. The test instruments used are obviously testing different functions.

Like intrauterine growth and development, normal development during the first year of life may depend to a considerable degree on a biological timetable, with but relatively slight impact from the postnatal environment. However, the environment becomes increasingly important in determining the level of intellectual function as the child grows through the preschool years (2).

The observations presented here emphasize the complexity of the relationships between variables affecting the development of children, and the difficulties in the elucidation of the importance of various factors. More sophisticated techniques are being employed in analyses now under way.

REFERENCES

(1) N. Bayley. 1968. Behavioral correlates of mental growth: Birth to thirty-six months. *American Psychologist* 23: 1–17.

(2) H. Knobloch and B. Pasamanick. 1963. Predicting intellectual potential in infancy. *American Journal of Diseases of Children* 106: 43–51.

(3) T. R. Boggs, J. B. Hardy, and T. M. Frazier. 1967. Correlation of neonatal serum total bilirubin concentrations and developmental status at age eight months. *Journal of Pediatrics* 71: 553–60.

(4) D. W. Welcher, E. D. Mellits, and J. B. Hardy. 1971. A multivariate analysis of factors affecting psychological performance. *Johns Hopkins Medical Journal* 129: 19–35.

(5) S. H. Broman, P. L. Nichols, and W. A. Kennedy. 1975. *Preschool IQ: Prenatal and Early Developmental Correlates*. Hillsdale, N.J.: Lawrence Erlbaum Associates (distributed by Halsted Press of John Wiley & Sons).

(6) N. Bayley. 1933. Mental growth during the first three years: A developmental study of sixty-one children by repeated tests. *Genetic Psychology Monographs* 14: 1–92. (As modified in 1958 for use in the NCPP.)

(7) N. Bayley. 1969. *Manual for the Bayley Scales of Infant Development*. New York: Psychological Corporation.

(8) H. Knobloch, R. Rider, P. Harper, and B. Pasamanick. 1956. Neuropsychiatric sequelae of prematurity; a longitudinal study. *Journal of the American Medical Association* 161: 581–85.

(9) K. R. Niswander and M. Gordon (eds.). 1972. *The Women and Their Pregnancies*. Philadelphia: W. B. Saunders Co.

14

NEUROLOGICAL STATUS
AT ONE YEAR

The *One-Year Neurological Examination* (PED–11) of study children was carried out by a specially trained pediatrician or neurologist. The children were examined as close to their first birthday as possible, within the time span of forty-eight to sixty weeks. The evaluation involved a complete pediatric examination, including a detailed assessment of neurological function and of developmental skills. In addition, the physician made a judgment as to whether the child was normal, suspect, or abnormal in each of two categories; neurological status, and nonneurological status, which included all other aspects of the pediatric evaluation. The child was rated separately in each category and might, for example, be normal in one category and abnormal or suspect in the other.

The data to be presented in this chapter include the physician's impressions, based on this examination of the child, both neurological and nonneurological; and the performance of children with respect to a number of specific developmental items included to ascertain development. Three items of general interest have been selected. Observations of this type on the large numbers of white and black children studied provide an important body of normative data. In order to maximize the usefulness of the developmental data, the age range for the data presented here has been restricted to those children examined between forty-eight and fifty-six weeks of age.

Physical growth parameters for the children in this study are not presented here. These data are currently under study and will be presented in a monograph describing physical growth.

NEUROLOGICAL STATUS

Because of the strong association of birthweight with neurological outcome, neurological status was examined in three birthweight groupings, those infants who weighed 2000 grams and below at birth, those who weighed 2001 to 2500 grams,

Table 14-1. Neurological and Nonneurological Status at One Year by Birthweight by Race

	WHITE				BLACK			
	Under 2001	2001–2500	2501+	Total	Under 2001	2001–2500	2501+	Total
Number*								
Neurological status								
Normal	110	536	10968	11614	277	1237	12338	13852
Suspect	33	72	780	885	92	151	810	1053
Abnormal	16	23	165	204	38	37	162	237
Total	159	631	11913	12703	407	1425	13310	15142
Nonneurological status								
None	90	371	8068	8529	251	966	9573	10790
Minor	48	191	3063	3302	108	341	3075	3524
Questionable	12	49	600	661	28	75	482	585
Definite	9	20	176	205	20	42	167	229
Total	159	631	11907	12697	407	1424	13297	15128
Percent								
Neurological status								
Normal	69.18	84.94	92.07	91.43	68.06	86.81	92.70	91.48
Suspect	20.75	11.41	6.55	6.97	22.60	10.60	6.09	6.95
Abnormal	10.06	3.65	1.39	1.61	9.34	2.60	1.22	1.57
Total	100.00	100.00	100.00	100.00	100.00	100.00	100.00	100.00
Nonneurological status								
None	56.60	58.80	67.76	67.17	61.67	67.84	71.99	71.32
Minor	30.19	30.27	25.72	26.01	26.54	23.95	23.13	23.29
Questionable	7.55	7.77	5.04	5.21	6.88	5.27	3.62	3.87
Definite	5.66	3.17	1.48	1.61	4.91	2.95	1.26	1.51
Total	100.00	100.00	100.00	100.00	100.00	100.00	100.00	100.00

*With known birthweight, examined at 48–56 weeks of age.

and those who weighed more than 2500 grams. The distributions are shown in Table 14–1.

The lowest birthweight group (2000 grams and below) in both racial groups yielded the highest rate of definite abnormalities and the lowest proportion of neurologically normal children. In this group, among white infants, 69 percent were considered normal, 21 percent were rated suspect, and 10 percent were reported to be definitely abnormal. Among blacks, 68 percent were normal, 23 percent were suspect, and 9 percent were definitely abnormal.

Among those infants weighing 2001 to 2500 grams, a larger proportion of children were neurologically normal (85 percent of the whites and 87 percent of the blacks). Approximately 11 percent of infants of both races were considered suspect, and 4 percent of the white and 3 percent of the black infants were rated abnormal.

As expected, the infants weighing over 2500 grams showed the largest normal proportion (92 percent) and the smallest numbers of suspect (7 percent) and abnormal (1.4 percent). There were no significant differences by race.

NONNEUROLOGICAL STATUS

The percentages of children with diagnoses other than neurological are tabulated for the three birthweight categories in Table 14–1. The children were reported to be normal (nonneurologically), to have minor abnormalities, to be questionable or suspect, or to have definite and significant abnormalities.

Overall, 67 percent of the white infants and 71 percent of the black had no nonneurological abnormalities reported. As birthweight decreased, the proportion of normal children decreased. In the lower-birthweight group (below 2001 grams), 57 percent of white and 62 percent of black infants were normal. The intermediate-birthweight group showed intermediate proportions of normal children. Among white infants, the proportion of infants with minor abnormalities was quite high in each birthweight group (30, 30, and 26 percent, respectively), while among black infants, it was 27, 24, and 23 percent. The proportions of questionable abnormalities by weight group for white infants were 8, 8, and 5 percent, respectively, and for black infants, 7, 5, and 4 percent, respectively. Definite nonneurological abnormalities showed a clearer relationship to birthweight and were also slightly more frequent among white infants, as compared with black infants. Among white babies, 6 percent weighing below 2001 grams, 3 percent weighing between 2001 and 2500 grams, and 1.5 percent of those above 2500 grams, at birth, were reported to have definite nonneurological abnormalities at the one-year examination. Among blacks, the frequencies were 5, 3, and 1.3 percent.

Comment

The importance of birthweight in relationship to the presence of abnormalities, particularly neurological abnormalities, at one year of age is clear. The very minor differences in the distribution of abnormalities by race should be noted.

Specific diagnoses have not been considered in this section. They are reported in Chapter 15.

DEVELOPMENTAL STATUS

Hand Preference at One Year of Age

During the one-year neurological examination, the child was tested for definite expression of hand preference. As a rough guideline, if more than three-quarters of the reaching and fine motor activity during the examination was performed by one hand, it was judged to be an expression of strong preference for that hand. The reporting was on the basis of observation during the examination, not on history. The examiners were specifically instructed not to let any reported information influence their own reporting of this item.

It will be noted from Table 14–2 that for both races from 85 percent to 90 percent of the children had variable hand preference, approximately 10 percent strongly right, and about 3 percent strongly left. Hand preference varied little by either race or sex.

Table 14-2. Hand Preference at One Year by Race

	WHITE		BLACK	
	Number*	Percent	Number*	Percent
Variable	11234	89.05	12875	85.67
Strongly right	1071	8.49	1664	11.07
Strongly left	311	2.47	489	3.25
Total	12616	100.00	15028	100.00
Unknown	87	0.68	114	0.75
Grand total	12703	100.00	15142	100.00

*With known birthweight, examined at 48-56 weeks of age.

Table 14-3. Prehensile Grasp at One Year by Birthweight — White

	Under 2001 gm		2001-2500 gm		2501+ gm		Total*	
	No.	%	No.	%	No.	%	No.	%
Grasps with thumb and fingers	125	91.24	528	94.96	10139	97.56	10792	97.35
Grasps with palm	9	6.57	24	4.32	216	2.08	249	2.25
Raking without grasp	1	0.73	1	0.18	1	0.01	3	0.03
Other	2	1.46	3	0.54	37	0.36	42	0.38
Total	137	100.00	556	100.00	10393	100.00	11086	100.00
Unknown	22	13.84	75	11.88	1520	12.76	1617	12.73
Grand total	159	100.00	631	100.00	11913	100.00	12703	100.00

*With known birthweight, examined at 48-56 weeks of age.

Prehensile Grasp

Prehensile grasp was determined by observing the child's handling of a one-inch plastic cube. At least three trials were made; the most mature pattern was reported. Many possible distinctions in grasp patterns were grouped into three categories. Examiners were given a diagrammatic scheme to assist them in classifying the three patterns observed, i.e., grasping with thumb and forefinger, palm free; grasping with palm; or raking without grasp.

By one year of age, over 90 percent of both black and white children in each birthweight group were able to grasp with thumb and fingers. However, as shown in Tables 14-3 and 14-4, there was a threefold difference in the proportion of children in the lowest-birthweight group who could not perform this task (9 percent) and those in the highest-birthweight group (3 percent).

Locomotor Development

The examiner was asked to observe the child's locomotor ability and report the highest level of development attained according to the categories shown in Table 14-5. The reported levels are those actually observed in the examining situation. It was recommended that a history of the child's locomotor development, including

Table 14-4. Prehensile Grasp at One Year by Birthweight — Black

	Under 2001 gm		2001–2500 gm		2501+ gm		Total*	
	No.	%	No.	%	No.	%	No.	%
Grasps with thumb and fingers	327	91.60	1217	96.74	11497	98.12	13041	97.82
Grasps with palm	24	6.72	34	2.70	179	1.53	237	1.78
Raking without grasp	0	0	1	0.08	1	0.01	2	0.02
Other	6	1.68	6	0.48	40	0.34	52	0.39
Total	357	100.00	1258	100.00	11717	100.00	13332	100.00
Unknown	50	12.29	167	11.72	1593	11.97	1810	11.96
Grand total	407	100.00	1425	100.00	13310	100.00	15142	100.00

*With known birthweight, examined at 48–56 weeks of age.

Table 14-5. Highest Locomotor Development Observed at One Year by Birthweight by Race

	Number Examined*							
	WHITE				BLACK			
	Birthweight (gm)				Birthweight (gm)			
Locomotor Development	Under 2001	2001–2500	2501+	Total	Under 2001	2001–2500	2501+	Total
Walks unaided	9	131	4448	4588	32	402	5937	6371
Walks supported	67	285	4384	4736	200	664	4717	5581
Stands unaided	7	17	319	343	13	25	204	242
Pulls to standing	12	49	509	570	35	61	362	458
Stands supported	21	42	457	520	51	59	328	438
Creeps	7	5	69	81	5	8	45	58
None of the above	14	20	129	163	21	37	114	172
Total	137	549	10315	11001	357	1256	11707	13320
	Percent							
Walks unaided	6.57	23.86	43.12	41.71	8.96	32.01	50.71	47.83
Walks supported	48.91	51.91	42.50	43.05	56.02	52.87	40.29	41.90
Stands unaided	5.11	3.10	3.09	3.12	3.64	1.99	1.74	1.82
Pulls to standing	8.76	8.93	4.93	5.18	9.80	4.86	3.09	3.44
Stands supported	15.33	7.65	4.43	4.73	14.29	4.70	2.80	3.29
Creeps	5.11	0.91	0.67	0.74	1.40	0.64	0.38	0.44
None of the above	10.22	3.64	1.25	1.48	5.88	2.95	0.97	1.29
Total	100.00	100.00	100.00	100.00	100.00	100.00	100.00	100.00

*With known birthweight, examined at 48–56 weeks of age.

creeping, be obtained, if the child did not at least walk with support during the examination. However, the item reported here is the highest level of motor development observed by the examiner during the period of the examination.

As shown in Figures 14–1 and 14–2, there is considerable range in the locomotor performance of one-year old children. Infants in the highest-birthweight group showed a distinctly greater achievement than those in the lowest group. A slightly

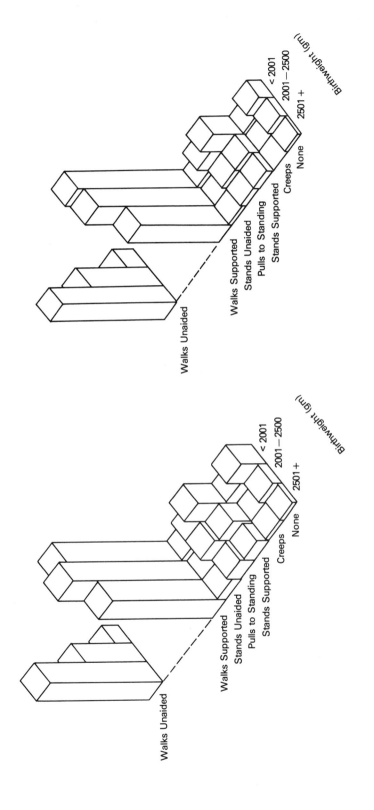

Figure 14-2. Highest Locomotor Development Observed at One Year by Birthweight—Black

Figure 14-1. Highest Locomotor Development Observed at One Year by Birthweight—White

higher percentage of black than white children in each birthweight group were walking unaided at one year. Approximately 51 percent of the black and 43 percent of the white children weighing over 2500 grams walked unaided, but only 9 percent of the black and 7 percent of the white infants weighing 2000 grams and below had achieved this level of development. However, approximately 50 percent of these low-weight infants were able to walk with support. As may be seen in Table 14–5, approximately 6 percent of the children were unable to pull to stand.

These data were examined by sex, and there appeared to be little difference between males and females in respect to the ability to walk either unaided or with support at one year. However, the number of males in the two lowest-achievement groups, "creeping" and "not yet creeping," is somewhat larger than the number of females. These results are not presented in tabular form.

15

SELECTED ABNORMALITIES, DISEASE CONDITIONS, AND EVENTS DURING THE FIRST YEAR

DIAGNOSTIC SUMMARY FOR FIRST YEAR OF LIFE

The *Summary of the First Year of Life* (PED–12) represents one of the milestones in the NCPP pediatric data. This form provided for a comprehensive summary of the diagnoses and major events from the time when the infant was discharged alive from the newborn nursery through the first birthday. Thus, the information recorded picks up at the point of the *Newborn Diagnostic Summary* (PED–8) which was completed upon the infant's discharge from the nursery. For most infants, nursery discharge was at a few days of age, but those who remained longer, because of low birthweight or the presence of some pathological condition, may have been considerably older at the time of discharge.

To insure an independent and unbiased assessment of diagnoses during the first year, a separate summary when the infant was one year old was made, without reference to the neonatal diagnosis. The NCPP is unusual in that it permits evaluation of neurological function or malfunction in a developmental sequence as the child grows. Observations made at specific time periods by study personnel with different professional backgrounds (pediatricians, neurologists, psychologists, etc.) provided an unusually well-rounded view of the developmental process.

The *Summary of the First Year of Life* (PED–12) was completed on all cases following the *One-Year Neurological Examination* (PED–11) (age range 48 to 60 weeks), after a brief interval to permit completion of any diagnostic studies initiated by that examination. In those instances where a one-year neurological evaluation could not be completed because the child had died since nursery discharge, the PED–12 was completed for the duration of the child's life. Similarly, when the child had been lost to follow-up in some other manner, the PED–12 was completed on the basis of whatever information was available, when the child was sixty weeks of age (the outside limit for performance of the *One-Year Neurological Examination*).

The *One-Year Summary* was completed by a senior pediatrician or neurologist, or under his immediate supervision. In order to fill in the form, it was necessary to review the study records, particularly the Four-Month Pediatric, the Eight-Month Developmental and the Twelve-Month Pediatric-Neurological Evaluations, their accompanying *Interval Medical Histories* (PED–20), *Summaries of Medical Records of Illness or Hospitalization* (PED–29), and reports of medical care, including physicians' visits, clinic visits, and diagnostic studies. Much of this latter information was obtained from direct review of hospital records.

To obtain precision and consistency in the reporting of diagnostic conditions, the development of a somewhat complex form with an accompanying manual was necessary. (See the Appendix for copy of PED–12.) As in other NCPP examinations, provision was made for differentiating diagnoses that were clear-cut and *definite* from those rated *suspect*, i.e., those in which there was some doubt about the presence of the condition or of its existence in significant degree. The diagnoses or events reported, in addition to being classified as definite or suspect, were further qualified, on the basis of source of information, in three categories: (1) the twelve-month pediatric-neurological evaluation and any findings from specialty clinic referral or diagnostic procedures initiated as a result of the neurological examination; (2) prior NCPP evaluation or a *Summary of Medical Records of Illness or Hospitalization* (PED–29) or other medical documentation; (3) "History Only" was used where diagnostic conditions or events were based on historical information without medical documentation.

The coding procedure provided for the recording of multiple abnormalities, even when these were present within one organ system. Therefore, one must bear in mind that the numbers listed in the accompanying tables pertain to abnormalities rather than to children; one child may have several diagnoses within one organ system and be normal with respect to other organ systems, or may have abnormalities within more than one organ system.

A diagnosis coded on PED–12 does not mean necessarily that the diagnosis was present at one year of age. It means that the diagnosis was reported at some point between the discharge of the child from the newborn nursery and his reaching one year of age. A discussion of the possible relationships between certain diagnoses reported during the newborn period and on the PED–12 summary is presented in the following chapter. Such information has special relevance to the understanding of the evaluation of neurological abnormalities and to the identification and frequency of occurrence of congenital malformation.

SUMMARY DATA FOR FIRST YEAR (EXCLUSIVE OF NEWBORN PERIOD)

General

The extensive tables that accompany this section (Tables 15–1 through 15–23) present the frequency of certain *definite* diagnostic conditions and events as reported on PED–12. Because of recognized or suspected relationships existing between birthweight and certain conditions, the distributions are presented for infants weighing more than 2500 grams at birth and for those weighing 2500 grams or less. Additionally, the mean birthweight has been computed for the children within each diagnostic category.

Again, it must be stressed that only definite diagnoses according to the criteria defined in the manual are included and that the children with suspect diagnoses are included among those considered normal with respect to the particular organ system under review.

Neurological Abnormality

General Comment. Of the 16,521 white children for whom a PED–12 *Diagnostic Summary* was submitted, 15,383 (93 percent) were considered to be free of definite abnormality within the central nervous system. Among the 18,121 black infants, 17,007 (94 percent) were reported to be without definite abnormality.

The important relationship of birthweight to frequency of neurological problems is clearly seen within each ethnic group. Among white infants, only 86 percent of those of low birthweight were reported to be without definite abnormalities, as compared with 94 percent of those weighing more than 2500 grams at birth. Among blacks, only 88 percent of the low-birthweight babies were without definite neurological abnormality, as compared with 95 percent of the larger infants. These findings from the PED–12 are generally in accord with those reported at one year and described in the preceding chapter.

The frequency of neurological abnormalities during the first year (exclusive of the newborn nursery period) is higher than generally reported. There are perhaps several reasons for this. As is apparent from the detailed listing of neurological conditions presented in the accompanying tables, it is clear that the overall diagnosis of neurological abnormality included a broad spectrum of conditions. In addition to the traditional range of neuromotor, neurosensory, peripheral nerve and spinal cord abnormalities, seizure states and developmental delays were included to assure completeness of reporting. The careful and repeated examinations of each child by trained staff, using a predetermined protocol, was also a factor.

It is important to note that the data show the frequency with which specific diagnostic conditions were observed. In general, there was considerable similarity between black and white infants with respect to the frequency of specific neurological abnormalities, and apparent differences often tend to disappear when the data within birthweight groups are examined. (Table 15–1.)

Table 15-1. Summary Data for First Year Neurologic Abnormality

Condition	WHITE All Birthweights No.	%	Mean Bwt.	Under 2501 gm No.	%	Over 2500 gm No.	%	BLACK All Birthweights No.	%	Mean Bwt.	Under 2501 gm No.	%	Over 2500 gm No.	%
Cerebral spastic paresis														
Hemi – right	11	0.07	3203	1	0.09	10	0.06	6	0.03	2537	2	0.09	4	0.03
Hemi – left	4	0.02	3126	1	0.09	3	0.02	9	0.05	2687	4	0.18	5	0.03
Tetra	20	0.12	2929	5	0.47	15	0.10	47	0.26	2630	19	0.85	28	0.18
Para	7	0.04	2948	1	0.09	6	0.04	25	0.14	2860	4	0.18	21	0.13
Other	11	0.07	3088	1	0.09	10	0.06	20	0.11	3093	3	0.13	17	0.11
Hypotonia														
With deep tendon reflex	152	0.92	3107	23	2.17	129	0.83	71	0.39	2944	15	0.67	56	0.35
Without deep tendon reflex	21	0.13	3118	3	0.28	18	0.12	9	0.05	2838	3	0.13	6	0.04
Dyskinesia	35	0.21	3067	7	0.66	28	0.18	12	0.07	2698	4	0.18	8	0.05
Ataxia	7	0.04	3005	1	0.09	6	0.04	4	0.02	1878	3	0.13	1	0.01
Other motor disorders	147	0.89	3136	22	2.07	125	0.81	109	0.60	2916	23	1.02	86	0.54
Delayed development														
Motor	331	2.00	2982	68	6.41	263	1.70	384	2.12	2686	141	6.28	243	1.53
Mental	136	0.82	2865	37	3.49	99	0.64	226	1.25	2618	90	4.01	136	0.86
Regression in motor activity	2	0.01	3204	0	0	2	0.01	2	0.01	3530	0	0	2	0.01
Cord disease														
Spastic	1	0.01	2920	0	0	1	0.01	1	0.01	3118	0	0	1	0.01
Flaccid	4	0.02	3225	0	0	4	0.03	4	0.02	3012	1	0.04	3	0.02
No neurologic abnormality	15383	93.11	3300	915	86.24	14468	93.58	17007	93.85	3074	1982	88.32	15025	94.63
Total	16521	100.00	3291	1061	100.00	15460	100.00	18121	100.00	3063	2244	100.00	15877	100.00

Table 15-1. (Continued)

Condition	WHITE All Birthweights No.	%	Mean Bwt.	WHITE Under 2501 gm No.	%	WHITE Over 2500 gm No.	%	BLACK All Birthweights No.	%	Mean Bwt.	BLACK Under 2501 gm No.	%	BLACK Over 2500 gm No.	%
Visual impairment														
Bilateral (total)														
Ocular	3	0.02	2523	2	0.19	1	0.01	12	0.07	2637	5	0.22	7	0.04
Non-ocular	1	0.01	3714	0	0	1	0.01	1	0.01	3005	0	0	1	0.01
Unilateral (total)														
Ocular	1	0.01	2863	0	0	1	0.01	1	0.01	2410	1	0.04	0	0
Non-ocular	0	0	–	0	0	0	0	0	0	–	0	0	0	0
Bilateral (partial)														
Ocular	3	0.02	3288	0	0	3	0.02	10	0.06	2889	4	0.18	6	0.04
Non-ocular	3	0.02	2929	1	0.09	2	0.01	2	0.01	2892	0	0	2	0.01
Unilateral (partial)														
Ocular	1	0.01	2722	0	0	1	0.01	0	0	–	0	0	0	0
Non-ocular	0	0	–	0	0	0	0	0	0	–	0	0	0	0
Extra ocular movements														
Esotropia														
Unilateral	222	1.34	3242	18	1.70	204	1.32	110	0.61	2960	25	1.11	85	0.54
Bilateral	76	0.46	3132	12	1.13	64	0.41	42	0.23	2917	6	0.27	36	0.23
Alt. int. strabismus	131	0.79	3272	10	0.94	121	0.78	105	0.58	2962	19	0.85	86	0.54
Exotropia														
Unilateral	14	0.08	3100	3	0.28	11	0.07	5	0.03	2637	1	0.04	4	0.03
Bilateral	4	0.02	3097	0	0	4	0.03	5	0.03	3101	1	0.04	4	0.03
Alt. ext. strabismus	6	0.04	3378	0	0	6	0.04	6	0.03	2972	1	0.04	5	0.03
Other	31	0.19	3123	4	0.38	27	0.17	31	0.17	2915	7	0.31	24	0.15
No neurologic abnormality	15383	93.11	3300	915	86.24	14468	93.58	17007	93.85	3074	1982	88.32	15025	94.63
Total	16521	100.00	3291	1061	100.00	15460	100.00	18121	100.00	3063	2244	100.00	15877	100.00

Table 15–1. (Continued)

Condition	WHITE All Birthweights No.	%	Mean Bwt.	Under 2501 gm No.	%	Over 2500 gm No.	%	BLACK All Birthweights No.	%	Mean Bwt.	Under 2501 gm No.	%	Over 2500 gm No.	%
Nystagmus involvement														
Unilateral	4	0.02	3423	0	0	4	0.03	16	0.09	3028	3	0.13	13	0.08
Unilateral with gaze only	0	0	—	0	0	0	0	3	0.02	2750	1	0.04	2	0.01
Bilateral	25	0.15	3022	5	0.47	20	0.13	57	0.31	2990	9	0.40	48	0.30
Bilateral with gaze only	5	0.03	3453	0	0	5	0.03	19	0.10	2810	5	0.22	14	0.09
Cranial nerve abnormality														
Facial (VII)	38	0.23	3384	6	0.57	32	0.21	30	0.17	2932	6	0.27	24	0.15
Other	9	0.05	3137	1	0.09	8	0.05	12	0.07	3036	2	0.09	10	0.06
Hearing impairment	9	0.05	2756	2	0.19	7	0.05	20	0.11	2682	7	0.31	13	0.08
Peripheral nerve abnormality														
Brachial plexus	6	0.04	3789	1	0.09	5	0.03	9	0.05	4019	0	0	9	0.06
Other	6	0.04	3194	1	0.09	5	0.03	3	0.02	3440	1	0.04	2	0.01
Seizure states														
Generalized — only with fever and under 15 min. duration	67	0.41	3332	3	0.28	64	0.41	97	0.54	3066	12	0.53	85	0.54
Generalized — other	50	0.30	3268	3	0.28	47	0.30	66	0.36	2978	10	0.45	56	0.35
Focal motor	9	0.05	3355	1	0.09	8	0.05	22	0.12	3193	1	0.04	21	0.13
Infantile myoclonic seizures	12	0.07	3159	1	0.09	11	0.07	3	0.02	2731	1	0.04	2	0.01
Other	10	0.06	2991	1	0.09	9	0.06	16	0.09	2899	4	0.18	12	0.08
Coma	6	0.04	3157	0	0	6	0.04	3	0.02	3147	1	0.04	2	0.01
Other	33	0.20	3152	4	0.38	29	0.19	24	0.13	3146	3	0.13	21	0.13
No neurologic abnormality	15383	93.11	3300	915	86.24	14468	93.58	17007	93.85	3074	1982	88.32	15025	94.63
Total	16521	100.00	3291	1061	100.00	15460	100.00	18121	100.00	3063	2244	100.00	15877	100.00

Specific Motor Abnormalities. Because cerebral palsy was of particular interest in this study, special attention was paid to this diagnosis. The term cerebral spastic paresis was used to refer to upper motor neuron paresis of presumed cerebral origin, with hyperreflexia but not necessarily hypertonus at one year of age. A total of 53 white children and 107 black children were reported to have cerebral palsy of some type during the first year. The cases of cerebral palsy were further classified as described below.

Cerebral Spastic Hemiparesis. This category included children with any unilateral cerebral paresis of the type usually associated with involvement of the corticospinal tract. By one year, some cases were not obviously spastic and were manifest only by asymmetry of function and of automatisms, with the additional observation perhaps of less obvious degrees of hyperreflexia, stretch reflexes on passive movement, and the like.

There were 15 white and 15 black children for whom a diagnosis of hemiparesis was reported. Among the whites there was a predominance of right-sided hemiparesis (11 cases to 4 left-sided cases), which is in accord with the prevailing concept that involvement of the left cerebral hemisphere (with malfunction of the right side of the body) is more frequent than the right. However, among the blacks, the ratio of right- to left-sided signs was reversed (6 right-sided to 9 left-sided).

Cerebral Spastic Tetraparesis. This category included such diagnoses as spastic quadriplegia, tetraplegia, double hemiparesis, and diplegia. No distinction was made as to whether the upper extremities or the legs were more severely involved. Twenty white infants and forty-seven black infants were reported to have conditions that justified their inclusion in this group. The frequency in the blacks was twice that of the whites. A marked association with low birthweight was observed in both ethnic groups and very likely accounts, at least in part, for the overall difference in frequency observed between white and black children.

Cerebral Spastic Paraparesis. This diagnostic category included children with neurological signs limited to the lower extremities only, without evidence of malfunction, such as hyperreflexia in the upper extremities. There were more cases reported among black infants [25] as compared with white infants [7]. Rather surprisingly, birthweight did not appear to be a major factor. The mean birthweight for both white and black babies was only slightly lower for children with the diagnosis.

Other. There was a group of cerebral palsies designated "other." Eleven white and twenty black babies were reported to have diagnoses in this category, which included monoplegias and other spastic conditions that did not fit the criteria for the more specific diagnoses listed above.

Comment. Cerebral palsy, a central issue in the NCPP, is the subject of detailed investigations that will be reported as they are completed.

Hypotonia, Dyskinesia, Ataxia, and Other Motor Disorders. As indicated in the accompanying tables, disorders of motor function, particularly hypotonia, were reported in 173 (1 percent) white and 80 (0.4 percent) black infants.

Delayed Development. Delayed development, either motor or mental or both, was reported with equal frequency in both white and black infants. The diagnostic category of delayed motor development was used to report the child with significant delay in the acquistion of "developmental milestones," regardless of the presence or absence of a diagnosis of cerebral palsy. For motor delay the frequency was approximately 2 percent for infants of each race. There was, as expected, a strong relationship with low birthweight. In the whites, 6.4 percent, and in the blacks, 6.3 percent of low-birthweight infants were reported to have delayed motor development.

Delayed mental development was the criterion used for the reporting of children with retardation in mental functioning for age. Because the array of mental skills that can be measured in young infants is very limited, a definite diagnosis in this area required a fairly marked degree of retardation. Most children thought to have delayed mental development were reported as suspct at this age. Slightly less than 1 percent of white children and slightly more than 1 percent of black children received this diagnosis. A strong relationship with birthweight was observed.

Spinal Cord Disease. This diagnostic category included conditions resulting from primary lesions in the spinal cord. For example, meningomyelocele, myelodysplasia, diastematomyelia, Werdnig–Hoffmann disease, and other specific cord lesions were included. These conditions were rarely encountered in the young children. Only 5 white and 5 black infants were reported to have primary cord lesions.

Nystagmus. This abnormality was related to birthweight, occurring approximately five times more frequently among the larger babies. Among the 34 white babies reported to have nystagmus, only 5 weighed 2500 grams or less at birth, and among the 95 black infants, 18 were in the low-weight category.

Nystagmus occurred in one eye only in 4 white and 19 black infants.

Cranial Nerve Abnormalities. Abnormalities of cranial nerves were reported in 47 white and 42 black infants. As expected, most infants with the condition weighed more than 2500 grams at birth; 40 of the 47 whites and 34 of the 42 blacks.

Most of the cranial nerve abnormalities reported involved the facial nerve; among whites, 38 facial nerve palsies were reported, as compared with 9 cases involving other nerves. Among blacks, 30 of the 42 cases reported involved the facial nerve.

Peripheral Nerve Abnormality. Abnormalities of peripheral nerves were infrequently reported after the newborn period. Six brachial plexus nerve injuries were reported at one year in whites (average birthweight 3789 grams) and 9 black infants (average birthweight 4019 grams). Only one white infant and no black infants with birthweight of 2500 grams or less were reported at one year to have brachial palsy.

Other peripheral nerve injuries were also infrequent.

Seizure States. Definite seizure disorders were reported with some frequency. Among whites, 148, and among blacks, 204 were reported. Seizure disorders were strongly related to birthweight and occurred very infrequently among low-weight infants.

Most seizure disorders were generalized in their manifestations (117 in whites and 163 in blacks). However, more than 50 percent of these were associated with fever and were of less than 15-minutes duration.

Seizure disorders, an important neurological disability, are the subject of an intensive investigation within the NCPP data and will be the subject of a separate report.

Eye Conditions

A number of ophthalmological conditions are tabulated with the neurological abnormalities in Table 15–1. Others are listed under eye conditions in Table 15–2.

Twelve white and 26 black infants were reported to be visually impaired, of whom 4 whites and 13 blacks were totally blind.

As may be seen in Table 15–1, abnormalities of extraocular movements were quite frequently reported, as was to be expected in this age group.

Chorioretinitis was reported in only 3 white and 4 black infants. Cataracts were more frequent, occurring in 12 white and 15 black infants, reflecting, at least in part, the effect of the rubella epidemic of 1963–64. Retrolental fibroplasia was not reported at all among white infants. It was reported only twice among blacks, and in one of these infants, when serological data became available, it was clearly a misdiagnosis. The child in all probability had congenital toxoplasmosis.

Other noninfectious eye conditions were reported in 224 white and 139 black children. Table 15–3 shows a further breakdown of selected abnormalities within this group.

Ear Conditions

Like eye problems, ear conditions were reported with low frequency in this age group. (Table 15–4.) The difference in frequency of branchial cleft anomalies, by race, is a well-recognized fact and the difference observed here, 25 in whites, 251 in black infants, may reflect either an unusual frequency of the condition in the study population of one participating institution or particular interest among examiners there.

Fifty-eight white and 29 black children were reported to have perforations of the ear drum. Because of the difficulties involved in evaluating historical data with respect to upper respiratory infections, with or without otitis media, these data have not been tabulated. It is well known that conductive hearing losses may accompany respiratory infections with middle-ear involvement. That so many young infants were reported to have perforated drums is a matter of concern. This is an age when the learning of language is proceeding at a rapid rate and adequate hearing is important.

Under "Neurological Abnormality," Table 15–1, 9 white and 20 black infants were reported to have definite hearing impairments. We do not know at this stage of the analysis whether these were conductive or neurosensory losses. Subsequent follow-up, with specific evaluation of speech, language, and hearing will have pinpointed these diagnoses more precisely.

Table 15-2. Summary Data for First Year Eye Conditions

Condition	WHITE							BLACK						
	All Birthweights			Under 2501 gm		Over 2500 gm		All Birthweights			Under 2501 gm		Over 2500 gm	
	No.	%	Mean Bwt.	No.	%	No.	%	No.	%	Mean Bwt.	No.	%	No.	%
Chorioretinitis	3	0.02	2722	1	0.09	2	0.01	4	0.02	2672	2	0.09	2	0.01
Retrolental fibroplasia	0	0	-	0	0	0	0	2	0.01	1078	2	0.09	0	0
Cataract	12	0.07	2844	4	0.38	8	0.05	15	0.08	2502	9	0.40	6	0.04
Corneal opacity	3	0.02	2958	0	0	3	0.02	8	0.04	2998	3	0.13	5	0.03
Microphthalmia	1	0.01	2410	1	0.09	0	0	4	0.02	2332	3	0.13	1	0.01
Other, non-infectious	224	1.36	3190	23	2.17	201	1.30	139	0.77	3015	22	0.98	117	0.74
No eye conditions	16285	98.57	3292	1034	97.46	15251	98.65	17963	99.13	3064	2212	98.57	15751	99.21
Total	16521	100.00	3291	1061	100.00	15460	100.00	18121	100.00	3063	2244	100.00	15877	100.00

Table 15-3. Selected Conditions Included in Other Non-Infectious Eye Conditions at One Year by Race

Condition	WHITE	BLACK
Megalocornea	0	2
Optic atrophy	1	2
Retinal hemorrhage	1	1
Wedge defect-superior palpebra	0	1
Exophthalmos, proptosis	2	9
Removal of eye	0	1
Synechiae	2	2
Anisocoria	16	0
Ptosis	19	30
Nasolacrimal duct stenosis	31	17
Coloboma	4	2
Glaucoma	2	5
Detached retina	1	0
Aniridia	0	1

SELECTED CONDITIONS DURING FIRST YEAR 269

Table 15-4. Summary Data for First Year Ear Conditions

| | WHITE | | | | | | | BLACK | | | | | | |
| | All Birthweights | | | Under 2501 gm | | Over 2500 gm | | All Birthweights | | | Under 2501 gm | | Over 2500 gm | |
Condition	No.	%	Mean Bwt.	No.	%	No.	%	No.	%	Mean Bwt.	No.	%	No.	%
Low-set ears	18	0.11	2987	2	0.19	16	0.10	41	0.23	3040	4	0.18	37	0.23
Deformed ear pinna	72	0.44	3250	3	0.28	69	0.45	79	0.44	3080	9	0.40	70	0.44
Branchial cleft anomaly	25	0.15	3314	3	0.28	22	0.14	251	1.39	3010	37	1.65	214	1.35
Perforated ear drum	58	0.35	3267	3	0.28	55	0.36	29	0.16	3180	1	0.04	28	0.18
Other, non-infectious	44	0.27	3336	2	0.19	42	0.27	39	0.22	2982	6	0.27	33	0.21
No ear condition	16322	98.80	3291	1047	98.68	15275	98.80	17708	97.72	3064	2192	97.68	15516	97.73
Total	16521	100.00	3291	1061	100.00	15460	100.00	18121	100.00	3063	2244	100.00	15877	100.00

Other Central Nervous System Conditions

A variety of skeletal conditions were reported in this section. Their frequency was approximately the same for children of both races, being slightly less than 3 percent in each. (Table 15–5.)

Most of the abnormalities reported concerned *skull shape*. Among white infants 2.2 percent and among black infants 1.5 percent were reported to have abnormally shaped skulls. It is of interest to note that abnormally shaped skulls were almost as frequent among the larger babies as among the smaller.

Pilonidal sinus was reported in 35 white and 20 black babies.

Meningomyelocele (meningocele) was diagnosed very infrequently after the newborn period, being reported for only 6 white and 7 black infants.

Atypical Behavior

This category included a number of behaviors sufficiently deviant from the normal pattern to be considered definitely abnormal and likely to be related to neurological malfunction. The frequency of the various types of abnormal behavior reported in Table 15–6 was essentially similar between whites and blacks. Breathholding without unconsciousness was the most frequent abnormality reported in the behavioral area, occurring in 147 (0.9 percent) of white and 128 (0.7 percent) of black babies.

No abnormalities of behavior were reported in 98 percent of infants of both races.

Musculoskeletal Abnormality

A variety of musculoskeletal conditions were reported in approximately 5 percent of both white and black infants during the first year (Table 15–7).

Metatarsus adductus was the most frequent abnormality reported in this category, occurring in approximately 1.5 percent of white and 2.5 percent of black children. It was not related to birthweight.

Congenital dislocation or dysplasia of the hip was reported in 59 white and only 9 black children, and, on the other hand, *polydactyly* was reported in 50 black but only 9 white children.

Thoracic Conditions

Anomaly of the diaphragm was very unusual, occurring in one of the 16,521 white infants and two of the 18,121 black infants. Pectus excavatum was reported in 73 (0.44 percent) white infants and only 7 (0.04 percent) black babies. The mean birthweight of 3451 grams for whites with the condition was substantially greater than the 3290 gram average of those with no thoracic abnormality, indicating that this condition represents a true developmental abnormality and is not related to low birthweight and immaturity of the thoracic cage. (Table 15–8.)

Upper Respiratory Tract and Mouth Conditions

As in other sections, infectious processes are summarized later in this chapter.

Cleft malformations were reported more frequently among white infants [66]

Table 15-5. Summary Data for First Year
Other Central Nervous System Conditions

Condition	WHITE							BLACK						
	All Birthweights			Under 2501 gm		Over 2500 gm		All Birthweights			Under 2501 gm		Over 2500 gm	
	No.	%	Mean Bwt.	No.	%	No.	%	No.	%	Mean Bwt.	No.	%	No.	%
Macrocephaly	18	0.11	3465	1	0.09	17	0.11	11	0.06	3492	0	0	11	0.07
Microcephaly	23	0.14	2644	9	0.85	14	0.09	35	0.19	2390	20	0.89	15	0.09
Hydranencephaly	0	0	–	0	0	0	0	1	0.01	3090	0	0	1	0.01
Hydrocephaly	18	0.11	3304	1	0.09	17	0.11	21	0.12	2917	4	0.18	17	0.11
Craniosynostosis	11	0.07	3051	2	0.19	9	0.06	6	0.03	2882	1	0.04	5	0.03
Other abnormal shape of skull	359	2.17	3192	34	3.20	325	2.10	272	1.50	2983	45	2.01	227	1.43
Porencephaly	1	0.01	2778	0	0	1	0.01	0	0	–	0	0	0	0
Encephalocele	0	0	–	0	0	0	0	0	0	–	0	0	0	0
Meningomyelocele/meningocele	6	0.04	3062	1	0.09	5	0.03	7	0.04	2677	3	0.13	4	0.03
Pilonidal sinus	35	0.21	3403	3	0.28	32	0.21	20	0.11	2756	7	0.31	13	0.08
Other midline sinuses	1	0.01	2948	0	0	1	0.01	3	0.02	2637	2	0.09	1	0.01
Subdural hematoma or effusion	12	0.07	3170	2	0.19	10	0.06	19	0.10	3135	2	0.09	17	0.11
Other intracranial hemorrhage	3	0.02	2977	0	0	3	0.02	5	0.03	2829	1	0.04	4	0.03
Other	46	0.28	2956	10	0.94	36	0.23	40	0.22	3104	1	0.04	39	0.25
No other CNS conditions	16038	97.08	3293	1008	95.00	15030	97.22	17717	97.77	3065	2168	96.61	15549	97.73
Total	16521	100.00	3291	1061	100.00	15460	100.00	18121	100.00	3063	2244	100.00	15877	100.00

Table 15-6. Summary Data for First Year
Atypical Behavior

| | WHITE | | | | | | | BLACK | | | | | | |
| Condition | All Birthweights | | | Under 2501 gm | | Over 2500 gm | | All Birthweights | | | Under 2501 gm | | Over 2500 gm | |
	No.	%	Mean Bwt.	No.	%	No.	%	No.	%	Mean Bwt.	No.	%	No.	%
Maladaptive responses	18	0.11	3221	2	0.10	16	0.10	9	0.05	2948	1	0.04	8	0.05
Inappropriate social behavior for age	101	0.61	3049	20	1.89	81	0.52	118	0.65	2916	29	1.29	89	0.56
Failure to form rhythmic patterns	20	0.12	3114	4	0.38	16	0.10	26	0.14	3027	2	0.09	24	0.15
Disruption of rhythmic patterns	7	0.04	3345	0	0	7	0.05	26	0.14	3243	1	0.04	25	0.16
Regression in behavior	4	0.02	3090	0	0	4	0.03	2	0.01	3317	0	0	2	0.01
Breath holding with unconsciousness	32	0.19	3172	3	0.28	29	0.19	11	0.06	2701	5	0.22	6	0.04
Breath holding without unconsciousness	147	0.89	3242	15	1.41	132	0.85	128	0.71	3047	18	0.80	110	0.69
Hyper-reactivity to sensory stimuli	18	0.11	3207	2	0.19	16	0.10	8	0.04	3048	2	0.09	6	0.04
Apathy	16	0.10	3069	3	0.28	13	0.08	22	0.12	2710	7	0.31	15	0.09
Other	5	0.03	3317	0	0	5	0.03	15	0.08	2945	1	0.04	14	0.09
No atypical behavior	16184	97.96	3293	1016	95.76	15168	98.11	17791	98.18	3064	2187	97.46	15604	98.28
Total	16521	100.00	3291	1061	100.00	15460	100.00	18121	100.00	3063	2244	100.00	15877	100.00

Table 15-7. Summary Data for First Year
Musculoskeletal Abnormality

	WHITE							BLACK						
	All Birthweights			Under 2501 gm		Over 2500 gm		All Birthweights			Under 2501 gm		Over 2500 gm	
Condition	No.	%	Mean Bwt.	No.	%	No.	%	No.	%	Mean Bwt.	No.	%	No.	%
Vertebral abnormality	9	0.05	2898	1	0.09	8	0.05	8	0.04	2824	4	0.18	4	0.03
Talipes equinovarus	30	0.18	3265	2	0.19	28	0.18	50	0.28	3016	9	0.40	41	0.26
Metatarsus adductus	251	1.52	3373	11	1.04	240	1.55	450	2.48	3121	51	2.27	399	2.51
Talipes calcaneo valgus	39	0.24	3114	7	0.66	32	0.21	83	0.46	3021	15	0.67	68	0.43
Congenital dislocation or dysplasia of the hip	59	0.36	3295	5	0.47	54	0.35	9	0.05	3122	0	0	9	0.06
Absence or hypoplasia of extremity or part	23	0.14	2874	5	0.47	18	0.12	15	0.08	3258	0	0	15	0.09
Polydactyly	9	0.05	3213	1	0.09	8	0.05	50	0.28	3171	2	0.09	48	0.30
Syndactyly	58	0.35	3161	7	0.66	51	0.33	19	0.10	3172	2	0.09	17	0.11
Torticollis	31	0.19	3175	2	0.19	29	0.19	20	0.11	2909	4	0.18	16	0.10
Arthrogryposis multiplex	1	0.01	3203	0	0	1	0.01	0	0	–	0	0	0	0
Other, non-infectious	370	2.24	3212	36	3.39	334	2.16	501	2.76	3073	67	2.99	434	2.73
No musculoskeletal abn.	15738	95.26	3292	999	94.16	14739	95.34	17075	94.23	3062	2110	94.03	14965	94.26
Total	16521	100.00	3291	1061	100.00	15460	100.00	18121	100.00	3063	2244	100.00	15877	100.00

than black [26], with a ratio of greater than 2:1. Abnormalities of the teeth were more frequent in blacks [126] as compared with whites [43]. (Table 15–9.)

Cleft defects are discussed in greater detail in Chapter 16.

Lower Respiratory Tract Abnormality

Reports of noninfectious conditions of the lower respiratory tract were infrequent (Table 15–10). Asthma was the most common, with 32 cases among whites and 49 among blacks.

Cardiovascular Conditions

The frequency of cardiac abnormalities reported during the first year is less than 1 percent in children of both races (Table 15–11). Findings with respect to the frequency of congenital heart disease (CHD) in the NCPP have been reported in some detail by Mitchell et al. (1,2). They identified 457 cases of congenital heart disease among 56,109 study children whose records were examined. The frequency of cardiac malformation per 1000 births was 8.14 for white infants and 8.30 for black. These rates are not only similar by race but are in accord with those reported in this volume.

In the studies by Mitchell and her colleagues, 93 percent of the infants classified as having definite CHD had been examined by a pediatric cardiologist. The average period of follow-up for the 272 survivors was 3 years. Among the 457 infants with cardiac malformations, 37 were stillborn, 78 died during the neonatal period, and an additional 50 failed to survive the first year. Among the 185 infants who died, 86 (46 percent) had additional, i.e., extra cardiac, malformations. With respect to the cardiac anomalies, ventricular septal defect (VSD) was by far the most common, occurring in 133 cases. Isolated pulmonic stenosis (PS) with 37 cases, isolated patent ductus arteriosus (PDA) with 35 cases, and auricular septal defect secundum (ASD) with 34 cases were next most frequent. A sizable variety of other less frequent abnormalities was described. Tetralogy of Fallot, for example, occurred in only 16 patients, 3.5 percent of those with cardiac malformations. Of the 16 patients with tetralogy, 5 died, but none as a result of the cardiac defect. Of the 11 survivors, 6 were cyanotic from birth, while the other 5 evolved gradually into clinically recognizable tetralogy; all five had previously been diagnosed as having VSD or PDA.

Possible genetic relationships were examined by Mitchell and colleagues. Among 443 of the children identified with CHD, 4 mothers also had CHD. Among 80 mothers with a diagnosis of CHD, 4 (5 percent) had infants with CHD. Maternal age (older mothers, thirty-five years and above), maternal diabetes, twinning, and Down's syndrome were identified as risk factors with respect to the occurrence of CHD in the infants.

Comparisons between findings reported on the newborn and one-year diagnostic summaries are presented in Chapter 16.

Table 15-8. Summary Data for First Year Thoracic Conditions

	WHITE							BLACK						
Condition	All Birthweights			Under 2501 gm		Over 2500 gm		All Birthweights			Under 2501 gm		Over 2500 gm	
	No.	%	Mean Bwt.	No.	%	No.	%	No.	%	Mean Bwt.	No.	%	No.	%
Anomaly of diaphragm	1	0.01	2920	0	0	1	0.01	2	0.01	3034	1	0.04	1	0.01
Anomaly of ribs	5	0.03	3748	0	0	5	0.03	1	0.01	2325	1	0.04	0	0
Pectus excavatum	73	0.44	3451	3	0.28	70	0.45	7	0.04	2997	1	0.04	6	0.04
Pigeon breast	5	0.03	3646	0	0	5	0.03	4	0.02	3048	1	0.04	3	0.02
Other	21	0.13	3077	3	0.28	18	0.12	22	0.12	3094	4	0.18	18	0.11
No thoracic conditions	16418	99.38	3290	1055	99.43	15363	99.37	18085	99.80	3063	2236	99.64	15849	99.82
Total	16521	100.00	3291	1061	100.00	15460	100.00	18121	100.00	3063	2244	100.00	15877	100.00

Table 15-9. Summary Data for First Year Upper Respiratory Tract and Mouth Conditions

	WHITE							BLACK						
Condition	All Birthweights			Under 2501 gm		Over 2500 gm		All Birthweights			Under 2501 gm		Over 2500 gm	
	No.	%	Mean Bwt.	No.	%	No.	%	No.	%	Mean Bwt.	No.	%	No.	%
Cleft palate	19	0.12	3224	3	0.28	16	0.10	11	0.06	2601	4	0.18	7	0.04
Cleft uvula	22	0.13	3189	1	0.09	21	0.14	8	0.04	3058	2	0.09	6	0.04
Cleft lip	19	0.12	3172	2	0.19	17	0.11	6	0.03	2916	2	0.09	4	0.03
Cleft gum	6	0.04	3544	0	0	6	0.04	1	0.01	3062	0	0	1	0.01
Micrognathia	18	0.11	3048	1	0.09	17	0.11	4	0.02	2332	2	0.09	2	0.01
Malformation of the epiglottis and larynx	8	0.05	3284	0	0	8	0.05	11	0.06	2652	3	0.13	8	0.05
Abnormality of teeth	43	0.26	3235	3	0.28	40	0.26	126	0.70	2815	32	1.43	94	0.59
Other, non-infectious	81	0.49	3180	8	0.75	73	0.47	61	0.34	2939	12	0.53	49	0.31
No upper respiratory tract/mouth conditions	16339	98.90	3292	1045	98.49	15294	98.93	17902	98.79	3066	2191	97.64	15711	98.95
Total	16521	100.00	3291	1061	100.00	15460	100.00	18121	100.00	3063	2244	100.00	15877	100.00

Table 15-10. Summary Data for First Year
Lower Respiratory Tract Abnormality

| | WHITE | | | | | | | BLACK | | | | | | |
| | All Birthweights | | | Under 2501 gm | | Over 2500 gm | | All Birthweights | | | Under 2501 gm | | Over 2500 gm | |
Condition	No.	%	Mean Bwt.	No.	%	No.	%	No.	%	Mean Bwt.	No.	%	No.	%
Asthma	32	0.19	3364	1	0.09	31	0.20	49	0.27	2967	7	0.31	42	0.26
Emphysema	6	0.04	3137	1	0.09	5	0.03	4	0.02	2495	2	0.09	2	0.01
Pneumothorax	2	0.01	2878	1	0.09	1	0.01	3	0.02	2646	1	0.04	2	0.01
Anomaly of lung	5	0.03	2926	1	0.09	4	0.03	4	0.02	3048	1	0.04	3	0.02
Other, non-infectious	20	0.12	3182	5	0.47	15	0.10	19	0.10	2722	5	0.22	14	0.09
No lower resp. tract abn.	16461	99.64	3291	1054	99.34	15407	99.66	18048	99.60	3064	2231	99.42	15817	99.02
Total	16521	100.00	3291	1061	100.00	15460	100.00	18121	100.00	3063	2244	100.00	15877	100.00

Table 15-11. Summary Data for First Year
Cardiovascular Conditions

| | WHITE | | | | | | | BLACK | | | | | | |
| | All Birthweights | | | Under 2501 gm | | Over 2500 gm | | All Birthweights | | | Under 2501 gm | | Over 2500 gm | |
Condition	No.	%	Mean Bwt.	No.	%	No.	%	No.	%	Mean Bwt.	No.	%	No.	%
Acyanotic CHD	53	0.32	2993	9	0.85	44	0.28	76	0.42	2864	21	0.94	55	0.35
Cyanotic CHD	19	0.12	3245	2	0.19	17	0.11	5	0.03	2620	3	0.13	2	0.01
Fibroelastosis	1	0.01	4137	0	0	1	0.01	2	0.01	2693	1	0.04	1	0.01
Disorders of rhythm	5	0.03	3481	0	0	5	0.03	11	0.06	2750	3	0.13	8	0.05
Disorders of rate	12	0.07	3298	5	0.47	12	0.08	18	0.10	2800	7	0.31	11	0.07
Cardiac enlargement	29	0.18	2980	3	0.28	24	0.16	19	0.10	2801	8	0.36	11	0.07
Decompensation	22	0.13	3003	0	0	19	0.12	22	0.12	2785	9	0.40	13	0.08
Severe cyanotic episodes	4	0.02	3097			4	0.03	2	0.01	1942	2	0.09	0	0
Specific C-V diagnosis	55	0.33	3071	10	0.94	45	0.29	54	0.30	2838	16	0.71	38	0.24
Other	21	0.13	3241	1	0.09	20	0.13	13	0.07	2892	2	0.09	11	0.07
No cardiovascular cond.	16407	99.31	3292	1046	98.59	15361	99.36	17972	99.18	3065	2202	98.13	15770	99.33
Total	16521	100.00	3291	1061	100.00	15460	100.00	18121	100.00	3063	2244	100.00	15877	100.00

Alimentary Tract Conditions

While a large variety of gastrointestinal diagnoses were reported on PED–12, individually they were of infrequent occurrence (Table 15–12). Hernias (of all types) occurred in 248 (1.5 percent) of white and 296 (1.6 percent) of black infants. Pyloric stenosis, as expected, occurred in more whites than blacks; 63 white and only 16 black infants had this condition.

Abnormality of Liver, Bile Ducts, and Spleen

Abnormalities of these types were rare, though slightly more common among whites than blacks (Table 15–13). Eighteen white and 8 black infants experienced jaundice that persisted beyond the new-born period. Only 2 white and 11 black infants were reported to have jaundice acquired later during the first year.

Genitourinary Conditions

Conditions in this category were infrequent in both white and black infants. Bladder outflow or urethral obstruction were reported in 12 white and 30 black children. Upper tract obstruction, hydroureter or hydronephrosis, and cystic kidney were very rare. (Table 15–14.)

Hematological Conditions

As was to be expected, the frequency of hematological problems was higher among black infants than among the white (Table 15–15). In the group of hemoglobinopathies, 46 (0.25 percent) black babies were reported to be affected, as compared with only 2 (0.01 percent) whites. A twofold difference was observed, with more black babies having severe (Hb under 5 gms%) and moderate anemias (Hb 5–8 gms%), both iron deficiency and other, than white infants. Furthermore, the anemias may well have been underreported, as the diagnosis was made on the basis of clinical indication rather than by routine screening of infants.

Skin Conditions and Malformations

Abnormalities related to the skin were commonly reported in children of both races (8.65 percent of the whites and 7.51 percent of the blacks). There appeared to be no particular relationship with birthweight. Hemangiomas appeared to be more frequent among white infants and café au lait spots and eczema more commonly reported among blacks (Table 15–16.)

Neoplastic Disease

Definite neoplastic conditions occurred during the first year in 45 white and 19 black children. While these are small frequencies (0.3 percent and 0.1 percent, respectively) they represent difficult and serious problems. (Table 15–17.)

Syndromes

Most of the syndromes listed in Table 15–18 were rare. However, mongolism occurred in 18 white and 13 black infants. Failure to thrive, while not a classical

Table 15–12. Summary Data for First Year Alimentary Tract Conditions

Condition	WHITE							BLACK						
	All Birthweights			Under 2501 gm		Over 2500 gm		All Birthweights			Under 2501 gm		Over 2500 gm	
	No.	%	Mean Bwt.	No.	%	No.	%	No.	%	Mean Bwt.	No.	%	No.	%
Hernia	248	1.50	3052	48	4.52	200	1.29	296	1.63	2847	77	3.43	219	1.38
Volvulus	2	0.01	3629	0	0	2	0.01	2	0.01	3090	0	0	2	0.01
Intussusception	7	0.04	3410	0	0	7	0.05	5	0.03	3357	0	0	5	0.03
Persistent vomiting	43	0.26	3096	5	0.47	38	0.25	20	0.11	2997	4	0.18	16	0.10
Megacolon	6	0.04	3180	0	0	6	0.04	1	0.01	2750	0	0	1	0.01
Pyloric stenosis	63	0.38	3280	5	0.47	58	0.38	16	0.09	2934	5	0.22	11	0.07
Visceral perforation	2	0.01	3742	0	0	2	0.01	1	0.01	3317	0	0	1	0.01
Malrotation	2	0.01	3601	0	0	2	0.01	3	0.02	3062	0	0	3	0.02
Intestinal obstruction	1	0.01	3175	0	0	1	0.01	7	0.04	3021	1	0.04	6	0.04
Chalasia	3	0.02	3024	0	0	3	0.02	2	0.01	2977	1	0.04	1	0.01
Other, non-infectious	66	0.40	3203	5	0.47	61	0.39	57	0.31	3072	12	0.53	45	0.28
No alimentary tract cond.	16107	97.49	3295	1000	94.25	15107	97.72	17730	97.84	3067	2146	95.63	15584	98.15
Total	16521	100.00	3291	1061	100.00	15460	100.00	18121	100.00	3063	2244	100.00	15877	100.00

Table 15-13. Summary Data for First Year
Abnormality of Liver, Bile Ducts and/or Spleen

| | WHITE | | | | | | | BLACK | | | | | | |
| | All Birthweights | | | Under 2501 gm | | Over 2500 gm | | All Birthweights | | | Under 2501 gm | | Over 2500 gm | |
Condition	No.	%	Mean Bwt.	No.	%	No.	%	No.	%	Mean Bwt.	No.	%	No.	%
Biliary atresia	3	0.02	2882	1	0.09	2	0.01	1	0.01	2863	0	0	1	0.01
Jaundice														
Persistent beyond nursery period	18	0.11	3079	3	0.28	15	0.10	8	0.04	2647	4	0.18	4	0.03
Acquired after nursery period	2	0.01	3048	0	0	2	0.01	11	0.06	2935	2	0.09	9	0.06
Other, non-infectious	116	0.70	3211	12	1.13	104	0.67	57	0.31	3032	10	0.45	47	0.30
No liver, bile ducts or spleen abnormality	16385	99.18	3291	1047	98.68	15338	99.21	18049	99.60	3063	2229	99.33	15820	99.64
Total	16521	100.00	3291	1061	100.00	15460	100.00	18121	100.00	3063	2244	100.00	15877	100.00

Table 15-14. Summary Data for First Year
Genitourinary Conditions

| | WHITE | | | | | | | BLACK | | | | | | |
| | All Birthweights | | | Under 2501 gm | | Over 2500 gm | | All Birthweights | | | Under 2501 gm | | Over 2500 gm | |
Condition	No.	%	Mean Bwt.	No.	%	No.	%	No.	%	Mean Bwt.	No.	%	No.	%
Bladder outflow or urethral obstruction	12	0.07	3220	2	0.19	10	0.06	30	0.17	3122	3	0.13	27	0.17
Upper tract obstruction, hydronephrosis or hydroureter	5	0.03	3073	2	0.19	3	0.02	3	0.02	3071	0	0	3	0.02
Cystic kidney	2	0.01	2552	1	0.09	1	0.01	2	0.01	3345	0	0	2	0.01
Other, non-infectious	41	0.25	3093	11	1.04	30	0.19	30	0.17	3104	4	0.18	26	0.16
No genitourinary abn.	16470	99.69	3291	1049	98.87	15421	99.75	18056	99.64	3063	2237	99.69	15819	99.63
Total	16521	100.00	3291	1061	100.00	15460	100.00	18121	100.00	3063	2244	100.00	15877	100.00

Table 15-15. Summary Data for First Year Hematologic Conditions

Condition	WHITE							BLACK						
	All Birthweights			Under 2501 gm		Over 2500 gm		All Birthweights			Under 2501 gm		Over 2500 gm	
	No.	%	Mean Bwt.	No.	%	No.	%	No.	%	Mean Bwt.	No.	%	No.	%
Hemoglobinopathy	2	0.01	1970	2	0.19	0	0	46	0.25	2955	8	0.36	38	0.24
Hemolytic disease														
Congenital	5	0.03	3090	0	0	5	0.03	7	0.04	3074	1	0.04	6	0.04
Acquired	1	0.01	4111	0	0	1	0.01	2	0.01	3416	0	0	2	0.01
Coagulation defect	3	0.02	3279	0	0	3	0.02	5	0.03	2767	1	0.04	4	0.03
Major hemorrhage	10	0.06	3399	1	0.09	9	0.06	4	0.02	2771	1	0.04	3	0.02
Anemia, under 5 gm %														
Iron deficiency	11	0.07	3335	1	0.09	10	0.06	16	0.09	2658	7	0.31	9	0.06
Other	2	0.01	2807	1	0.09	1	0.01	8	0.04	3108	2	0.09	6	0.04
Anemia, 5–8 gm %														
Iron deficiency	59	0.36	2924	14	1.32	45	0.29	159	0.88	2664	50	2.23	109	0.69
Other	21	0.13	2931	6	0.57	15	0.10	49	0.27	2699	16	0.71	33	0.21
Other	17	0.10	3075	1	0.09	16	0.10	38	0.21	3030	4	0.18	34	0.21
No hematologic cond.	16399	99.26	3293	1035	97.55	15364	99.38	17810	98.28	3068	2160	96.26	15650	98.57
Total	16521	100.00	3291	1061	100.00	15460	100.00	18121	100.00	3063	2244	100.00	15877	100.00

Table 15-16. Summary Data for First Year Skin Conditions and Malformations

	WHITE							BLACK						
	All Birthweights			Under 2501 gm		Over 2500 gm		All Birthweights			Under 2501 gm		Over 2500 gm	
Condition	No.	%	Mean Bwt.	No.	%	No.	%	No.	%	Mean Bwt.	No.	%	No.	%
Portwine hemangioma	168	1.02	3284	10	0.94	158	1.02	45	0.25	2765	7	0.31	38	0.24
Strawberry hemangioma	431	2.61	3230	36	3.39	395	2.55	111	0.61	2894	25	1.11	86	0.54
Cavernous hemangioma	171	1.04	3249	16	1.51	155	1.00	80	0.44	3130	11	0.49	69	0.43
Hairy pigmented nevus	11	0.07	3237	1	0.09	10	0.06	7	0.04	3082	1	0.04	6	0.04
Pigmented nevus	47	0.28	3328	0	0	47	0.30	113	0.62	3195	9	0.40	104	0.66
Lymphangioma	3	0.02	3525	0	0	3	0.02	2	0.01	3544	0	0	2	0.01
Café au lait spots	64	0.39	3334	5	0.47	59	0.38	209	1.15	3099	20	0.87	189	1.19
Eczema	271	1.64	3385	11	1.04	260	1.68	343	1.89	3172	31	1.38	312	1.97
Other, non-infectious	314	1.90	3286	19	1.79	295	1.91	508	2.80	3079	62	2.76	446	2.81
No skin conditions	15092	91.35	3291	970	91.42	14122	91.35	16761	92.49	3060	2082	92.78	14679	92.45
Total	16521	100.00	3291	1061	100.00	15460	100.00	18121	100.00	3063	2244	100.00	15877	100.00

Table 15-17. Summary Data for First Year Neoplastic Disease and/or Other Tumors

	WHITE							BLACK						
	All Birthweights			Under 2501 gm		Over 2500 gm		All Birthweights			Under 2501 gm		Over 2500 gm	
Condition	No.	%	Mean Bwt.	No.	%	No.	%	No.	%	Mean Bwt.	No.	%	No.	%
Specified type and organ	45	0.27	3329	2	0.19	43	0.28	19	0.10	3002	2	0.09	17	0.11
No neo. dis./other tumors	16476	99.73	3290	1059	99.81	15417	99.72	18102	99.90	3063	2242	99.91	15860	99.89
Total	16521	100.00	3291	1061	100.00	15460	100.00	18121	100.00	3063	2244	100.00	15877	100.00

diagnostic entity, was reported here only if the underlying etiology could not be identified. This condition was more common than the others in the group, occurring in 92 (0.56 percent) of the white and 169 (0.93 percent) of the black babies.

Other Endocrine and Metabolic Disease

Conditions listed in Table 15–19 were remarkable for their rarity. Hypothyroidism was reported in only 2 white infants and one black. Fibrocystic disease of the pancreas occurred in 7 white infants and no black babies.

Infection and Inflammation

Reported in this section were a variety of definite, acute and chronic infections and specific childhood diseases occurring during the first year, exclusive of the neonatal period. (Table 15–20.) Infections were reported in 14.82 percent of the white and 16.59 percent of the black children.

Septicemia and *central nervous system infections* were strikingly more frequent among blacks than whites. There were 13 cases of septicemia among whites, 28 among blacks. There were 19 cases of bacterial and 7 nonbacterial meningitis among whites, as compared with 59 and 14, respectively, among blacks.

Pneumonia, also, was reported twice as frequently among blacks, 888 cases, as compared with 434 among whites. *Severe croup*, on the other hand, was diagnosed 56 times among whites, as compared with 12 among blacks. The frequency of *genitourinary infection* was essentially the same for both races, 38 in whites, 36 in blacks.

Gastrointestinal infections requiring hospitalization occurred with somewhat higher frequency among blacks [304] as compared with whites [200].

Specific Childhood Diseases. *Roseola* was reported more frequently in whites [326], as might have been expected because of the difficulty in ascertaining fine rashes in the black skin [38].

Measles occurred with some frequency, in 195 (1.18 percent) of the whites and 420 (2.32 percent) of the black children. Several of the children died from what is essentially a preventable disease. It has not been determined how many of these infants (born between 1959–66) were immunized during the early months of life.

Whooping cough was reported in only 20 white and 38 black infants during the first year.

Trauma, Physical Agents and Intoxications

Table 15–21 shows that about one percent of the children experienced trauma or intoxication during the first year. Skull fractures were reported in 71 white and 27 black children, and other fractures in 68 white and 41 black infants. Burns requiring hospitalization were more frequent among blacks [23], as compared with whites [13]. Symptomatic intoxications occurred in 10 white, as compared with 30 black infants. These are all potentially serious problems that are largely preventable.

Table 15-18. Summary Data for First Year Syndromes

| | WHITE | | | | | | | BLACK | | | | | | |
| | All Birthweights | | | Under 2501 gm | | Over 2500 gm | | All Birthweights | | | Under 2501 gm | | Over 2500 gm | |
Condition	No.	%	Mean Bwt.	No.	%	No.	%	No.	%	Mean Bwt.	No.	%	No.	%
Mongolism	18	0.11	2726	6	0.57	12	0.08	13	0.07	3110	3	0.13	10	0.06
Gonadal dysgenesis	2	0.01	2208	2	0.19	0	0	0	0	-	0	0	0	0
Adrenogenital	2	0.01	3909	0	0	2	0.01	1	0.01	2523	0	0	0	0.01
Marfan's	0	0	-	0	0	0	0	0	0	-	0	0	0	0
Pierre robin	2	0.01	3105	0	0	2	0.01	1	0.01	2608	0	0	1	0.01
Spasmus nutans	3	0.02	3487	0	0	3	0.02	31	0.17	2923	6	0.27	25	0.16
Hurler's	0	0	-	0	0	0	0	0	0	-	0	0	0	0
Failure to thrive	92	0.56	2985	19	1.79	73	0.47	169	0.93	2681	52	2.32	117	0.74
Other	28	0.17	3075	7	0.66	21	0.14	21	0.12	2979	6	0.27	15	0.09
No syndromes	16381	99.15	3293	1024	96.48	15352	99.30	17888	98.71	3067	2177	97.01	15711	98.95
Total	16521	100.00	3291	1061	100.00	15460	100.00	18121	100.00	3063	2244	100.00	15877	100.00

Table 15-19. Summary Data for First Year Other Endocrine and Metabolic Diseases

| | WHITE | | | | | | | BLACK | | | | | | |
| | All Birthweights | | | Under 2501 gm | | Over 2500 gm | | All Birthweights | | | Under 2501 gm | | Over 2500 gm | |
Condition	No.	%	Mean Bwt.	No.	%	No.	%	No.	%	Mean Bwt.	No.	%	No.	%
Hypothyroidism	2	0.01	2736	0	0	2	0.01	1	0.01	3487	0	0	1	0.01
Fibrocystic disease of pancreas	7	0.04	3358	0	0	7	0.05	0	0	-	0	0	0	0
Inborn errors of metabolism	2	0.01	2637	1	0.09	1	0.01	4	0.02	3239	1	0.04	3	0.02
Other	14	0.08	3161	3	0.28	11	0.07	23	0.13	3163	1	0.04	22	0.14
No endo./metab. disease	16498	99.86	3291	1057	99.62	15441	99.88	18093	99.85	3063	2242	99.91	15851	99.84
Total	16521	100.00	3291	1061	100.00	15460	100.00	18121	100.00	3063	2244	100.00	15877	100.00

Table 15-20. Summary Data for First Year Infection and Inflammation

Condition	WHITE All Birthweights No.	%	Mean Bwt.	WHITE Under 2501 gm No.	%	WHITE Over 2500 gm No.	%	BLACK All Birthweights No.	%	Mean Bwt.	BLACK Under 2501 gm No.	%	BLACK Over 2500 gm No.	%
Septicemia	13	0.08	3454	1	0.09	12	0.08	28	0.15	3003	3	0.13	25	0.16
Central nervous system														
Bacterial meningitis	19	0.12	3430	1	0.09	18	0.12	59	0.33	2963	9	0.40	50	0.31
Non-bacterial meningitis	7	0.04	3297	1	0.09	6	0.04	14	0.08	2987	2	0.09	12	0.08
Encephalitis	1	0.01	3289	0	0	1	0.01	3	0.02	3052	0	0	3	0.02
Other CNS	2	0.01	3530	0	0	2	0.01	9	0.05	2854	3	0.13	6	0.04
Respiratory														
Pneumonia	434	2.63	3180	49	4.62	385	2.49	888	4.90	2967	152	6.77	736	4.64
Severe croup	56	0.34	3329	5	0.47	51	0.33	12	0.07	3085	0	0	12	0.08
Bronchiolitis	168	1.02	3272	21	1.98	147	0.95	222	1.23	2967	38	1.69	184	1.16
Other respiratory	278	1.68	3218	28	2.64	250	1.62	249	1.37	3085	36	1.60	213	1.34
Genitourinary tract	38	0.23	3059	9	0.85	29	0.19	36	0.20	2988	7	0.31	29	0.18
Bone and joint	4	0.02	2913	1	0.09	3	0.02	12	0.07	2991	2	0.09	10	0.06
Heart	5	0.03	3402	0	0	5	0.03	5	0.03	2761	2	0.09	3	0.02
Gastrointestinal														
Diarrhea requiring hospitalization	200	1.21	3125	23	2.17	177	1.14	304	1.68	2972	57	2.54	247	1.56
Other G.I.	46	0.28	3238	4	0.38	42	0.27	51	0.28	2983	9	0.40	42	0.26
Liver	1	0.01	2722	0	0	1	0.01	2	0.01	2651	1	0.04	1	0.01
Eye	42	0.25	3494	2	0.19	40	0.26	52	0.29	3006	9	0.40	43	0.27
Ear	403	2.44	3299	24	2.26	379	2.45	424	2.34	3084	46	2.05	378	2.38
Skin	86	0.52	3305	3	0.28	83	0.54	121	0.67	3030	18	0.80	103	0.65
No. inf./inflam.	14073	85.18	3295	854	80.49	13219	85.50	15114	83.41	3070	1813	80.79	13301	83.78
Total	16521	100.00	3291	1061	100.00	15460	100.00	18121	100.00	3063	2244	100.00	15877	100.00

Table 15-20. (Continued)

Condition	WHITE							BLACK						
	All Birthweights			Under 2501 gm		Over 2500 gm		All Birthweights			Under 2501 gm		Over 2500 gm	
	No.	%	Mean Bwt.	No.	%	No.	%	No.	%	Mean Bwt.	No.	%	No.	%
Specific childhood diseases														
Roseola	326	1.97	3261	18	1.70	308	1.99	38	0.21	3117	5	0.22	33	0.21
German measles	88	0.53	3291	8	0.75	80	0.52	84	0.46	3088	11	0.49	73	0.46
Measles	195	1.18	3302	11	1.04	184	1.19	420	2.32	3044	54	2.41	366	2.31
Mumps	24	0.15	3181	3	0.28	21	0.14	26	0.14	3108	3	0.13	23	0.14
Chickenpox	312	1.89	3337	22	2.07	290	1.88	395	2.18	3074	46	2.05	349	2.20
Whooping cough	20	0.12	3369	1	0.09	19	0.12	38	0.21	3054	3	0.13	35	0.22
Other	10	0.06	2943	3	0.28	7	0.05	11	0.06	3015	2	0.09	9	0.06
Unusually recurrent or chronic infections	88	0.53	3181	6	0.57	82	0.53	56	0.31	2966	10	0.45	46	0.29
Other	65	0.39	3377	3	0.28	62	0.40	80	0.44	3121	6	0.27	74	0.47
No inf./inflam.	14073	85.18	3295	854	80.49	13219	85.50	15114	83.41	3070	1813	80.79	13301	83.78
Total	16521	100.00	3291	1061	100.00	15460	100.00	18121	100.00	3063	2244	100.00	15877	100.00

Table 15-21. Summary Data for First Year Trauma, Physical Agents, and Intoxication

Condition	WHITE All Birthweights No.	%	Mean Bwt.	Under 2501 gm No.	%	Over 2500 gm No.	%	BLACK All Birthweights No.	%	Mean Bwt.	Under 2501 gm No.	%	Over 2500 gm No.	%
Head trauma														
Unconsciousness	16	0.10	3241	1	0.09	15	0.10	12	0.07	3166	1	0.04	11	0.07
Fractured skull	71	0.43	3261	8	0.75	63	0.41	27	0.15	3087	2	0.09	25	0.16
Bloody spinal fluid	1	0.01	3232	0	0	1	0.01	2	0.01	2821	1	0.04	1	0.01
Vomiting - 3 times	11	0.07	3314	0	0	11	0.07	7	0.04	2900	2	0.09	5	0.03
Subgaleal hematoma	17	0.10	3309	0	0	17	0.11	3	0.02	3496	0	0	3	0.02
Fractures, other	68	0.41	3329	2	0.19	66	0.43	41	0.23	3051	8	0.36	33	0.21
Burns leading to hospitalization	13	0.08	3286	2	0.19	11	0.07	23	0.13	3075	5	0.22	18	0.11
Symptomatic intoxication														
Salicylate	0	0	—	0	0	0	0	4	0.02	3090	1	0.04	3	0.02
Hydrocarbon kerosene	1	0.01	2863	0	0	1	0.01	3	0.02	3307	0	0	3	0.02
Other hydrocarbon	0	0	—	0	0	0	0	3	0.02	3241	0	0	3	0.02
Lead	0	0	—	0	0	0	0	4	0.02	2736	1	0.04	3	0.02
Other	9	0.05	3311	0	0	9	0.06	16	0.09	2950	2	0.09	14	0.09
No trauma, physical agents, and intox,	16330	98.84	3291	1048	98.77	15282	98.85	17990	99.28	3063	2225	99.15	15765	99.29
Total	16521	100.00	3291	1061	100.00	15460	100.00	18121	100.00	3063	2244	100.00	15877	100.00

Table 15-22. Summary Data for First Year Disturbances in Homeostasis

	WHITE							BLACK						
	All Birthweights			Under 2501 gm		Over 2500 gm		All Birthweights			Under 2501 gm		Over 2500 gm	
Condition	No.	%	Mean Bwt.	No.	%	No.	%	No.	%	Mean Bwt.	No.	%	No.	%
Shock requiring hospitalization	10	0.06	3266	2	0.19	8	0.05	8	0.04	2732	3	0.13	5	0.03
Dehydration requiring parenteral fluid therapy	137	0.83	3187	13	1.23	124	0.80	226	1.25	2952	43	1.92	183	1.15
Electrolyte imbalance	57	0.35	3187	7	0.66	50	0.32	129	0.71	2903	28	1.25	101	0.64
Hyperthermia	59	0.36	3217	3	0.28	56	0.36	41	0.23	3074	4	0.18	37	0.23
Hypothermia	1	0.01	2637	0	0	1	0.01	1	0.01	2948	0	0	1	0.01
Episode of hypoxia														
with unconsciousness	30	0.18	3016	4	0.38	26	0.17	12	0.07	2769	4	0.18	8	0.05
without unconsciousness	25	0.15	3200	2	0.19	23	0.15	10	0.06	2824	3	0.13	7	0.04
Other	20	0.12	3123	3	0.28	17	0.11	19	0.10	2811	4	0.18	15	0.09
No homeostasis disturb.	16246	98.34	3293	1032	97.27	15214	98.41	17797	98.21	3065	2179	97.10	15618	98.37
Total	16521	100.00	3291	1061	100.00	15460	100.00	18121	100.00	3063	2244	100.00	15877	100.00

Table 15-23. Summary Data for First Year Procedures

Condition	WHITE							BLACK						
	All Birthweights			Under 2501 gm		Over 2500 gm		All Birthweights			Under 2501 gm		Over 2500 gm	
	No.	%	Mean Bwt.	No.	%	No.	%	No.	%	Mean Bwt.	No.	%	No.	%
Blood transfusions	64	0.39	3182	5	0.47	59	0.38	97	0.54	2837	26	1.16	71	0.45
Parenteral fluid	243	1.47	3222	23	2.17	220	1.42	345	1.90	2928	74	3.30	271	1.71
Spinal puncture	244	1.48	3220	18	1.70	226	1.46	396	2.19	2981	64	2.85	332	2.09
Subdural puncture	36	0.22	3299	1	0.09	35	0.23	61	0.34	2969	14	0.62	47	0.30
Ventricular puncture	11	0.07	3399	0	0	11	0.07	11	0.06	2724	4	0.18	7	0.04
General anesthesia	398	2.41	3189	45	4.24	353	2.28	336	1.85	2891	80	3.57	256	1.61
Surgery	510	3.09	3193	62	5.84	448	2.90	434	2.40	2908	98	4.37	336	2.12
Chromosome studies	15	0.09	3056	3	0.28	12	0.08	6	0.03	2646	3	0.13	3	0.02
EEG	738	4.47	3314	50	4.71	688	4.45	419	2.31	2929	83	3.70	336	2.12
Other	270	1.63	3238	30	2.83	240	1.55	245	1.35	3034	35	1.56	210	1.32
No procedures	14820	89.70	3294	912	85.96	13408	89.96	16599	91.60	3073	1951	86.94	14648	92.26
Total	16521	100.00	3291	1061	100.00	15460	100.00	18121	100.00	3063	2244	100.00	15877	100.00

Disturbances in Homeostasis

A number of definite conditions potentially compromising neurological integrity were reported in this section. (Table 15–22.) Hypoxic episodes were more frequent among white infants, whereas electrolyte imbalance and dehydration were reported with considerably greater frequency among the blacks. Overall, almost 2 percent of the children were reported to have disturbances of homeostasis during the first year.

Procedures

The study protocol required reporting of a number of diagnostic procedures. These are listed in Table 15–23. Among white children, 89.7 percent had no procedures reported and among blacks, a slightly larger number, 91.6 percent.

REFERENCES

(1) S. C. Mitchell, S. B. Korones, and H. W. Berendes. 1971. Congenital Heart Disease in 56,109 Births. *Circulation* 43: 323–32.

(2) S. C. Mitchell, A. H. Sellmann, M. C. Westphal, and J. Park. 1971. Etiologic correlates in a study of congenital heart disease in 56,109 births. *American Journal of Cardiology* 28: 653–57.

16

COMPARISON OF NEWBORN AND
LATER DIAGNOSES

For many years there has been speculation about the true frequency of certain congenital malformations and other conditions of young infants. Data has of necessity been somewhat fragmentary because some conditions are not compatible with long survival; the presence of some is not recognized until later in childhood; others may be recognized early and corrected by surgical or other means, so that they are no longer present when the child is seen at a later age. Thus, there may be a change over time in the reported presence or absence of specific conditions for individual children. The longitudinal data from the NCPP are unusually well suited to identifying the changing frequency of certain malformations and conditions identified during the first year of life.

In this project, where each child was examined at a number of specified ages according to a predetermined protocol, assessment of the consistency of diagnosis between birth and one year of age was possible and a better understanding of the frequency of certain conditions could be developed. The children were examined by the physician without the benefit of the traditional prior historical enquiry. This approach was used to reduce bias and to encourage the physician to proceed without information about predetermined normalcy or abnormality, so that a "pre set" to any given system or set of findings was prevented insofar as possible. During the first year, children were examined by project physicians in the nursery and at four and twelve months of age, and by a developmental psychologist at eight months. Independently, at each visit, trained interviewers collected interval medical histories and records of medical care, including hospitalization. Similarly, the *Newborn Diagnostic Summary* (PED–8) and the *One-Year Summary* (PED–12) were completed independently of each other. The PED–8 Summary reported diagnoses identified during the nursery period and the PED–12 Summary those reported during the remainder of the first year and summarized immediately following the one-year neurological examination.

Table 16–1 displays data comparing selected diagnoses from the nursery examinations reported on the *Newborn Diagnostic Summary* (PED–8) and those reported on the *One-Year Summary* (PED–12). The diagnoses examined included those that might reasonably be expected to persist through the first year and those where sufficient numbers of cases permitted comparisons. The comparisons are limited to those diagnoses considered *definite*; suspect diagnoses have been combined with the normal for this table. Because of small numbers in most individual diagnostic categories, black and white children have been grouped together.

The intent of the analysis presented here is to provide a comparison between findings reported in the nursery and those reported during the remainder of the first year. As a result, analysis is limited to children who had both PED–8 and PED–12 forms. Children who died during the nursery period and those who were not available for follow-up during the first year have been excluded.

This analysis included the records of 18,121 black and 16,521 white infants for a total of 34,642 children. The results are presented in Table 16–1. For purposes of comparison, there were three possibilities with respect to specific diagnosis. First (column a), a diagnosis may have been reported in the nursery period only (i.e., on PED–8) and not have been reported on the *One-Year Summary* (PED–12). Second (column b), the diagnosis may have been reported at one year only (PED–12) and not during the nursery period; and third (column c), the diagnosis may have been reported at both times, i.e., an overlap of both periods.

Microcephaly (62 Cases). In this cohort of 34,642 children, there were 62 reported to have had a definite diagnosis of microcephaly. Of these 62, 8 were reported during the nursery period, and of the 8, 4 were not considered to be microcephalic at one year, leaving 4 who were reported at both times. There were 54 reported at one year only, plus the 4 reported at both periods, bringing the total to 58 children considered microcephalic at one year. Thus, of the 62 children (100 percent) designated at one time or another to be microcephalic, 6.5 percent were noted only in the nursery, 87.1 percent only at one year, 6.5 percent at both times (overlap). There were 12.9 percent of the total noted in the nursery and 93.5 percent of the total noted at one year (this adds up to more than 100 percent, as some children were reported at both times).

Why were 4 children thought to be microcephalic in the nursery not so designated at one year? All 4 were reported to have small head size in the nursery, but later were considered to be within normal limits.

Among the 54 children not diagnosed as microcephalic during the nursery period, several were considered suspect for microcephaly during the nursery period. Four were recognized later to have congenital rubella, another had Pierre robin syndrome, and another had Down's syndrome. Several others had other malformations. Twenty-nine of the 54 children weighed less than 2500 grams and only 8 were over 3000 grams at birth.

Hydrocephaly (43 Cases). There were 43 children reported to have hydrocephaly at either or both of the diagnostic periods; 4 of these were reported only in the nursery, 7 at both nursery and one year, for a total of 11 in the nursery. There

Table 16-1. Comparison of Newborn and Later Diagnoses
N = 34,642 (White 16,521; Black 18,121)

Diagnosis	Frequency						Percent					
	Nursery Only	1-Year Only	Nursery and 1-Year	Total Nursery	Total 1-Year	Total	Nursery Only	1-Year Only	Nursery and 1-Year	Total Nursery	Total 1-Year	Total
	a	b	c	(a+c)	(b+c)	a+b+c	$\frac{a}{a+b+c}$	$\frac{b}{a+b+c}$	$\frac{c}{a+b+c}$	$\frac{(a+c)}{a+b+c}$	$\frac{(b+c)}{a+b+c}$	$\frac{a+b+c}{a+b+c}$
Microcephaly	4	54	4	(8)	(58)	62	6.5	87.1	6.5	(12.9)	(93.5)	100.0
Hydranencephaly	2	0	1	(3)	(1)	3	66.7	0	33.3	(100.0)	(33.3)	100.0
Hydrocephaly	4	32	7	(11)	(39)	43	9.3	74.4	16.3	(25.6)	(90.7)	100.0
Craniosynostosis	0	11	6	(6)	(17)	17	0	64.7	35.3	(35.3)	(100.0)	100.0
Abnormal shape of skull	35	624	7	(42)	(631)	666	5.3	93.7	1.1	(6.3)	(94.7)	100.0
Encephalocele	2	0	0	(2)	(0)	2	100.0	0	0	(100.0)	(0)	100.0
Meningomyelocele	3	3	10	(13)	(13)	16	18.8	18.8	62.5	(81.3)	(81.3)	100.0
Pilonidal sinus	21	41	14	(35)	(55)	76	27.6	53.9	18.4	(46.1)	(72.4)	100.0
Vertebral abnormality	6	13	4	(10)	(17)	23	26.1	56.5	17.4	(43.5)	(73.9)	100.0
Talipes equinovarus	18	58	22	(40)	(80)	98	18.4	59.2	22.4	(40.8)	(81.6)	100.0
Metatarsus adductus	37	686	15	(52)	(701)	738	5.0	93.0	2.0	(7.0)	(95.0)	100.0
Calcaneo valgus	10	116	6	(16)	(122)	132	7.6	87.9	4.5	(12.1)	(92.4)	100.0
Congenital dislocation or dysplasia — hip	8	55	13	(21)	(68)	76	10.5	72.4	17.1	(27.6)	(89.5)	100.0
Absence or hypoplasia (extremity or part)	6	20	18	(24)	(38)	44	13.6	45.5	40.9	(54.5)	(86.4)	100.0
Polydactyly	220	7	52	(272)	(59)	279	78.9	2.5	18.6	(97.5)	(21.1)	100.0
Syndactyly	22	51	26	(48)	(77)	99	22.2	51.5	26.3	(48.5)	(77.8)	100.0
Torticollis	2	50	1	(3)	(51)	53	3.8	94.3	1.9	(5.7)	(96.2)	100.0
Cataract	0	9	18	(18)	(27)	27	0	33.3	66.7	(66.7)	(100.0)	100.0
Microphthalmia	2	5	0	(2)	(5)	7	28.6	71.4	0	(28.6)	(71.4)	100.0

Table 16-1. (Continued)

Diagnosis	Frequency Nursery Only a	1-Year Only b	Nursery and 1-Year c	Total Nursery (a+c)	Total 1-Year (b+c)	Total a+b+c	Percent Nursery Only a/(a+b+c)	1-Year Only b/(a+b+c)	Nursery and 1-Year c/(a+b+c)	Total Nursery (a+c)/(a+b+c)	Total 1-Year (b+c)/(a+b+c)	Total (a+b+c)/(a+b+c)
Low-set ears	55	55	4	(59)	(59)	114	48.2	48.2	3.5	(51.7)	(51.7)	100.0
Deformed ear pinna	59	137	14	(73)	(151)	210	28.1	65.2	6.7	(34.8)	(71.9)	100.0
Branchial cleft anomaly	107	118	158	(265)	(276)	383	27.9	30.8	41.3	(69.2)	(72.1)	100.0
Cleft palate	2	4	26	(28)	(30)	32	6.3	12.5	81.3	(87.5)	(93.8)	100.0
Cleft uvula (bifid)	8	28	2	(10)	(30)	38	21.1	73.7	5.3	(26.4)	(78.9)	100.0
Cleft lip	2	0	25	(27)	(25)	27	7.4	0	92.6	(100.0)	(92.6)	100.0
Cleft gum	87	2	5	(92)	(7)	94	92.6	2.1	5.3	(97.9)	(7.4)	100.0
Micrognathia	8	17	5	(13)	(22)	30	26.7	56.7	16.7	(43.3)	(73.3)	100.0
Anomaly of diaphragm	5	2	1	(6)	(3)	8	62.5	25.0	12.5	(75.0)	(37.5)	100.0
Pectus excavatum	8	80	0	(8)	(80)	88	9.1	90.9	0	(9.1)	(90.9)	100.0
Acyanotic CHD	13	121	8	(21)	(129)	142	9.2	85.2	5.6	(14.8)	(90.8)	100.0
Cyanotic CHD	1	18	6	(7)	(24)	25	4.0	72.0	24.0	(28.0)	(96.0)	100.0
Hernia, inguinal and femoral	19	531	12	(31)	(543)	562	3.4	94.5	2.1	(5.5)	(96.6)	100.0
Hypospadias	33	38	67	(100)	(105)	138	23.9	27.5	48.6	(72.5)	(76.1)	100.0
Chordee	5	11	1	(6)	(12)	17	29.4	64.7	5.9	(35.3)	(70.6)	100.0
Bladder outflow obstruction	3	41	1	(4)	(42)	45	6.7	91.1	2.2	(8.9)	(93.3)	100.0
Upper urinary tract obstruction	6	6	2	(8)	(8)	14	42.9	42.9	14.3	(57.1)	(57.1)	100.0
Strawberry-portwine hemangioma	122	700	46	(168)	(746)	868	14.1	80.6	5.3	(19.4)	(85.9)	100.0
Cavernous hemangioma	24	243	8	(32)	(251)	275	8.7	88.4	2.9	(11.6)	(91.3)	100.0
Café au lait spots	30	267	6	(36)	(273)	303	9.9	88.1	2.0	(11.9)	(90.1)	100.0
Mongolism	1	8	23	(24)	(31)	32	3.1	25.0	71.9	(75.0)	(96.9)	100.0

were 32 reported only at one year, plus the 7 at both periods, for a total of 39 noted at one year. Thus, of the 43 cases identified at one time or another as definite hydrocephaly, 25.6 percent were noted in the nursery, 90.7 percent were noted at one year, the overlap between the two periods being 16.3 percent. Follow-up of the 4 children thought to have hydrocephaly in the nursery period but not at one year showed that 2 were thought to have arrested hydrocephaly and one was suspect at one year. The remaining child was macrocephalic.

Craniosynostosis (17 Cases). There were 6 newborn infants who received this diagnosis during the nursery stay and retained the diagnosis during the first year. There were no instances where the diagnosis was made in the nursery, but not confirmed at a later time. Eleven children with craniosynostosis were identified after the nursery period, bringing the total to 17 children with craniosynostosis during the first year of life.

Abnormal Shape of Skull (666 Cases). A total of 666 children were reported to have had an abnormally shaped skull during the first year. Thirty-five were so diagnosed in the nursery period, but were not confirmed on later examination. Only 7 children were thought to have the condition both in the nursery and at one year. The relative infrequency of the diagnosis during the nursery period, in comparison to the number reported during the remainder of the first year, is noteworthy. This difference is undoubtedly related to the nursery examiners acceptance of delivery molding as an explanation for unusual shape, and positional effects on skull shape during the remainder of the first year; for example, occipital flattening in the infant who spends most of his time lying on his back.

Encephalocele (2 Cases). Two cases of encephalocele were noted in the nursery. These were surgically corrected and therefore were not noted on later examination.

Meningomyelocele (16 Cases). There were 3 children reported to have had a meningomyelocele in the nursery, but not during the remainder of the first year; 2 received surgical intervention and in 1 child the diagnosis was changed to spina bifida. The 3 children noted to have the definite condition only after the nursery period were classified as suspect in the nursery. There were an additional 10 children reported with meningomyelocele noted in the nursery and during the remainder of the first year, or 62.5 percent reported at both periods.

Pilonidal Sinus (Not Dimple) (76 Cases). From a total of 76 children reported at one time or another to have pilonidal sinus, only 14 (18.4 percent) were so identified during both the nursery period and during the remainder of the first year of life. There were 21 children reported during the nursery period to have had pilonidal sinus who actually had "dimples" or "deep dimples." The pilonidal sinuses of 41 children were missed or not reported as definite during the nursery period, the diagnosis being reported as definite later in the first year.

Talipes Equinovarus (98 Cases). There were a total of 98 children reported to have talipes equinovarus during the entire first year of life, of whom 22 (22.4 percent) were reported during both the nursery period and the remainder of the first year. The 18 reported only during the nursery period were noted as "mild," "self-correcting," and "positional," or at a later date thought to be suspect. There were

58 cases not reported as definite during the nursery period that later were thought to warrant such a diagnosis.

Metatarsus Adductus (738 Cases). The reporting of this condition shows that only a very small proportion, 15 (2 percent), were reported during both the nursery period and at one year. A slightly larger proportion, 37 (5 percent), were reported only during the nursery period. These were often noted to be "mild" and were not reported on later examinations. The great majority, 686 (93 percent), were reported after the nursery period.

Calcaneovalgus (132 Cases). There were 132 cases of calcaneovalgus reported. The reporting of this condition is similar to that for metatarsus adductus, with 87.9 percent being reported only on PED–12. Very few were reported during the nursery period only, 10 (7.6 percent), and only 6 were reported in the nursery and at one year.

Congenital Dislocation or Dysplasia of the Hip (76 Cases). The diagnosis of congenital hip dislocation or dysplasia is difficult to make with assurance during the newborn period. As early X-ray findings are unreliable, the physician must depend primarily on physical signs. Of the 21 infants reported to have a definite diagnosis in the nursery, in 8 the diagnosis did not continue on later follow-up. In 13 the diagnosis was also present on the one-year summary. There were 55 children who had a definite diagnosis made after nursery discharge (72.4 percent of the total number of cases). These 55, plus the 13 (17.1 percent) in whom the diagnosis was present at both times, bring to 68 the number reported at one year. It is of interest that the condition was noted six times more frequently among whites than blacks; 65 whites and 11 blacks being reported to have the abnormality.

Absence or Hypoplasia of Extremity or Part (44 Cases). Among the 44 cases of absence or hypoplasia of an extremity or part thereof, 18 were reported at both time periods. Thirty-eight were noted both in the nursery and at one year. Of the 6 cases noted in the nursery, but not at later ages, 2 concerned absence of muscle mass, others a hypoplastic mandible, rudimentary toes, ulnar deviation of toes, and slight but definite shortening of femur and tibia.

Polydactyly (279 Cases). Most of the children (97.5 percent) with this condition were detected in the nursery, and only 2.5 percent of the cases reported were not observed in this period, but were noted at one year. Most abnormalities noted in the nursery were "nubbins" or "post mini," which were ligated, excised, or not noted to be present at one year.

Syndactyly (99 Cases). Of the 99 children with syndactyly, 22.2 percent were detected in the nursery, 26.3 percent in the nursery and at one year, and 51.5 percent only at one year. A number of the cases reported in the nursery, but not on later examinations, represented mild webbing of hands or webbing of toes not noted on later examinations.

Torticollis (53 Cases). This diagnosis was made in only 3 instances in the nursery period and was not confirmed in 2 cases on later examinations. There were 50 cases identified during the remainder of the first year of life.

Cataract (27 Cases). There were 27 children noted to have cataracts at some time during the nursery period or during the remainder of the first year of life. None were noted only in the nursery, 9 only at one year, and 18 noted at both times.

Microphthalmia (7 Cases). There were 7 children noted to have this condition during the first year. Five were reported at one year only, and 2 in the nursery only, and no cases were reported at both times.

Low-set Ears (114 Cases). The diagnosis of low-set ears was inconsistent, with 55 children reported from the nursery only, 55 reported at one year only, with 4 cases reported at both times (3.5 percent).

Deformed Ear Pinna (210 Cases). At some time during the first year, there were 210 children reported to have deformed ear pinnae. There were 59 in the nursery only, 14 in both the nursery and at one year, and 137 at one year only. The 14 reported at both examinations represent only 6.7 percent of the cases identified. The 59 cases reported only in the nursery were not so identified at later examinations. This diagnosis is somewhat subjective, and there seems to be little consistency between the nursery period and the remainder of the first year of life. Some of the deformities noted in the nursery may have been the result of fetal position and fold-overs that in time were self-correcting.

Branchial Cleft Anomaly (383 Cases). Of the total of 383 definite cases reported, 107 or 27.9 percent were noted in the nursery, 118 or 30.8 percent noted only at one year, and 158 or 41.3 percent noted in both periods. Most of these malformations were preauricular sinuses and preauricular skin tags, which are easily overlooked when hair is abundant.

Cleft Palate (32 Cases). Among the 28 children reported to have cleft palate in the nursery period, 26 were reported both in the nursery period and at one year and 2 reported only in the nursery period. One of these 2 had had a surgical repair and the cleft was not noted at one year and the other had a mild cleft of the soft palate not noted on the one-year examination. Of the 4 cleft palates not noted in the nursery, 2 children had cleft lips noted in the nursery, 1 an absent uvula with partial soft palate cleft not noted in the nursery, and the last was a child with a cleft gum reported in the nursery and later discovered to have a submucous cleft palate.

Cleft Uvula (Bifid) (38 Cases). This malformation was noted only in the nursery in 8 newborns and in 2 additional children both in the nursery and at one year. The majority of cases, 28, were noted at one year only.

Cleft Lip (27 Cases). All cases were reported in the nursery. Of the 2 children reported to have cleft lip in the nursery but not at one year, both had had surgical repair.

Cleft Gum (94 Cases). There were 94 children with this malformation identified during the first year, with 87 noted only in the nursery, 5 at both times, and only 2 at one year only. Most of these clefts were midline clefts of the alveolar ridge of the maxilla and undoubtedly ceased to be readily detectable after eruption of the two upper central incisors.

Micrognathia (30 Cases). There were 8 children with this condition noted only in the nursery, and 5 more noted in the nursery and at one year. Seventeen children were identified only at one year. The overlap between the nursery and one year was 16.7 percent. Among the 8 noted only in the nursery, one child was reported to have Turner's syndrome and in 6 the condition was slight or mild and not noted on later examinations.

Anomaly of Diaphragm (8 Cases). A malformation of the diaphragm was noted in 5 children during the nursery stay, in one child in the nursery and at one year, and in 2 at the later time only. Among the 5 reported during the newborn period, 4 had a diaphragmatic hernia, one had a thoracic cage malformation affecting the diaphragm with 13 ribs on one side and 8 on the other.

Pectus Excavatum (88 Cases). There were 8 cases of pectus excavatum reported in the nursery only, and 80 cases reported at one year only. No cases were reported at both times. Thus, 90.9 percent of the cases reported during the entire first year were reported after the nursery period and only 9.1 percent during the nursery period. Six of the 8 infants with the diagnosis reported during the newborn period weighed less than 2700 grams. As noted in the previous chapter, the mean birthweight of children with the condition reported at one year was considerably higher than that of those without.

Acyanotic Congenital Heart Disease (142 Cases). Of the 142 children, only 21 (14.8 percent) were reported during the nursery period. Thirteen of those reported in the newborn period were not reported as definite subsequently, although 3 were considered suspect. There were 121 children (85.2 percent) reported to have definite acyanotic congenital heart disease after the newborn period.

Cyanotic Congenital Heart Disease (25 Cases). Twenty-five children were reported to have definite cyanotic heart disease during the first year. All but one were reported on the one-year-summary. Of the 25, one was reported in the nursery and not later, and 6 others noted in the nursery were also reported at one year. In 18 infants a definite diagnosis was not made during the nursery stay.

Hernia (562 Cases). A total of 562 children were noted to have had hernias (inguinal, femoral, complicated umbilical, and other) during the first year of life. The bulk of these, 531 (or 94.5 percent) were noted only at one year, and an additional 12 (or 2.1 percent) were noted in the nursery and at one year. Nineteen (or 3.4 percent) were noted in the nursery only, and 8 of these were noted to have had surgical repair.

Hypospadias (138 Cases). Hypospadias was reported for 100 newborn children, but 33 of these were during the nursery period only, of which 9 were described as minimal or mild. There were 67 diagnosed both in the nursery and during the remainder of the first year. An additional 38 children were noted only at one year. Thus, during the entire first year, 138 definite cases were reported, with a 48.6 percent overlap between the nursery period and the remainder of the first year.

Chordee (17 Cases). Among the 17 cases reported as definite during the first year, 5 were from the nursery period only, 11 were noted later only, and one case was from both examination periods.

Bladder Outflow Obstruction (45 Cases). There were 45 children identified to have bladder outflow obstruction. Four of these were identified during the nursery stay, and 41 during the remainder of the first year of life. One child was reported to have the condition during both time intervals. Of the 3 cases with nursery-only diagnosis, all three had corrective surgery.

Upper Urinary Tract Obstruction (14 Cases). Fourteen children were noted to have had this condition during the first year of life, 6 in the nursery only, 6 at one year only, and 2 at both times.

Strawberry-Port Wine Hemangioma (868 Cases). While 868 children were reported during the entire first year to have had this type of hemangioma, only 5.3 percent of the cases were reported both in the nursery and at one year. The vast majority (700, or 80.6 percent) were noted only at one year.

Cavernous Hemangioma (275 Cases). Of the 275 cases, 243 were noted only at one year, representing 88.4 percent of the total cases for the entire year.

Café au Lait Spots (303 Cases). The reporting pattern for café au lait spots is similar in number and in distribution between examining periods to that seen for cavernous hemangioma, with the bulk of the cases reported only at one year and just 2 percent reported at both times.

Mongolism (32 Cases). There were 32 children identified as having Down's syndrome during the first year of life. Twenty-four or 75 percent were identified as definite in the nursery, but one of these was not considered to be definite at age one. An additional 8 cases were identified during the remainder of the first year.

SUMMARY

Comparisons between selected specific diagnoses reported during the newborn period and later during the first year show differences between the two reports that vary with the condition under consideration. Consistency for the diagnoses reviewed varies from essentially zero (abnormal shape of skull and encephalocele) to 92.6 percent (cleft lip). The variation is dependent upon the complexity and severity of the malformation, its ease of detection, and its amenability to correction.

These analyses show that simple addition of cases identified at one year to those reported during the newborn period may well provide slightly inflated frequencies when neonatal diagnoses are not confirmed later.

17

SUMMARY AND CONCLUSIONS

The purpose of this volume is to describe the many medical and developmental characteristics reported, from the moment of birth through the first birthday, for the 18,481 white and 19,504 black, single, liveborn infants with known birthweight in the NINCDS Collaborative Perinatal Project. The intent has been to provide a broad description of the children, the mortality experience, and the neurological and developmental problems identified during the neonatal period and the remainder of the first year.

The data were collected prospectively in twelve university medical centers across the United States, using a standard examination schedule and structured data forms and manuals. The material presented here is complementary to that in *The Women and Their Pregnancies* (published in 1972), which describes the characteristics of the study populations, the maternal conditions of pregnancy, labor, and delivery, and their relationship to immediate pregnancy outcome.

A Comprehensive Plan for Analysis and Interpretation of Collaborative Perinatal Project Data is well under way. These comprehensive analyses will relate specific outcomes identified at seven and eight years of age to data collected earlier, especially during pregnancy, labor, delivery, and the neonatal period. The developmental disabilities to be covered by these comprehensive analyses include cerebral palsy, mental retardation, seizure disorders, and disorders of learning, communication, and behavior. This volume provides information on many of the characteristics of the neonatal period and first year of life that are being used in the Comprehensive Analyses. The volume also displays some of the range and detail of data available for future research analysis efforts.

Characteristics described in this volume provide a global view of an extensive spectrum of neonatal problems studied in a single large population of infants. The frequency of diagnostic entities and medical procedures, both during the nursery period and later during the first year, is described. A high rate of successful completion of required follow-up examinations of surviving children was maintained, and little bias could be discerned with respect to those who could not be followed (see Chapter 2). The study protocol provided for a repeated, systematic search for abnormal findings and, as these infants were examined in university teaching hospitals, it is unlikely that major diagnoses were missed. Autopsies, carried out on approximately 90 percent of perinatal and 70 percent of later deaths, provided additional diagnostic information. The data presented are thought to be unusually complete and reliable.

A brief outline describing the organization of the volume follows in the next few paragraphs. A few comments are made in passing on specific observations, but comment on major observations is reserved for the last section of the chapter.

The first six chapters present background material important to the understanding and assessment of the main body of data presented in Chapters 7 through 16. *Chapters 1 through 4* provide a basic description of the study, its populations and procedures. *Chapter 5* consists of a brief summary, from *The Women and Their Pregnancies*, of maternal characteristics, with demonstrated effects on pregnancy outcome. *Chapter 6* presents a brief overview of population characteristics with respect to outcome for the project infants in terms of birthweight, death, and neurological abnormalities at twelve months, in order that these may serve as a basis for the assessment and interpretation of the large amount of specific information that follows.

In *Chapter 7*, the birthweight-gestational age relationships are discussed and their effect on outcome examined in some detail (see comment below).

Chapter 8 includes data on body length and head circumference. A strong relationship was observed between neurological abnormality at one year and neonatal head circumference at both extremes of the distribution. Children with either unusually small or large heads had higher risks of abnormality than those whose head circumference was within the normal range at birth.

In *Chapter 9*, Apgar scores are discussed. The Apgar score at 1 and 5 minutes was used as an indication of stress at birth. Apgar scores below 7 were found to be related to both low birthweight and short gestational age. In general, the lower the score the higher the mortality and the greater the risk of neurological abnormality at one year.

In *Chapter 10*, the distributions of neonatal hematocrit levels show what appear to be increased risks of neonatal death and neurological abnormality at one year, associated with levels outside the normal neonatal range, i.e., with levels below 40 and above 60 mm.

Chapter 11 contains a detailed discussion of maximum neonatal serum bilirubin levels and their relationships. Differences in the frequency of elevated levels (i.e., 12 mg% and above) are related to birthweight, gestational age, and to risk of neurological abnormality at one year of age.

Chapter 12, Specific Neonatal Diagnoses, is one of the major chapters in the book. The summary tables catalogue an important range of neonatal diagnoses in relation to frequency, birthweight, and mortality for both white and black infants. In addition, the analyses were extended and the discussion amplified for the two important areas of neurological and respiratory abnormalities.

Chapter 13 describes the developmental findings in these large populations, at eight months of age, as observed by a psychologist, using modified Bayley Scales. Developmental status at this age (eight months ± two weeks) is strongly related to birthweight and gestational age, and when these variables are controlled, maternal education and race appear to have little effect on developmental performance.

In *Chapter 14*, findings are reported from the one-year pediatric neurological examination, pertaining to overall status both neurological and nonneurological and to certain key developmental items. Among white infants, definite neurological abnormalities were reported in 1.4 percent of those weighing more than 2500 grams, 4 percent of those weighing between 2001 and 2500 grams, and 10 percent of those weighing less than 2001 grams. Among black infants the risks were 1.2, 3, and 9 percent, respectively.

Chapter 15 contains a major and detailed diagnostic summary for the remainder of the first year. It provides an important information source for those concerned with the health and developmental status of young infants (see comments below).

In *Chapter 16*, an attempt is made to provide an overview of the frequency in these populations of certain congenital malformations and neurological and other diagnostic conditions reported during the first year of life. It is clear that in many diagnostic categories simple addition of cases reported at one year to those identified during the neonatal period may well provide overestimates when neonatal conditions are not confirmed on later examination.

A primary purpose of the final chapter is to comment on some of the major findings during the first year of life. A number of striking points emerge. For the most part, these observations are not new, but the breadth and diversity of the data add new dimensions and permit a broad perspective.

The importance of birthweight to outcome and of low birthweight as a potent risk factor is evident throughout the volume. Approximately 7 percent of the white and 13 percent of the black infants were in that category. Death, developmental status, and neurological abnormality at one year are all strongly related to weight at birth, as are many neonatal problems. However, birthweight, while useful as an independent outcome measure, reflects underlying antecedent factors, maternal, demographic, genetic, obstetrical, etc. For example, low birthweight alone did not account for the higher neonatal mortality observed among black infants, as approximately 30 percent of those who died weighed over 2500 grams.

While very low birthweight, 1500 grams and below, carried a grave prognosis, only a small number of infants were in this group (0.77 percent of white and 1.65 percent of black infants). Even though the risk of mortality among babies in the 2001–2500 gram weight was much less than that of smaller infants, this group contributed a greater proportion of deaths because of the larger number in this weight group.

Low-birthweight infants had a greater likelihood of adverse outcome in most, but not all, diagnostic categories. The association between low birthweight and neurological and developmental abnormalities was quite striking, and a similar though less strong relationship was observed between low birthweight and nonneurological abnormalities at one year (Chapter 14). However, a small number of abnormalities were associated with high birthweight (e.g., facial and brachial plexus, injury, and skull fracture).

Birthweight is, of course, strongly correlated with gestational age at delivery (Chapter 7), and gestational age, when less than thirty-seven weeks or when of inappropriate duration for birthweight of the child, was also a risk factor. Generally speaking, within a given gestational age group, the higher the birthweight (within appropriate limits) the lower the risk of perinatal mortality and neurological abnormality at one year. Similarly, within birthweight groups, the longer the gestation (again within appropriate limits) the better the outcome. However, the unusually high risks for the "small-for-dates" babies clearly stood out, and higher than usual risks for the "large-for-dates" infants were suggested. A substantial difference in average gestational age at delivery was observed between the white and black infants, with the whites having a gestational age that was approximately nine days longer than the blacks.

Neonatal respiratory problems also represent major risk factors (Chapter 12). These problems were of several kinds. Resuscitation was required at birth to initiate and/or maintain respiration in 6 percent of all infants of both races and in 14 percent of those with low birthweight. The respiratory distress syndrome (RDS) occurred in approximately 1 percent of infants, males being affected almost twice as often as females. RDS occurred most often following breech delivery, and it was strongly related to both low birthweight and short gestation. Definite pneumonia was reported in approximately 0.5 percent of infants. The importance of respiratory problems is clear when one considers that the risk of death is markedly increased in their presence. When no respiratory problems were reported the neonatal death rate was only 2.1/1000 for white and 1.6/1000 for black infants.

The neonatal death rate was, in general, higher among black infants than white, and the rate of low birthweight among the former (134.2/1000) was almost twice that of the latter (71.4/1000); however, the rates of neurological abnormality at one year and those for many other diagnostic entities were little different for the children of both races. It must be remembered that the project infants were born between 1959 and 1966 and that in the ensuing years neonatal mortality rates have declined. The numbers of surviving but abnormal infants may also be declining as a result of the availability of prenatal diagnosis and abortion, on the one hand, and improved perinatal care, on the other.

Serious, life-threatening, specific neonatal conditions were rarely encountered. Review of the data from the extensive diagnostic summary completed for each infant indicates a striking diversity of reported abnormalities with but very small numbers in each category. (Neonatal diagnostic summary tables at the end of Chapter 12.) For example, tracheo-esophageal fistula occurred once in 18,029 white and three times in 19,259 black infants. Similarly, there were 9 white infants and 6 black infants with anomalies of the diaphragm and 3 white and 4 black infants with malrotation of the gut. Also, 167 white and 105 black children had erythroblastosis. In all, 172 exchange transfusions were performed on white and 136 on black infants. Congenital heart disease was reported in only 40 white (0.2 percent) and 21 black infants (0.1 percent). Major surgical procedures were carried out in only 64 white and 100 black babies, and general anesthesia was administered to 38 of the former and 33 of the latter.

The findings with respect to the neonatal period strongly reinforce the importance, on every obstetrical service, of proper provisions for initiating and maintaining respiration at birth under optimal environmental conditions for the infant during the immediate postnatal period; and the need for special planning for sophisticated and efficient perinatal care for the relatively small number of infants with life-threatening conditions. The information about the diversity and relative infrequency of major diagnostic entities presented here may be helpful in planning for concentration of sophisticated equipment and experienced personnel with special training and experience to provide effective care without unnecessary duplication of expensive facilities. Assessment of maternal, fetal, and neonatal risk factors, prenatally and perinatally, with referral, where indicated, to special perinatal centers may be an efficient way of providing superior care and reducing both perinatal mortality and the continuum of handicapping conditions in survivors.

Relationships between birthweight, gestational age, and developmental performance were quite strong at eight months (Chapter 13) and less so at twelve months. Unfortunately, the data presented do not answer the question of whether normal low-birthweight infants have caught up developmentally by one year. We suspect that relationships observed at one year may, at least in part, reflect the higher proportion of low-weight infants with neurological and intellectual defects, but we have not documented this. The question of when the normal but low-birthweight/short-gestation infant catches up requires further analysis beyond the scope of this volume.

Perusal of the diagnostic data gathered between nursery discharge and one year of age (Chapter 15) provides an opportunity to examine the frequency of postnatal trauma and illness. The reader should be impressed by the relatively high frequency, in what should be a well-protected age group, of serious accidents and burns and serious childhood diseases, such as measles, in both white and black infants. These conditions are generally preventable.

This large volume of descriptive information pertaining to 18,029 white and 19,259 black infants followed through the first year of life has been presented because of the useful information it provides about infants as a basis for understanding a number of more detailed studies in progress focused on specific pathological, neurological, intellectual, neurosensory, and other aspects of the overall seven- to eight-year follow-up of children in the NINCDS Collaborative Perinatal Project.

APPENDIX

SELECTED PEDIATRIC FORMS

305

1. PATIENT IDENTIFICATION

DELIVERY ROOM OBSERVATION
OF THE NEONATE

2. OBSERVED BY	3. TITLE OR POSITION

4. DATE OF BIRTH Mo.	Day	Year	5. TIME OF BIRTH (24-hr clock)

Time all events below as age before or after delivery

		Age Begun	Age Ended

6. CORD CLAMPED (Age) Min. Sec.
☐ Before Delivery
☐ After Delivery

7. FIRST BREATH (Age) Min. Sec.
☐ Before Delivery
☐ After Delivery

8. FIRST CRY (Age) Min. Sec.
☐ Before Delivery
☐ After Delivery

9. PROCEDURES (*Omit uncomplicated oral-pharyngeal suction*)
☐ None 0
☐ Gastric Suction 1
☐ Tracheal Suction 2
☐ Drugs (*Give type & Dose*) 3

☐ Open Oxygen 4 — Min. / Min.
☐ Positive Pressure Oxygen or Air 5 — Min. / Min.
☐ Intubation 6 — Min. / Min.
☐ Other (*Specify*) 8 — Min. / Min.

10. APGAR SCORE (*Score infant at 1, 2 and 5 minutes of age. If score of 8 is not attained, score at 10, 15 and 20 minutes.*)

1) AGE AT TIME OF SCORING

				11. Min. Sec.	12. Min. Sec.	13. Min. Sec.	14. Min. Sec.	15. Min. Sec.	16. Min. Sec.
2) HEART RATE	0 – Absent	1 – Slow – Less Than 100	2 – 100 or over						
3) RESPIRATORY EFFORT	0 – Absent	1 – Weak Cry Hypoventilation	2 – Crying Lustily						
4) MUSCLE TONE	0 – Flaccid	1 – Some Flexion Extremities	2 – Well Flexed						
5) REFLEX IRRI-TABILITY	0 – No Response	1 – Some Motion	2 – Cry						
6) COLOR	0 – Blue Pale	1 – Blue Hands and Feet	2 – Entirely Pink						
7) TOTAL									

PHYSICAL EXAMINATION

17. Begun at _____ min. of age	18. EXAMINED BY	19. TITLE OR POSITION

20. RESPIRATION ☐ Normal 0 ☐ Other 8

21. MOTOR ACTIVITY AND TONE ☐ Normal and Symmetrical 0 ☐ Other 8

22. TONE OF NECK ☐ Normal and Symmetrical 0 ☐ Other 8

23. MOLDING ☐ Absent or Minimal 0 ☐ Moderate or Marked 1

24. FORCEPS MARKS ☐ Absent 0 ☐ Present 1

25. UMBILICAL CORD ☐ Unstained 0 ☐ Stained 1

26. LENGTH OF CORD (*Include all segments*)

On Body _____ Cm. Other _____ Cm.

On Placenta _____ Cm. Total _____ Cm.

27. SKIN (*Acute or transient findings*)
☐ Normal (*Including peripheral cyanosis*) 0
☐ Pallor 1
☐ General Cyanosis 2
☐ Petechiae 3
☐ Stained 4
☐ Other 8

28. CRY
☐ Present 0
☐ Present, Abnormal 1
☐ Absent After Maximal Stimulation 2

29. MORO REFLEX
☐ Flexor and Extensor Components Present and Symmetrical 0
☐ Other Pattern 8
☐ Not Evaluated 9

30. COMMENTS AND OTHER FINDINGS

(Continue on CP-5, Continuation Sheet)

31. RACE (*Copy from AR-1. Optional*)
☐ W 1 ☐ N 2 ☐ Or 3 ☐ PR 4 ☐ Other 8

32. SEX
☐ Male 1 ☐ Female 2 ☐ Undetermined 9

33. BIRTH WEIGHT

Collaborative Research
Perinatal Research Branch, NINDB, NIH
Bethesda 14, Md.

(PĒD-1) (Rev. 1-61)

COLR-3004-8
1-63

NEWBORN DIAGNOSTIC SUMMARY

1. PATIENT IDENTIFICATION:

2. NAME CODER	4. SUMMARY DATE
3. TITLE	5. DISCHARGE DATE

7. DISCHARGE STATUS	8.	6. DISCHARGE TIME
☐ ALIVE ☐ DEAD	☐ AUTOPSY	

9. DYSMATURITY (Circle answer)

NONE   EQUIVOCAL   STAGE: I   II   III

10. *LOWEST APGAR	11. *HIGHEST BILIRUBIN	12. CHECK THIS BOX IF NO ITEMS ARE CODED IN CATEGORIES A THRU S. ☐ NONE
SCORE_____	Level _____ mgm. %	

13. DO NOT WRITE HERE

INSTRUCTIONS: Circle number in appropriate box.

A. NEUROLOGIC ABNORMALITY	SUSPECT	DEFINITE
☐ None		
I. Brain abnormality	001	002
manifested by:		
1. seizures (general and local)	003	004
2. myoclonus	005	006
3. hypertonia	007	008
4. jitteriness or tremulousness	009	010
5. hyperactivity	011	012
6. paralysis—paresis		
7. hemi-	013	014
8. para-	015	016
9. tetra-	017	018
10. other, specify	019	020
11. hypotonia	049	050
12. hypoactivity	051	052
13. lethargy	053	054
14. asymmetry of reflexes, activity, or tone	055	056
15. symmetrical, but abnormal reflexes	057	058
16. abnormal Moro	059	060
17. abnormal cry	061	062
18. abnormal suck	063	064
19. other, specify	065	066

Abnormal Brain Status:

a. transient	090
b. persistent	092
c. one or no exam	094

A. NEUROLOGIC ABNORMALITY (Cont.)	SUSPECT	DEFINITE
II. Peripheral or cranial nerve abnormality		
1. brachial	095	096
2. facial	097	098
3. ocular	099	100
4. other, specify	101	102
III. Other neurologic abnormality		
1. Fractured skull	119	120
2. Cephalhematoma	121	122
3. Intracranial hemorrhage	123	124
Specify site		
4. Spinal cord abnormality, specify	133	134
5. Other, specify	153	154

B. CENTRAL NERVOUS SYSTEM MALFORMATIONS: RELATED SKELETAL CONDITIONS	SUSPECT	DEFINITE
☐ None		
1. Anencephaly	▨	184
2. Microcephaly	185	186
3. Hydranencephaly	187	188
4. Hydrocephaly	189	190
5. Craniosynostosis	191	192
6. Abnormal separation of sutures	193	194
7. Abnormal shape of skull	195	196
8. Encephalocele	197	198
9. Meningomyelocele/meningocele	199	200
10. Pilonidal sinus (not dimple)	201	202
11. Other midline sinuses, specify	203	204
12. Other, specify (do not code spina bifida occulta or craniotabes)	223	224

C. MUSCULOSKELETAL ABNORMALITY (do not list diastasis recti)	SUSPECT	DEFINITE
☐ None		
1. Vertebral abnormality (do not code spina bifida occulta)	253	254
2. Talipes equinovarus	255	256
3. Metatarsus adductus (varus)	257	258
4. Calcaneo valgus	259	260
5. Congenital dislocation or dysplasia of the hip	261	262
6. Absence or hypoplasia of extremity or part, specify	263	264
7. Polydactyly	▨	294
8. Syndactyly	▨	296
9. Torticollis	297	298
10. Arthrogryposis multiplex (amyoplasia congenita)	299	300
11. Achondroplasia	301	302
12. Fractured clavicle	303	304
13. Fractures, other (specify)	305	306
14. Other (non-infectious), specify	333	334

D. EYE CONDITIONS	SUSPECT	DEFINITE
☐ None		
1. Chorio-retinitis	351	352
2. Retrolental fibroplasia	353	354
3. Cataract	355	356
4. Corneal opacity	357	358
5. Microphthalmia	359	360
6. Blindness	361	362
7. Nystagmus	363	364
8. Other (non-infectious), specify	365	366

COLLABORATIVE RESEARCH
PERINATAL RESEARCH BRANCH, NINDB, NIH
BETHESDA 14, MD.

*Optional

PAGE 1 OF 4
(1-63)

PED-8

308

NEWBORN DIAGNOSTIC SUMMARY

E. EAR CONDITIONS	SUSPECT	DEFINITE
☐ None		
1. Low set ears	391	392
2. Deformed ear pinna	393	394
3. Branchial cleft anomaly (pre-auricular sinus, etc.)	395	396
4. Deafness	397	398
5. Other (non-infectious), specify	399	400
_ _ _ _ _ _ _ _ _ _ _ _		
_ _ _ _ _ _ _ _ _ _ _ _		
_ _ _ _ _ _ _ _ _ _ _ _		
_ _ _ _ _ _ _ _ _ _ _ _		

F. UPPER RESPIRATORY TRACT AND MOUTH CONDITIONS	SUSPECT	DEFINITE
☐ None		
1. Choanal atresia	419	420
2. Cleft palate	▨	422
3. Cleft uvula (bifid)	▨	424
4. Cleft lip	▨	426
5. Cleft gum	▨	428
6. Micrognathia	429	430
7. Malformation of epiglottis and larynx	431	432
8. Other (non-infectious), specify (T-E fistula listed under J-1.)	433	434
_ _ _ _ _ _ _ _ _ _ _ _		
_ _ _ _ _ _ _ _ _ _ _ _		
_ _ _ _ _ _ _ _ _ _ _ _		
_ _ _ _ _ _ _ _ _ _ _ _		

G. THORACIC ABNORMALITY (except neoplasms and cardiovascular conditions)	SUSPECT	DEFINITE
☐ None		
1. Anomaly of diaphragm	447	448
2. Anomaly of lung, specify	449	450
_ _ _ _ _ _ _ _ _ _ _ _		
3. Anomaly of chest wall, specify	459	460
_ _ _ _ _ _ _ _ _ _ _ _		
4. Pectus excavatum	467	468
5. Other, specify	469	470
_ _ _ _ _ _ _ _ _ _ _ _		
_ _ _ _ _ _ _ _ _ _ _ _		

H. RESPIRATORY ABNORMALITY	SUSPECT	DEFINITE
☐ None		
respiratory abnormality associated with:		
1. Respiratory distress syndrome (Hyaline membrane disease)	479	480
2. Primary atelectasis	481	482
3. Pneumonia	483	484
4. Aspiration <u>before</u> or <u>during</u> delivery	485	486
5. Aspiration <u>after</u> delivery	487	488
6. Pulmonary hemorrhage	489	490
7. Cardiac conditions	491	492
8. C.N.S. abnormality	493	494
9. Metabolic imbalance	495	496
10. Other, specify	497	498
_ _ _ _ _ _ _ _ _ _ _ _		
_ _ _ _ _ _ _ _ _ _ _ _		
11. Unknown condition	511	512

associated degree of respiratory distress

a. None	514
b. Slight	516
c. Moderate	518
d. Marked	520

significant respiratory events

12. Primary apnea	522
13. Single apneic episode	524
14. Multiple apneic episodes	526
15. Resuscitation—during first 5 minutes of life	528
16. Resuscitation—after first 5 minutes of life	530

I. CARDIOVASCULAR CONDITIONS	SUSPECT	DEFINITE
☐ None		
1. Acyanotic CHD	531	532
2. Cyanotic CHD	533	534
3. Fibroelastosis	535	536
4. Disorders of rhythm	537	538
5. Disorders of rate	539	540
6. Cardiac enlargement	541	542
7. Decompensation	543	544
8. Specific C-V diagnosis	▨	546
_ _ _ _ _ _ _ _ _ _ _ _		
_ _ _ _ _ _ _ _ _ _ _ _	▨	
9. Other, specify (list hemangiomata under skin, O.)	573	574
_ _ _ _ _ _ _ _ _ _ _ _		
_ _ _ _ _ _ _ _ _ _ _ _		

J. ALIMENTARY TRACT MALFORMATIONS AND OTHER CONDITIONS	SUSPECT	DEFINITE
☐ None		
1. Tracheo-esophageal fistula	601	602
2. Duodenal atresia	603	604
3. Malrotation	605	606
4. Omphalocele	▨	608
5. Visceral perforation	609	610
6. Imperforate anus	▨	612
7. Hernia, specify (omit uncomplicated umbilical, code diaphragmatic under G-1.)		
8. Inguinal	613	614
9. Femoral	615	616
10. Other, specify	617	618
_ _ _ _ _ _ _ _ _ _ _ _		
11. Other (non-infectious), specify	621	622
_ _ _ _ _ _ _ _ _ _ _ _		
_ _ _ _ _ _ _ _ _ _ _ _		

COLLABORATIVE RESEARCH
PERINATAL RESEARCH BRANCH, NINDB, NIH
BETHESDA 14, MD.

PAGE 2 OF 4
(1-63)

309

NEWBORN DIAGNOSTIC SUMMARY

K. ABNORMALITY OF LIVER, BILE DUCTS, AND/OR SPLEEN

☐ None

	SUSPECT	DEFINITE
1. Specify (non-infectious)	641	642
_ _ _ _ _ _ _ _ _ _ _		
_ _ _ _ _ _ _ _ _ _ _		
_ _ _ _ _ _ _ _ _ _ _		
_ _ _ _ _ _ _ _ _ _ _		

L. GENITOURINARY CONDITIONS
(do not list hydrocele, phimosis, or cryptorchidism)

☐ None

	SUSPECT	DEFINITE
1. Hypospadias	▨	658
2. Chordee	659	660
3. Other abnormalities of external genitalia (include pseudohermaphroditism), specify	661	662
_ _ _ _ _ _ _ _ _ _		
_ _ _ _ _ _ _ _ _ _		
4. Bladder outflow or urethral obstruction	677	678
5. Upper tract obstruction—hydronephrosis or hydro-ureter (megalo-ureter)	679	680
6. Cystic kidney	681	682
7. Other (non-infectious), specify	683	684
_ _ _ _ _ _ _ _		
_ _ _ _ _ _ _ _		

M. NEOPLASTIC DISEASE AND/OR OTHER TUMORS (list hemangiomata and lymphangiomata under skin, O.)

☐ None

	SUSPECT	DEFINITE
1. Specify type and organ	701	702
a._ _ _ _ _ _ _ _ _ _		
b._ _ _ _ _ _ _ _ _ _		
c._ _ _ _ _ _ _ _ _ _		
d._ _ _ _ _ _ _ _ _ _		

N. HEMATOLOGIC CONDITIONS

☐ None

	SUSPECT	DEFINITE
1. Erythroblastosis	719	720
2. Rh	721	722
3. ABO	723	724
4. Other, specify	725	726
_ _ _ _ _ _ _ _ _		
5. Other hemolytic disease, specify	741	742
_ _ _ _ _ _ _ _ _		
6. Coagulation defect, specify	751	752
_ _ _ _ _ _ _ _ _		
7. Intra-uterine blood loss	761	762
8. Other major hemorrhage, specify site	763	764
_ _ _ _ _ _ _ _ _		
9. Other, specify	783	784
_ _ _ _ _ _ _ _ _		

O. SKIN CONDITIONS AND MALFORMATIONS

☐ None

	SUSPECT	DEFINITE
1. Strawberry/portwine hemangioma	815	816
2. Cavernous hemangioma	817	818
3. Hairy nevus	▨	820
4. Lymphangioma	821	822
5. Sclerema	823	824
6. Severe ecchymosis	▨	826
7. Significant petechiae	▨	828
8. Supernumerary nipples	829	830
9. Café au lait spots (six or more)	▨	832
10. Other (non-infectious), specify (do not list skin tags)	833	834
_ _ _ _ _ _ _ _ _		
_ _ _ _ _ _ _ _ _		

P. INFECTION (specify (a) condition and (b) agent under appropriate symbol)

☐ None

	SUSPECT	DEFINITE
1. Septicemia	863	864
b._ _ _ _ _ _ _ _ _		
2. Central nervous system	865	866
a._ _ _ _ _ _ _ _ _		
b._ _ _ _ _ _ _ _ _		
3. Respiratory (upper and lower, including mouth)	867	868
a._ _ _ _ _ _ _ _ _		
b._ _ _ _ _ _ _ _ _		
4. Urinary tract	869	870
a._ _ _ _ _ _ _ _ _		
b._ _ _ _ _ _ _ _ _		
5. Bone and joint	871	872
a._ _ _ _ _ _ _ _ _		
b._ _ _ _ _ _ _ _ _		
6. Heart	873	874
a._ _ _ _ _ _ _ _ _		
b._ _ _ _ _ _ _ _ _		
7. Gastrointestinal (including diarrhea)	875	876
a._ _ _ _ _ _ _ _ _		
b._ _ _ _ _ _ _ _ _		
8. Eye	877	878
a._ _ _ _ _ _ _ _ _		
b._ _ _ _ _ _ _ _ _		
9. Ear	879	880
a._ _ _ _ _ _ _ _ _		
b._ _ _ _ _ _ _ _ _		
10. Cutaneous (including umbilical stump)	881	882
a._ _ _ _ _ _ _ _ _		
b._ _ _ _ _ _ _ _ _		
11. Mucous membranes	883	884
a._ _ _ _ _ _ _ _ _		
b._ _ _ _ _ _ _ _ _		
12. Other, specify	885	886
a._ _ _ _ _ _ _ _ _		
b._ _ _ _ _ _ _ _ _		

COLLABORATIVE RESEARCH
PERINATAL RESEARCH BRANCH, NINDB, NIH
BETHESDA 14, MD.

PAGE 3 OF 4
(1-63)

PED-8

310

NEWBORN DIAGNOSTIC SUMMARY

Q. SYNDROMES	SUSPECT	DEFINITE
□ None		
1. Mongolism	887	888
2. Gonadal dysgenesis	889	890
3. Adrenogenital	891	892
4. Marfan's	893	894
5. Pierre Robin	895	896
6. Other syndromes, specify	897	898
_ _ _ _ _ _ _ _ _ _ _		
_ _ _ _ _ _ _ _ _ _ _		

R. OTHER ENDOCRINE OR METABOLIC DISEASE	SUSPECT	DEFINITE
□ None		
1. Cretinism	915	916
2. Fibrocystic disease of pancreas	917	918
3. Presumed symptomatic hypocalcemia	919	920
4. Presumed symptomatic hypoglycemia	921	922
5. Inborn errors of metabolism, specify	923	924
_ _ _ _ _ _ _ _ _ _ _		
_ _ _ _ _ _ _ _ _ _ _		
6. Other, specify	937	938
_ _ _ _ _ _ _ _ _ _ _		
_ _ _ _ _ _ _ _ _ _ _		
_ _ _ _ _ _ _ _ _ _ _		

S. OTHER CONDITIONS	SUSPECT	DEFINITE
□ None		
1. Specify	951	952
_ _ _ _ _ _ _ _ _ _ _		
_ _ _ _ _ _ _ _ _ _ _		
_ _ _ _ _ _ _ _ _ _ _		
_ _ _ _ _ _ _ _ _ _ _		
_ _ _ _ _ _ _ _ _ _ _		

T. PROCEDURES □ None	
1. Simple blood transfusions	965
2. Exchange transfusions	966
3. Parenteral fluids	967
4. Spinal puncture	968
5. Subdural puncture	969
6. Ventricular puncture	970
7. General anesthesia	971
8. Surgery, specify (do not list circumcision)	972
_ _ _ _ _ _ _ _ _ _ _	
_ _ _ _ _ _ _ _ _ _ _	
9. Chromosome studies	982
10. X-ray and/or fluoroscopy	983
11. Antibiotics (Internal only)	984
_ _ _ _ _ _ _ _ _ _ _	
_ _ _ _ _ _ _ _ _ _ _	
_ _ _ _ _ _ _ _ _ _ _	
_ _ _ _ _ _ _ _ _ _ _	

T. PROCEDURES (Cont.)	
12. E.E.G.	985
13. Other, specify	986
_ _ _ _ _ _ _ _ _ _ _	
_ _ _ _ _ _ _ _ _ _ _	
_ _ _ _ _ _ _ _ _ _ _	
_ _ _ _ _ _ _ _ _ _ _	

U. PRESUMPTIVE ETIOLOGIC IMPRESSIONS	
□ None	
1. Presumed anoxia	987
2. Presumed trauma	988

V. INFORMATION SOURCE (Check applicable boxes)

1. Study Record □
2. Nursery Record □
3. Additional records □
4. CP-5 attached □

COMMENTS (For Local Use Only)

COLLABORATIVE RESEARCH
PERINATAL RESEARCH BRANCH, NINDB, NIH
BETHESDA 14, MD.

PAGE 4 OF 4
(1-63)

PED-8

311

ONE-YEAR NEUROLOGICAL EXAMINATION

1. PATIENT IDENTIFICATION

2. NAME OF EXAMINER

3. TITLE OR POSITION

4. DATE OF EXAM.
Mo. | Day | Year

*5. AGE OF CHILD (Weeks Completed)

6. WEIGHT_____

7. BODY LENGTH (crown-heel) _____ cm.

*8. LOWER SEGMENT (Symphysis-heel) _____ cm.

9. HEAD CIRCUMFERENCE_____cm.

*10. CHEST CIRCUMFERENCE _____ cm.

11. HEAD – SHAPE AND CONTOUR
☐ Normal   ☐ Other (describe)
0   8

12. ANTERIOR FONTANELLE
☐ Closed (1 cm. or less)   ☐ Open (complete items 13, 14, 15)
0 x

SIZE   15. TENSION
                        ☐ Normal
13. AP_____cm.   0
                        ☐ Other
14. LAT_____cm.   8 (Specify)

*16. TRANSILLUMINATION
☐ Normal   ☐ Other (describe)
0   8

17. FACIES
☐ Normal   ☐ Hypertelorism
0   3

  ☐ Epicanthal folds   ☐ Other (describe)
  1   8

  ☐ Cleft lip
  2

18. EYES – STRUCTURE – EXTERNAL EXAMINATION (lids, cornea, sclera, conjunctiva, iris, red reflex)
☐ Normal   ☐ Other (describe)
0   8

*19. EYES – STRUCTURE – OPHTHALMOSCOPIC EXAMINATION
(lens, media, macula, disk, vessels, posterior retina)
☐ Normal   ☐ Other (describe)
0   8

20. EARS – SIZE, SHAPE AND LOCATION
☐ Normal   ☐ Other (describe)
0   8

*21. EARS – OTOSCOPIC EXAMINATION
☐ Normal   ☐ Unable to evaluate (explain)
0   9

  ☐ Other (describe)
  8

22. NOSE, MOUTH AND PHARYNX
☐ Normal   ☐ Other (specify)
0   8

NOTE: Items marked with an asterisk * are required only if an abnormality is suspected on the basis of other tests. They are optional for otherwise normal cases. It is not necessary to comment "Not Evaluated" for these.
     All other items must be evaluated or a reason given for failure.

23. COMMENTS

Collaborative Research
Perinatal Research Branch, NINDB, NIH
Bethesda 14, Md.

PED–11 (Rev. 5-61)
Page 1 of 7

312

ONE-YEAR NEUROLOGICAL EXAMINATION
(Continued)

25. NECK

☐ Normal
0

    ☐ Restricted Range of Motion
    1

    ☐ Masses *(Other than lymph nodes)*
    2

    ☐ Other *(Specify)*
    8

NOTE: Items marked with an asterisk * are required only if an abnormality is suspected on the basis of other tests. They are optional for otherwise normal cases. It is not necessary to comment "Not Evaluated" for these.
    All other items must be evaluated or a reason given for failure.

26. THORAX

☐ Normal   ☐ Other *(Specify)*
0   8

39. COMMENTS

27. RESPIRATIONS

☐ Normal   ☐ Other *(Specify)*
0   8

28. LUNGS

☐ Normal   ☐ Other *(Specify)*
0   8

29. HEART

☐ Normal
0

    ☐ Irregular Rhythm *(do not*   ☐ Thrill
    1 *report sinus arrhythmia)*   4

    ☐ Murmur *(Describe)*   ☐ Other *(Specify)*
    2   8

*30. FEMORAL PULSES

☐ Strong and Equal Bilaterally   ☐ Other *(Specify)*
0   8

*31. BLOOD PRESSURE

Arm _____   Leg _____

32. ABDOMEN AND CONTENTS

☐ Normal *(Including Umbilical*   ☐ Other *(Specify)*
0   *Hernia)*   8

33. LIVER

☐ Normal   ☐ Other *(Specify)*
0   8

34. SPLEEN

☐ Normal   ☐ Other *(Specify)*
0   8

35. KIDNEYS

☐ Not Palpable
0

    ☐ Palpable *(Describe)*
    1

36. GENITALIA

☐ Normal   ☐ Other *(Specify)*
0   8

37. SKIN

☐ Normal *(Including Mongolian Spots, Stork Bites and diaper rash)*
0

    ☐ Pigmented Nevi   ☐ Cafe Au Lait Spots – approximate
    1   5

    ☐ Vascular Nevi   number _____
    2

    ☐ Other Rashes   ☐ Other *(Specify)*
    3   8

    ☐ Loose and Wrinkled   [All items other than normal
    4   must be described.]

38. SPINE

☐ Normal   ☐ Other *(Specify)*
0   8

Collaborative Research
Perinatal Research Branch, NINDB, NIH
Bethesda 14, Md.

PED–11 (Rev. 5-61)
Page 2 of 7

313

ONE-YEAR NEUROLOGICAL EXAMINATION
(Continued)

40. PATIENT IDENTIFICATION

41. MUSCULOSKELETAL SYSTEM

	Normal	Other (Specify)
42. Shoulder Girdle	☐ 0	☐ 8
43. Arms and Wrists	☐ 0	☐ 8
44. Hands	☐ 0	☐ 8
45. Pelvic Girdle	☐ 0	☐ 8
46. Legs and Ankles	☐ 0	☐ 8
47. Feet	☐ 0	☐ 8

NOTE: Items marked with an asterisk * are required only if an abnormality is suspected on the basis of other tests. They are optional for otherwise normal cases. It is not necessary to comment "Not Evaluated" for these.
   All other items must be evaluated or a reason given for failure.

48. STATE OF CONSCIOUSNESS

☐ Alert and responding appropriately
0

☐ Other (Specify)
8

49. AFFECTIVE RESPONSE

☐ Normal
0

☐ Other (Describe)
8

50. PHONATION

51. Observed

☐ Intelligible words
0

☐ Unintelligible sounds
1 other than crying

☐ Crying only
2

☐ Other (Describe)
8

*52. Reported

☐ Intelligible words
0

☐ Unintelligible sounds
1 other than crying

☐ Crying
2

☐ Other (Describe)
8

53. LOCOMOTOR AND POSTURAL DEVELOPMENT

54. Observed

☐ Walks unaided
0

☐ Walks supported
1

☐ Stands unaided
2

☐ Pulls to standing
3

☐ Stands supported
4

☐ Creeps
5

☐ None of the above
8

☐ Not evaluated (Explain)
9

*55. Reported

☐ Walks unaided
0

☐ Walks supported
1

☐ Stands unaided
2

☐ Pulls to standing
3

☐ Stands supported
4

☐ Creeps
5

☐ None of the above
8

56. ABNORMALITIES OF GAIT OR POSTURE

☐ None, locomotion and posture normal
0

☐ Retarded locomotor development (Describe)
1

☐ Hemiparesis — hemiplegia (Describe)
2

☐ Other weakness or paralysis (Describe)
4

☐ Other (Describe)
8

☐ Not evaluated (Explain)
9

57. PREHENSILE GRASP (1 inch cube or similar object)

☐ Grasp using thumb and finger(s), palm free
0

☐ Grasp with palm
1

☐ Unable to evaluate (Explain)
9

☐ Raking without grasp
2

☐ Other (Describe)
8

58. COMMENTS

Collaborative Research
Perinatal Research, Branch, NINDB, NIH
Bethesda 14, Md.

ONE-YEAR NEUROLOGICAL EXAMINATION
(Continued)

59. PATIENT IDENTIFICATION

60. REACHING COORDINATION

☐ Normal
0

☐ Unable to evaluate *(Explain)*
9

☐ Dyskinesia *(Describe)*
1

☐ Other *(Describe)*
8

61. HAND PREFERENCE

☐ Variable
0

☐ Unable to evaluate *(Explain)*
9

☐ Strongly right
1

☐ Strongly left
2

NOTE: Items marked with an asterisk * are required only if an abnormality is suspected on the basis of other tests. They are optional for otherwise normal cases. It is not necessary to comment "Not Evaluated" for these.
   All other items must be evaluated or a reason given for failure.

62. SENSATION – EXTREMITIES AND TRUNK – LIGHT TOUCH

☐ No abnormality detected
0

☐ Unable to evaluate *(Explain)*
9

☐ Other *(Describe, drawing preferred)*
8

70. COMMENTS

*63. SENSATION – EXTREMITIES AND TRUNK – PIN PRICK

☐ No abnormality detected
0

☐ Other *(Describe, drawing preferred)*
8

64. SPONTANEOUS MOVEMENTS OF FACE

☐ Present and symmetical
0

☐ Unable to evaluate *(Explain)*
9

☐ Other *(Describe)*
8

65. PALPEBRAL FISSURES

☐ Wide and equal
0

☐ Unable to evaluate *(Explain)*
9

☐ Other *(Describe)*
8

66. LID CLOSURE

☐ Normal and symmetrical
0

☐ Unable to evaluate *(Explain)*
9

☐ Other *(Describe)*
8

*67. CORNEAL REFLEX

☐ Present and symmetrical
0

☐ Other *(Describe)*
8

68. FOLLOWS LIGHT OR OBJECT

☐ Yes
0

☐ Unable to evaluate *(Explain)*
9

☐ Questionable
1

☐ No
8

69. OPTICOKINETIC NYSTAGMUS

☐ Present and symmetrical
0

☐ Unable to evaluate *(Explain)*
9

☐ Questionable *(Describe)*
1

☐ Absent
2

☐ Other *(Describe)*
8

Collaborative Research
Perinatal Research Branch, NIH, NINDB
Bethesda 14, Md.

PED-11 (Rev. 5-61)
Page 4 of 7

COLR-3004-11
REV. 5-61

ONE-YEAR NEUROLOGICAL EXAMINATION
(Continued)

72. VISUAL FIELDS BY CONFRONTATION

☐ No abnormality detected
0

☐ Unable to evaluate (*Explain*)
9

☐ Other (*Describe*)
8

73. POSITION OF EYES AT REST

☐ Normal
0

☐ Unable to evaluate (*Explain*)
9

☐ Other (*Describe*)
8

74. WEAKNESS OR PARALYSIS OF INDIVIDUAL EYE MOVEMENTS

75. Right Eye	76. Left Eye
☐ None (normal movements) 0	☐ None (normal movements) 0
☐ Right 1	☐ Right 1
☐ Left 2	☐ Left 2
☐ Upward 3	☐ Upward 3
☐ Downward 4	☐ Downward 4
☐ Other (*Describe*) 5	☐ Other (*Describe*) 5
☐ Unable to evaluate (*Explain*) 9	☐ Unable to evaluate (*Explain*) 9

77. SPONTANEOUS NYSTAGMUS

☐ None
0

☐ Unable to evaluate (*Explain*)
9

☐ Central, bilateral
1

☐ Other (*Describe*)
8

78. PUPILS – SHAPE AND SYMMETRY

☐ Normal
0

☐ Unable to evaluate (*Explain*)
9

☐ Other (*Describe*)
8

79. PUPILS – REACTION TO LIGHT – DIRECT

☐ Normal and symmetrical
0

☐ Unable to evaluate (*Explain*)
9

☐ Other (*Describe*)
8

*80. PUPILS – REACTION TO LIGHT – CONSENSUAL

☐ Present and symmetrical
0

☐ Other (*Describe*)
8

81. RESPONSE TO SOUND

☐ No abnormality detected
0

☐ Unable to evaluate (*Explain*)
9

☐ Other (*Describe*)
8

*82. GAG REFLEX

☐ Present
0

☐ Unable to evaluate (*Explain*)
9

☐ Other (*Describe*)
8

83. PALATE MOVEMENT

☐ Present and symmetrical
0

☐ Unable to evaluate (*Explain*)
9

☐ Other (*Describe*)
8

84. TONGUE

☐ Normal
0

☐ Unable to evaluate (*Explain*)
9

☐ Other (*Describe*)
8

NOTE: Items marked with an asterisk * are required only if an abnormality is suspected on the basis of other tests. They are optional for otherwise normal cases. It is not necessary to comment "Not Evaluated" for these.

All other items must be evaluated or a reason given for failure.

85. COMMENTS

Collaborative Research
Perinatal Research Branch, NIH, NINDB
Bethesda 14, Md.

ONE-YEAR NEUROLOGICAL EXAMINATION
(Continued)

86. PATIENT IDENTIFICATION

87. ABNORMAL INVOLUNTARY MOVEMENTS

☐ None
0

☐ Unable to evaluate (Explain)
9

☐ Choreoathetosis (Describe)
1

☐ Dystonia (Describe)
2

☐ Tremor (Describe)
3

☐ Other (Describe)
4

NOTE: Items marked with an asterisk * are required only if an abnormality is suspected on the basis of other tests. They are optional for otherwise normal cases. It is not necessary to comment "Not Evaluated" for these.

All other items must be evaluated or a reason given for failure.

88. TONE – Use the following code which will indicate a gradation from flaccid to rigid. Describe any asymmetry in right hand column.

1. Hypotonic
2. Questionable Hypotonicity
3. Normal

4. Questionable Hypertonicity
5. Hypertonic
9. Unable to evaluate

105. COMMENTS

	BILATERAL	RIGHT	LEFT
89. Upper Extremity			
90. Lower Extremity			
91. Neck Flexor			
92. Neck Extensor			
93. Trunk			

94. DEEP TENDON REFLEXES – Use the following code which will indicate a gradation from Absent to Increased with clonus.

0. Absent
1. Hypoactive
2. Normal

3. Increased
4. Increased with clonus
9. Unable to evaluate

	BILATERAL	RIGHT	LEFT
95. Biceps jerk			
96. Triceps jerk			
97. Knee jerk			
98. Ankle jerk			

99. PLANTAR RESPONSE

100. Right

☐ Variable
0

☐ Upward movement of
1 great toe

☐ Upward movement of great
2 toe and fanning of toes

☐ Flexion of toes
3

101. Left

☐ Variable
0

☐ Upward movement of
1 great toe

☐ Upward movement of great
2 toe and fanning of toes

☐ Flexion of toes
3

*102. SUPERFICIAL ABDOMINAL REFLEX

☐ Present and symmetrical
0

☐ Other (Describe)
8

*103. TONIC NECK REFLEX

☐ No constant pattern
0

☐ Obtained with difficulty
1

☐ Obtained with ease
2

☐ Other (Describe)
8

*104. MORO REFLEX

☐ No constant pattern
0

☐ Flexor and extensor components present and symmetrical
1

☐ Other (Describe)
8

Collaborative Research
Perinatal Research Branch, NIH, NINDB
Bethesda 14, Md.

PED-11 (Rev. 5-61)

Page 6 of 7

106. PATIENT IDENTIFICATION

ONE-YEAR NEUROLOGICAL EXAMINATION
(Continued)

107. PALMAR GRASP REFLEX

☐ Absent or variable ☐ Unable to evaluate
0   9

☐ Reflex present and symmetrical
1

☐ Other (Describe)
8

108. SWEATING

109. Observed   *110. Reported

☐ Present, normal   ☐ Present, normal
0   0

☐ Other (Describe)   ☐ Other (Describe)
8   8

☐ Unable to evaluate   ☐ Unable to evaluate
9   9

NOTE: Items marked with an asterisk * are required only if an abnormality is suspected on the basis of other tests. They are optional for otherwise normal cases. It is not necessary to comment "Not Evaluated" for these.

All other items must be evaluated or a reason given for failure.

111. URINARY STREAM

112. Observed   *113. Reported

☐ Good periodic stream   ☐ Good periodic stream
0   0

☐ Dribbling   ☐ Dribbling
1   1

☐ Other (Describe)   ☐ Other (Describe)
8   8

☐ Unable to evaluate   ☐ Unable to evaluate
9   9

*114. SUPERFICIAL ANAL REFLEX

☐ Present, normal   ☐ Unable to evaluate
0   9

☐ Other (Describe)
8

*115. RECTAL TONE

☐ Normal   ☐ Other (Describe)
0   8

116. OTHER SIGNS, REFLEXES, TESTS, ETC.

☐ No   ☐ Yes (Specify)
0   1

IMPRESSION

117. NEUROLOGICAL ABNORMALITIES

☐ None
0

☐ Neurologically Suspicious But No Definite Abnormalities
1 (Describe reasons for this statement in detail)

☐ Neurologically Abnormal Child
2 (Describe fully and give reasons)

118. NON-NEUROLOGICAL ABNORMALITIES (Check all that apply)

☐ None
0

☐ Minor Abnormalities or Deviations (Describe)
1

☐ Questionable Abnormalities (Describe)
2

☐ Definite Major Abnormalities (Describe)
4

119. UNSATISFACTORY CONDITIONS FOR EXAMINATION

☐ Absent   ☐ Present (Specify)
0   1

120. DISPOSITION

☐ – No Indication, At This Time, For Further Evaluation
0

☐ Further Evaluation Proposed Or Scheduled (Specify)
8

121. CP-5 ATTACHED (Medical editor's comments, report of further studies, etc.)

☐ No   ☐ Yes
0   1

122. COMMENTS

Collaborative Research
Perinatal Research Branch, NINDB, NIH
Bethesda 14, Md.

PED-11 (Rev. 5-61)

Page 7 of 7

318

COLR–3004-12
6-63

PED-12

SUMMARY OF THE FIRST YEAR OF LIFE AFTER THE DURATION SUMMARIZED ON THE PED-8

1. PATIENT IDENTIFICATION

2. NAME CODER		4. SUMMARY DATE	MO.	DAY	YEAR

3. TITLE

5. PED-4 ☐
AUTOPSY ☐

6. INFORMATION SOURCES
PED-10 ☐   PS-3 ☐   PED-11 ☐   PED-20 ☐   PED-29 ☐

7. DATE OF PED-11 EXAMINATION | MO. | DAY | YEAR

8. AGE OF CHILD AT PED-11 EXAMINATION | WEEKS

9. INFORMATION INADEQUATE ON CATEGORIES A-16 ☐ W ☐

10. CHECK THIS BOX IF NO ITEMS ARE CODED IN CATEGORIES A THRU W ☐ NONE

11. DO NOT WRITE HERE

A	B	C	D	E	F	G	H	I	J	K	L	M	N	O	P	Q	R	S	T	U	V	W	TOTAL	I	II	III

INSTRUCTIONS: Check appropriate box.

Columns: SUSPECT | DEFINITE | (1) PED-11 | (2) PRIOR EXAM OR PED-29 | (4) HISTORY ONLY

A. NEUROLOGIC ABNORMALITY

NONE ☐

1. CEREBRAL SPASTIC PARESIS

a. Hemi

RIGHT............ 001 ☐ 002 ☐   ☐ ☐ ☐

LEFT............ 003 ☐ 004 ☐   ☐ ☐ ☐

b. Tetra............ 005 ☐ 006 ☐   ☐ ☐ ☐

c. Para............ 007 ☐ 008 ☐   ☐ ☐ ☐

d. Other, specify............ 009 ☐ 010 ☐   ☐ ☐ ☐

– – – – – – – – – – – – – – – –

2. HYPOTONIA

a. Hypotonia with deep tendon reflexes............ 015 ☐ 016 ☐   ☐ ☐ ☐

b. Hypotonia without deep tendon reflexes............ 017 ☐ 018 ☐   ☐ ☐ ☐

3. DYSKINESIA (includes "extra-pyramidal" rigidity)............ 019 ☐ 020 ☐   ☐ ☐ ☐

4. ATAXIA............ 021 ☐ 022 ☐   ☐ ☐ ☐

5. OTHER MOTOR DISORDERS, SPECIFY............ 023 ☐ 024 ☐   ☐ ☐ ☐

– – – – – – – – – – – – – – – –

6. DELAYED DEVELOPMENT

a. Motor............ 031 ☐ 032 ☐   ☐ ☐ ☐

b. Mental............ 033 ☐ 034 ☐   ☐ ☐ ☐

7. REGRESSION IN MOTOR ACTIVITY....... 035 ☐ 036 ☐   ☐ ☐ ☐

A. NEUROLOGIC ABNORMALITY (Cont.)

Columns: SUSPECT | DEFINITE | (1) PED-11 | (2) PRIOR EXAM OR PED-29 | (4) HISTORY ONLY

8. CORD DISEASE

(include signs of meningomyelocele)

a. Spastic............ 037 ☐ 038 ☐   ☐ ☐ ☐

b. Flaccid............ 039 ☐ 040 ☐   ☐ ☐ ☐

9. VISUAL IMPAIRMENT

a. Total

(1) BILATERAL

(A) OCULAR............ 041 ☐ 042 ☐   ☐ ☐ ☐

(B) NON-OCULAR............ 043 ☐ 044 ☐   ☐ ☐ ☐

(2) UNILATERAL

(A) OCULAR............ 045 ☐ 046 ☐   ☐ ☐ ☐

(B) NON-OCULAR............ 047 ☐ 048 ☐   ☐ ☐ ☐

b. Partial

(1) BILATERAL

(A) OCULAR............ 049 ☐ 050 ☐   ☐ ☐ ☐

(B) NON-OCULAR............ 051 ☐ 052 ☐   ☐ ☐ ☐

(2) UNILATERAL

(A) OCULAR............ 053 ☐ 054 ☐   ☐ ☐ ☐

(B) NON-OCULAR............ 055 ☐ 056 ☐   ☐ ☐ ☐

COLLABORATIVE RESEARCH
PERINATAL RESEARCH BRANCH, NINDB, NIH
BETHESDA 14, MD.

6-63   PAGE 1 OF 8   **PED-12**

319

1. PATIENT IDENTIFICATION

PED-12

SUMMARY OF THE FIRST YEAR OF LIFE AFTER THE DURATION SUMMARIZED ON THE PED-8

A. NEUROLOGIC ABNORMALITY (Cont.)

	SUSPECT	DEFINITE	(1) PED-11	(2) PRIOR EXAM OR PED-29	(4) HISTORY ONLY
10. EXTRA OCULAR MOVEMENTS					
a. Esotropia					
(1) UNILATERAL	057 ☐	058 ☐	☐	☐	☐
(2) BILATERAL	059 ☐	060 ☐	☐	☐	☐
b. Alternating internal strabismus	061 ☐	062 ☐	☐	☐	☐
c. Exotropia					
(1) UNILATERAL	063 ☐	064 ☐	☐	☐	☐
(2) BILATERAL	065 ☐	066 ☐	☐	☐	☐
d. Alternating external strabismus	067 ☐	068 ☐	☐	☐	☐
e. Other, specify	069 ☐	070 ☐	☐	☐	☐

- - - - - - - - - - - - - -

	SUSPECT	DEFINITE	(1) PED-11	(2) PRIOR EXAM OR PED-29	(4) HISTORY ONLY
11. NYSTAGMUS					
a. Involvement					
(1) UNILATERAL	077 ☐	078 ☐	☐	☐	☐
(2) UNILATERAL WITH GAZE ONLY	079 ☐	080 ☐	☐	☐	☐
(3) BILATERAL	081 ☐	082 ☐	☐	☐	☐
(4) BILATERAL WITH GAZE ONLY	083 ☐	084 ☐	☐	☐	☐
b. Character					
(1) PENDULAR	085 ☐	086 ☐	☐	☐	☐
(2) JERKY	087 ☐	088 ☐	☐	☐	☐
c. Direction					
(1) HORIZONTAL	089 ☐	090 ☐	☐	☐	☐
(2) VERTICAL	091 ☐	092 ☐	☐	☐	☐
(3) ROTATORY	093 ☐	094 ☐	☐	☐	☐
d. Other, specify	095 ☐	096 ☐	☐	☐	☐

- - - - - - - - - - - - - -

	SUSPECT	DEFINITE	(1) PED-11	(2) PRIOR EXAM OR PED-29	(4) HISTORY ONLY
12. CRANIAL NERVE ABNORMALITY (other than II, III, IV, VI, VIII)					
a. Facial (VII)	101 ☐	102 ☐	☐	☐	☐
b. Other, specify	103 ☐	104 ☐	☐	☐	☐

- - - - - - - - - - - - - -

A. NEUROLOGIC ABNORMALITY (Cont.)

	SUSPECT	DEFINITE	(1) PED-11	(2) PRIOR EXAM OR PED-29	(4) HISTORY ONLY
13. HEARING IMPAIRMENT	113 ☐	114 ☐	☐	☐	☐
14. PERIPHERAL NERVE ABNORMALITY (other than cranial nerve)					
a. Brachial plexus	115 ☐	116 ☐	☐	☐	☐
b. Other, specify	117 ☐	118 ☐	☐	☐	☐

- - - - - - - - - - - - - -

	SUSPECT	DEFINITE	(1) PED-11	(2) PRIOR EXAM OR PED-29	(4) HISTORY ONLY
15. SEIZURE STATES					
a. Generalized (grand mal)					
Estimate total number _ _ _ _					
(1) ONLY WITH FEVER AND LESS THAN 15 MINUTES DURATION	129 ☐	130 ☐	☐	☐	☐
(2) OTHER	131 ☐	132 ☐	☐	☐	☐
b. Focal motor					
Estimate total number _ _ _ _	133 ☐	134 ☐	☐	☐	☐
c. Infantile myoclonic seizures	135 ☐	136 ☐	☐	☐	☐
d. Other, specify	137 ☐	138 ☐	☐	☐	☐

- - - - - - - - - - - - - -

	SUSPECT	DEFINITE	(1) PED-11	(2) PRIOR EXAM OR PED-29	(4) HISTORY ONLY
16. ATYPICAL BEHAVIOR INFORMATION INADEQUATE ☐					
a. Maladaptive responses	149 ☐	150 ☐	☐	☐	☐
b. Failure to develop social responses or inappropriate social behavior for age	151 ☐	152 ☐	☐	☐	☐
c. Failure to form rhythmic patterns	153 ☐	154 ☐	☐	☐	☐
d. Disruption of rhythmic patterns	155 ☐	156 ☐	☐	☐	☐
e. Regression in behavior	157 ☐	158 ☐	☐	☐	☐
f. Stereotyped behavior	159 ☐	160 ☐	☐	☐	☐
g. Abnormalities of behavior control, specify	161 ☐	162 ☐	☐	☐	☐

- - - - - - - - - - - - - -

	SUSPECT	DEFINITE	(1) PED-11	(2) PRIOR EXAM OR PED-29	(4) HISTORY ONLY
h. Breath holding (1) WITH UNCONSCIOUSNESS	173 ☐	174 ☐	☐	☐	☐
(2) WITHOUT UNCONSCIOUSNESS	175 ☐	176 ☐	☐	☐	☐
i. Hyper-reactivity to sensory stimuli	177 ☐	178 ☐	☐	☐	☐
j. Apathy	179 ☐	180 ☐	☐	☐	☐
k. Phobia	181 ☐	182 ☐	☐	☐	☐

COLLABORATIVE RESEARCH
PERINATAL RESEARCH BRANCH, NINDB, NIH
BETHESDA 14, MD.

6-63   PAGE 2 OF 8   PED-12

320

1. PATIENT IDENTIFICATION

PED-12   SUMMARY OF THE FIRST YEAR OF LIFE AFTER THE DURATION SUMMARIZED ON THE PED-8

A. NEUROLOGIC ABNORMALITY (Cont.)

	SUSPECT	DEFINITE	(1) PED-11	(2) PRIOR EXAM OR PED-29	(4) HISTORY ONLY
16. ATYPICAL BEHAVIOR *(Continued)*					
l. Pica					
(1) PAINT OR PLASTER	183 ☐	184 ☐	☐	☐	☐
(2) OTHER, SPECIFY	185 ☐	186 ☐	☐	☐	☐
m. Other, specify	195 ☐	196 ☐	☐	☐	☐
17. COMA, specify cause	205 ☐	206 ☐	☐	☐	☐
18. OTHER, SPECIFY	215 ☐	216 ☐	☐	☐	☐

B. RELATED CENTRAL NERVOUS SYSTEM AND SKELETAL CONDITIONS

NONE ☐

	SUSPECT	DEFINITE	(1) PED-11	(2) PRIOR EXAM OR PED-29	(4) HISTORY ONLY
1. MACROCEPHALY	225 ☐	226 ☐	☐	☐	☐
2. MICROCEPHALY	227 ☐	228 ☐	☐	☐	☐
3. HYDRANENCEPHALY	229 ☐	230 ☐	☐	☐	☐
4. HYDROCEPHALY	231 ☐	232 ☐	☐	☐	☐
a. Specify cause					
b. Specify anatomic lesion					
5. CRANIOSYNOSTOSIS Specify involved sutures	243 ☐	244 ☐	☐	☐	☐
6. OTHER ABNORMAL SHAPE OF SKULL Specify	249 ☐	250 ☐	☐	☐	☐
7. PORENCEPHALY	255 ☐	256 ☐	☐	☐	☐
8. ENCEPHALOCELE	257 ☐	258 ☐	☐	☐	☐
9. MENINGOMYELOCELE/ MENINGOCELE	259 ☐	260 ☐	☐	☐	☐
10. PILONIDAL SINUS *(not dimple)*	261 ☐	262 ☐	☐	☐	☐
11. OTHER MIDLINE SINUSES, SPECIFY	263 ☐	264 ☐	☐	☐	☐
12. SUBDURAL HEMATOMA OR EFFUSION	269 ☐	270 ☐	☐	☐	☐
13. OTHER INTRACRANIAL HEMORRHAGE Specify site	271 ☐	272 ☐	☐	☐	☐
14. OTHER, SPECIFY *(do not code spina bifida occulta or craniotabes)*	279 ☐	280 ☐	☐	☐	☐

C. MUSCULOSKELETAL ABNORMALITY

(do not list diastasis recti)

NONE ☐

	SUSPECT	DEFINITE	(1) PED-11	(2) PRIOR EXAM OR PED-29	(4) HISTORY ONLY
1. VERTEBRAL ABNORMALITY *(do not code spina bifida occulta)*	291 ☐	292 ☐	☐	☐	☐
2. TALIPES EQUINOVARUS	293 ☐	294 ☐	☐	☐	☐
3. METATARSUS ADDUCTUS *(varus)*	295 ☐	296 ☐	☐	☐	☐
4. TALIPES CALCANEOVALGUS	297 ☐	298 ☐	☐	☐	☐
5. CONGENITAL DISLOCATION OR DYSPLASIA OF THE HIP	299 ☐	300 ☐	☐	☐	☐
6. ABSENCE OR HYPOPLASIA OF EXTREMITY OR PART, SPECIFY	301 ☐	302 ☐	☐	☐	☐
7. POLYDACTYLY	▨	310 ☐	☐	☐	☐
8. SYNDACTYLY	▨	312 ☐	☐	☐	☐
9. TORTICOLLIS	313 ☐	314 ☐	☐	☐	☐
10. ARTHROGRYPOSIS MULTIPLEX *(amyoplasia congenita)*	315 ☐	316 ☐	☐	☐	☐
11. OTHER NON-INFECTIOUS, SPECIFY	317 ☐	318 ☐	☐	☐	☐

D. EYE CONDITIONS

NONE ☐

	SUSPECT	DEFINITE	(1) PED-11	(2) PRIOR EXAM OR PED-29	(4) HISTORY ONLY
1. CHORIO-RETINITIS	329 ☐	330 ☐	☐	☐	☐
2. RETROLENTAL FIBROPLASIA	331 ☐	332 ☐	☐	☐	☐
3. CATARACT	333 ☐	334 ☐	☐	☐	☐
4. CORNEAL OPACITY	335 ☐	336 ☐	☐	☐	☐
5. MICROPHTHALMIA	337 ☐	338 ☐	☐	☐	☐
6. OTHER NON-INFECTIOUS, SPECIFY	339 ☐	340 ☐	☐	☐	☐

E. EAR CONDITIONS

NONE ☐

	SUSPECT	DEFINITE	(1) PED-11	(2) PRIOR EXAM OR PED-29	(4) HISTORY ONLY
1. LOW SET EARS	349 ☐	350 ☐	☐	☐	☐
2. DEFORMED EAR PINNA	351 ☐	352 ☐	☐	☐	☐
3. BRANCHIAL CLEFT ANOMALY *(pre-auricular sinus, etc.)*	353 ☐	354 ☐	☐	☐	☐
4. PERFORATED EAR DRUM	355 ☐	356 ☐	☐	☐	☐
5. OTHER NON-INFECTIOUS, SPECIFY	357 ☐	358 ☐	☐	☐	☐

COLLABORATIVE RESEARCH
PERINATAL RESEARCH BRANCH, NINDB, NIH
BETHESDA 14, MD.

6-63   PAGE 3 OF 8   **PED-12**

321

1. PATIENT IDENTIFICATION

PED-12

SUMMARY OF THE FIRST YEAR OF LIFE AFTER THE DURATION SUMMARIZED ON THE PED-8

F. UPPER RESPIRATORY TRACT AND MOUTH CONDITIONS

NONE ☐

	SUSPECT	DEFINITE	(1) PED-11	(2) PRIOR EXAM OR PED-29	(4) HISTORY ONLY
1. CLEFT PALATE	▨	368 ☐	☐	☐	☐
2. CLEFT UVULA	▨	370 ☐	☐	☐	☐
3. CLEFT LIP	▨	372 ☐	☐	☐	☐
4. CLEFT GUM	▨	374 ☐	☐	☐	☐
5. MICROGNATHIA	375 ☐	376 ☐	☐	☐	☐
6. MALFORMATION OF THE EPIGLOTTIS AND LARYNX, SPECIFY	377 ☐	378 ☐	☐	☐	☐
- - - - - - - - - - - - - - -					
7. ABNORMALITY OF TEETH, SPECIFY	385 ☐	386 ☐	☐	☐	☐
- - - - - - - - - - - - - - -					
8. OTHER NON-INFECTIOUS, SPECIFY	393 ☐	394 ☐	☐	☐	☐
- - - - - - - - - - - - - - -					

G. THORACIC CONDITIONS (except neoplastic and cardiovascular conditions)

NONE ☐

	SUSPECT	DEFINITE	PED-11	PRIOR EXAM OR PED-29	HISTORY ONLY
1. ANOMALY OF DIAPHRAGM, SPECIFY	405 ☐	406 ☐	☐	☐	☐
- - - - - - - - - - - - - - -					
2. ANOMALY OF RIBS, SPECIFY	413 ☐	414 ☐	☐	☐	☐
- - - - - - - - - - - - - - -					
3. PECTUS EXCAVATUM	417 ☐	418 ☐	☐	☐	☐
4. PIGEON BREAST	419 ☐	420 ☐	☐	☐	☐
5. OTHER, SPECIFY	421 ☐	422 ☐	☐	☐	☐
- - - - - - - - - - - - - - -					

H. LOWER RESPIRATORY TRACT ABNORMALITY

NONE ☐

	SUSPECT	DEFINITE	PED-11	PRIOR EXAM OR PED-29	HISTORY ONLY
1. ASTHMA	431 ☐	432 ☐	☐	☐	☐
2. EMPHYSEMA	433 ☐	434 ☐	☐	☐	☐
3. PNEUMOTHORAX	435 ☐	436 ☐	☐	☐	☐
4. ANOMALY OF LUNG, SPECIFY	437 ☐	438 ☐	☐	☐	☐
- - - - - - - - - - - - - - -					
5. OTHER NON-INFECTIOUS, SPECIFY	445 ☐	446 ☐	☐	☐	☐
- - - - - - - - - - - - - - -					

I. CARDIOVASCULAR CONDITIONS

NONE ☐

	SUSPECT	DEFINITE	(1) PED-11	(2) PRIOR EXAM OR PED-29	(4) HISTORY ONLY
1. ACYANOTIC CHD	457 ☐	458 ☐	☐	☐	☐
2. CYANOTIC CHD	459 ☐	460 ☐	☐	☐	☐
3. FIBROELASTOSIS	461 ☐	462 ☐	☐	☐	☐
4. DISORDERS OF RHYTHM	463 ☐	464 ☐	☐	☐	☐
5. DISORDERS OF RATE	465 ☐	466 ☐	☐	☐	☐
6. CARDIAC ENLARGEMENT	467 ☐	468 ☐			
7. DECOMPENSATION	469 ☐	470 ☐			
8. SEVERE CYANOTIC EPISODES	471 ☐	472 ☐			
9. SPECIFIC C-V DIAGNOSIS (code also under I-1 or I-2)	▨	474 ☐	☐	☐	☐
- - - - - - - - - - - - - - -					
- - - - - - - - - - - - - - -					
10. OTHER (list hemangioma under skin, O.) SPECIFY	483 ☐	484 ☐	☐	☐	☐
- - - - - - - - - - - - - - -					

J. ALIMENTARY TRACT CONDITIONS

NONE ☐

	SUSPECT	DEFINITE	PED-11	PRIOR EXAM OR PED-29	HISTORY ONLY
1. HERNIA (omit uncomplicated umbilical, code diaphragmatic under G-1) SPECIFY	493 ☐	494 ☐	☐	☐	☐
- - - - - - - - - - - - - - -					
2. VOLVULUS	501 ☐	502 ☐	☐	☐	☐
3. INTUSSUSCEPTION	503 ☐	504 ☐	☐	☐	☐
4. PERSISTENT VOMITING	505 ☐	506 ☐	☐	☐	☐
5. MEGACOLON	507 ☐	508 ☐	☐	☐	☐
6. PYLORIC STENOSIS	509 ☐	510 ☐	☐	☐	☐
7. VISCERAL PERFORATION	511 ☐	512 ☐	☐	☐	☐
8. MALROTATION	513 ☐	514 ☐	☐	☐	☐
9. INTESTINAL OBSTRUCTION	515 ☐	516 ☐	☐	☐	☐
10. CHALASIA	517 ☐	518 ☐	☐	☐	☐
11. OTHER NON-INFECTIOUS, SPECIFY	519 ☐	520 ☐	☐	☐	☐
- - - - - - - - - - - - - - -					

COLLABORATIVE RESEARCH
PERINATAL RESEARCH BRANCH, NINDB, NIH
BETHESDA 14, MD.

6-63   PAGE 4 OF 8

PED-12

322

PED-12

SUMMARY OF THE FIRST YEAR OF LIFE AFTER THE DURATION SUMMARIZED ON THE PED-8

K. ABNORMALITY OF LIVER, BILE DUCTS, AND/OR SPLEEN

NONE ☐

	SUSPECT	DEFINITE	PED-11	PRIOR EXAM OR PED-29	HISTORY ONLY
			(1)	(2)	(4)
1. BILIARY ATRESIA............................	531 ☐	532 ☐	☐	☐	☐
2. JAUNDICE					
a. Persistent <u>beyond</u> duration summarized on PED-8.....................	533 ☐	534 ☐	☐	☐	☐
b. Acquired <u>after</u> duration summarized on PED-8.....................	535 ☐	536 ☐	☐	☐	☐
3. OTHER NON-INFECTIOUS, SPECIFY.	537 ☐	538 ☐	☐	☐	☐

- - - - - - - - - - - - - - - - - -

L. GENITOURINARY CONDITIONS
(do not code hydrocele or phimosis)

NONE ☐

1. UNDESCENDED TESTICLE					
a. Unilateral..............................	549 ☐	550 ☐	☐	☐	☐
b. Bilateral..............................	551 ☐	552 ☐	☐	☐	☐
2. HYPOSPADIAS	▨	554 ☐	☐	☐	☐
3. CHORDEE	555 ☐	556 ☐	☐	☐	☐
4. OTHER ABNORMALITY OF THE EXTERNAL GENITALIA *(include pseudohemaphroditism)*, SPECIFY........	557 ☐	558 ☐	☐	☐	☐

- - - - - - - - - - - - - - - - - -

5. BLADDER OUTFLOW OR URETHRAL OBSTRUCTION, SPECIFY	563 ☐	564 ☐	☐	☐	☐

- - - - - - - - - - - - - - - - - -

6. UPPER TRACT OBSTRUCTION, HYDRONEPHROSIS OR HYDRO-URETER *(megalo-ureter)*, SPECIFY.....	569 ☐	570 ☐	☐	☐	☐

- - - - - - - - - - - - - - - - - -

7. CYSTIC KIDNEY.................................	575 ☐	576 ☐	☐	☐	☐
8. OTHER NON-INFECTIOUS, SPECIFY.	577 ☐	578 ☐	☐	☐	☐

- - - - - - - - - - - - - - - - - -

M. NEOPLASTIC DISEASE AND/OR OTHER TUMORS *(code hemangioma and lymphangioma under skin, O.)*

NONE ☐

	SUSPECT	DEFINITE	PED-11	PRIOR EXAM OR PED-29	HISTORY ONLY
			(1)	(2)	(4)
1. SPECIFY TYPE AND ORGAN	589 ☐	590 ☐	☐	☐	☐
a. _ _ _ _ _ _ _ _ _ _ _ _ _ _					
b. _ _ _ _ _ _ _ _ _ _ _ _ _ _					
c. _ _ _ _ _ _ _ _ _ _ _ _ _ _					
d. _ _ _ _ _ _ _ _ _ _ _ _ _ _					

N. HEMATOLOGIC CONDITIONS

NONE ☐

1. HEMOGLOBINOPATHY, SPECIFY TYPE	601 ☐	602 ☐	☐	☐	☐

- - - - - - - - - - - - - - - -

2. HEMOLYTIC DISEASE					
a. Congenital..	609 ☐	610 ☐	☐	☐	☐
b. Acquired..	611 ☐	612 ☐	☐	☐	☐
3. COAGULATION DEFECT, SPECIFY..	613 ☐	614 ☐	☐	☐	☐

- - - - - - - - - - - - - - - -

4. MAJOR HEMORRHAGE, SPECIFY SITE *(code intracranial hemorrhage under B.)*..	619 ☐	620 ☐	☐	☐	☐

- - - - - - - - - - - - - - - -

5. ANEMIA					
a. Less than 5 gm. %					
(1) IRON DEFICIENCY..................	627 ☐	628 ☐	☐	☐	☐
(2) OTHER, SPECIFY..................	629 ☐	630 ☐	☐	☐	☐

- - - - - - - - - - - - -

b. 5 to *(but not including)* 8 gm. %....					
(1) IRON DEFICIENCY..................	635 ☐	636 ☐	☐	☐	☐
(2) OTHER, SPECIFY....................	637 ☐	638 ☐	☐	☐	☐

- - - - - - - - - - - - -

6. OTHER, SPECIFY...............................	645 ☐	646 ☐	☐	☐	☐

- - - - - - - - - - - - - - - -

COLLABORATIVE RESEARCH
PERINATAL RESEARCH BRANCH, NINDB, NIH
BETHESDA 14, MD.

6-63   PAGE 5 OF 8   **PED-12**

323

1. PATIENT IDENTIFICATION

PED-12   SUMMARY OF THE FIRST YEAR OF
LIFE AFTER THE DURATION
SUMMARIZED ON THE PED-8

O. SKIN CONDITIONS AND MALFORMATIONS

NONE ☐

	SUSPECT	DEFINITE		(1) PED-11	(2) PRIOR EXAM OR PED-29	(4) HISTORY ONLY
1. PORTWINE HEMANGIOMA	657 ☐	658 ☐		☐	☐	☐
2. STRAWBERRY HEMANGIOMA	659 ☐	660 ☐		☐	☐	☐
3. CAVERNOUS HEMANGIOMA	661 ☐	662 ☐		☐	☐	☐
4. HAIRY PIGMENTED NEVUS	663 ☐	664 ☐		☐	☐	☐
5. PIGMENTED NEVUS (6 or more that are 0.5 cms., or one larger than 3 cms.)	665 ☐	666 ☐		☐	☐	☐
6. LYMPHANGIOMA	667 ☐	668 ☐		☐	☐	☐
7. CAFÉ AU LAIT SPOTS (6 or more or one larger than 3 cms.)	669 ☐	670 ☐		☐	☐	☐
8. ECZEMA	671 ☐	672 ☐		☐	☐	☐
9. OTHER NON-INFECTIOUS, SPECIFY	673 ☐	674 ☐		☐	☐	☐

- - - - - - - - - - - - - - - -

P. SYNDROMES

NONE ☐

	SUSPECT	DEFINITE		PED-11	PRIOR EXAM OR PED-29	HISTORY ONLY
1. MONGOLISM (Down's syndrome)	685 ☐	686 ☐		☐	☐	☐
2. GONADAL DYSGENESIS	687 ☐	688 ☐		☐	☐	☐
3. ADRENOGENITAL	689 ☐	690 ☐		☐	☐	☐
4. MARFAN'S	691 ☐	692 ☐		☐	☐	☐
5. PIERRE ROBIN	693 ☐	694 ☐		☐	☐	☐
6. SPASMUS NUTANS	695 ☐	696 ☐		☐	☐	☐
7. HURLER'S (Gargoylism)	697 ☐	698 ☐		☐	☐	☐
8. FAILURE TO THRIVE	699 ☐	700 ☐		☐	☐	☐
9. OTHER, SPECIFY	701 ☐	702 ☐		☐	☐	☐

- - - - - - - - - - - - - - - -

Q. OTHER ENDOCRINE AND METABOLIC DISEASE

NONE ☐

	SUSPECT	DEFINITE		PED-11	PRIOR EXAM OR PED-29	HISTORY ONLY
1. HYPOTHYROIDISM, SPECIFY	713 ☐	714 ☐		☐	☐	☐

- - - - - - - - - - - - - - -

	SUSPECT	DEFINITE				
2. FIBROCYSTIC DISEASE OF PANCREAS	719 ☐	720 ☐		☐	☐	☐
3. INBORN ERRORS OF METABOLISM, SPECIFY	721 ☐	722 ☐		☐	☐	☐

- - - - - - - - - - - - - - - -

4. OTHER, SPECIFY	729 ☐	730 ☐		☐	☐	☐

- - - - - - - - - - - - - - - -

R. INFECTION AND INFLAMMATION (specify condition and agent)

NONE ☐

	SUSPECT	DEFINITE		(1) PED-11	(2) PRIOR EXAM OR PED-29	(4) HISTORY ONLY
1. SEPTICEMIA	739 ☐	740 ☐		☐	☐	☐
Agent _ _ _ _ _ _ _ _ _ _ _						
2. CENTRAL NERVOUS SYSTEM	741 ☐	742 ☐		☐	☐	☐
a. Bacterial meningitis	743 ☐	744 ☐		☐	☐	☐
Agent _ _ _ _ _ _ _ _ _ _						
b. Non-bacterial meningitis	745 ☐	746 ☐		☐	☐	☐
Agent _ _ _ _ _ _ _ _ _ _						
c. Encephalitis	747 ☐	748 ☐		☐	☐	☐
Agent _ _ _ _ _ _ _ _ _ _						
d. Other CNS, specify	749 ☐	750 ☐		☐	☐	☐
- - - - - - - - - - - - -						
Agent _ _ _ _ _ _ _ _ _						

3. RESPIRATORY (include upper and lower, mouth, retropharyngeal abscess and herpetic stomatitis; exclude, in general, common cold, pharyngitis, tonsillitis)

	SUSPECT	DEFINITE				
a. Pneumonia	761 ☐	762 ☐		☐	☐	☐
Agent _ _ _ _ _ _ _ _ _ _						
b. Severe croup	763 ☐	764 ☐		☐	☐	☐
Agent _ _ _ _ _ _ _ _ _ _						
c. Bronchiolitis	765 ☐	766 ☐		☐	☐	☐
Agent _ _ _ _ _ _ _ _ _ _						
d. Other respiratory, specify	767 ☐	768 ☐		☐	☐	☐
- - - - - - - - - - - - -						
Agent _ _ _ _ _ _ _ _ _ _						
4. GENITOURINARY TRACT	779 ☐	780 ☐		☐	☐	☐
a. _ _ _ _ _ _ _ _ _ _ _ _ _						
Agent _ _ _ _ _ _ _ _ _ _						
5. BONE AND JOINT	781 ☐	782 ☐		☐	☐	☐
a. _ _ _ _ _ _ _ _ _ _ _ _						
Agent _ _ _ _ _ _ _ _ _ _						
6. HEART	783 ☐	784 ☐		☐	☐	☐
a. _ _ _ _ _ _ _ _ _ _ _ _						
Agent _ _ _ _ _ _ _ _ _ _						

COLLABORATIVE RESEARCH
PERINATAL RESEARCH BRANCH, NINDB, NIH
BETHESDA 14, MD.

6-63   PAGE 6 OF 8   **PED-12**

324

PED-12 **SUMMARY OF THE FIRST YEAR OF LIFE AFTER THE DURATION SUMMARIZED ON THE PED-8**

R. INFECTION AND INFLAMMATION
(Continued)

	SUSPECT	DEFINITE	(1) PED-11	(2) PRIOR EXAM OR PED-29	(4) HISTORY ONLY
7. GASTROINTESTINAL					
a. Diarrhea requiring hospitalization....	785 ☐	786 ☐	☐	☐	☐
Agent_ _ _ _ _ _ _ _ _ _ _ _ _					
b. Other GI, specify	787 ☐	788 ☐	☐	☐	☐
_ _ _ _ _ _ _ _ _ _ _ _ _					
Agent_ _ _ _ _ _ _ _ _ _ _					
8. LIVER................................	799 ☐	800 ☐	☐	☐	☐
a._ _ _ _ _ _ _ _ _ _ _ _ _					
Agent_ _ _ _ _ _ _ _ _ _ _					
9. EYE *(exclude uncomplicated simple conjunctivitis)*............................	801 ☐	802 ☐	☐	☐	☐
a._ _ _ _ _ _ _ _ _ _ _ _ _					
Agent_ _ _ _ _ _ _ _ _ _ _					
10. EAR *(exclude external otitis and uncomplicated non-draining otitis media)*	803 ☐	804 ☐	☐	☐	☐
a._ _ _ _ _ _ _ _ _ _ _ _ _					
Agent_ _ _ _ _ _ _ _ _ _ _					
11. SKIN *(exclude impetigo, furunculosis, ecthyma, and diaper rashes)*..........	805 ☐	806 ☐	☐	☐	☐
a._ _ _ _ _ _ _ _ _ _ _ _ _					
Agent_ _ _ _ _ _ _ _ _ _ _					
12. SPECIFIC CHILDHOOD DISEASES					
a. Roseola	807 ☐	808 ☐	☐	☐	☐
b. German measles	809 ☐	810 ☐	☐	☐	☐
c. Measles	811 ☐	812 ☐	☐	☐	☐
d. Mumps	813 ☐	814 ☐	☐	☐	☐
e. Chickenpox	815 ☐	816 ☐	☐	☐	☐
f. Whooping cough...................	817 ☐	818 ☐	☐	☐	☐
g. Other, specify.....................	819 ☐	820 ☐	☐	☐	☐
_ _ _ _ _ _ _ _ _ _ _ _					
13. UNUSUALLY RECURRENT OR CHRONIC INFECTIONS, SPECIFY......	831 ☐	832 ☐	☐	☐	☐
_ _ _ _ _ _ _ _ _ _ _ _					
14. OTHER, SPECIFY	837 ☐	838 ☐	☐	☐	☐
a._ _ _ _ _ _ _ _ _ _ _ _					
Agent_ _ _ _ _ _ _ _ _ _ _					

S. TRAUMA, PHYSICAL AGENTS, AND INTOXICATION

NONE ☐

	SUSPECT	DEFINITE	(1) PED-11	(2) PRIOR EXAM OR PED-29	(4) HISTORY ONLY
1. HEAD TRAUMA					
a. Unconsciousness	849 ☐	850 ☐	☐	☐	☐
b. Fractured skull...................	851 ☐	852 ☐	☐	☐	☐
c. Bloody spinal fluid	853 ☐	854 ☐	☐	☐	☐
d. Vomiting x3.......................	855 ☐	856 ☐	☐	☐	☐
e. Subgaleal hematoma...........	857 ☐	858 ☐	☐	☐	☐
2. FRACTURES, OTHER, SPECIFY....	859 ☐	860 ☐	☐	☐	☐
_ _ _ _ _ _ _ _ _ _ _ _					
3. BURNS LEADING TO HOSPITALIZATION *(including lye and specify the location and agent)*........	871 ☐	872 ☐	☐	☐	☐
a._ _ _ _ _ _ _ _ _ _ _ _					
Agent_ _ _ _ _ _ _ _ _ _					
4. SYMPTOMATIC INTOXICATION					
a. Salicylate	883 ☐	884 ☐	☐	☐	☐
b. Hydrocarbon					
(1) KEROSENE......................	885 ☐	886 ☐	☐	☐	☐
(2) OTHER HYDROCARBON, SPECIFY..................	887 ☐	888 ☐	☐	☐	☐
_ _ _ _ _ _ _ _ _ _ _ _					
c. Lead.................................	893 ☐	894 ☐	☐	☐	☐
d. Other, specify....................	895 ☐	896 ☐	☐	☐	☐
_ _ _ _ _ _ _ _ _ _ _ _					

T. DISTURBANCES IN HOMEOSTASIS

NONE ☐

	SUSPECT	DEFINITE	(1) PED-11	(2) PRIOR EXAM OR PED-29	(4) HISTORY ONLY
1. SHOCK REQUIRING HOSPITALIZATION	901 ☐	902 ☐	☐	☐	☐
2. DEHYDRATION REQUIRING PARENTERAL FLUID THERAPY....	903 ☐	904 ☐	☐	☐	☐
3. ELECTROLYTE IMBALANCE, SPECIFY	905 ☐	906 ☐	☐	☐	☐
a._ _ _ _ _ _ _ _ _ _ _ _					
b._ _ _ _ _ _ _ _ _ _ _ _					
4. HYPERTHERMIA (106°F or over)....	911 ☐	912 ☐	☐	☐	☐
5. HYPOTHERMIA (below 94°F)..........	913 ☐	914 ☐	☐	☐	☐

COLLABORATIVE RESEARCH
PERINATAL RESEARCH BRANCH, NINDB, NIH
BETHESDA 14, MD.

6-63   PAGE 7 OF 8   **PED-12**

325

1. PATIENT IDENTIFICATION

PED-12   SUMMARY OF THE FIRST YEAR OF
LIFE AFTER THE DURATION
SUMMARIZED ON THE PED-8

T. DISTURBANCES IN HOMEOSTASIS (Continued)

	SUSPECT	DEFINITE	(1) PED-11	(2) PRIOR EXAM OR PED-29	(4) HISTORY ONLY
6. EPISODE OF "HYPOXIA"					
a. With unconsciousness	915 ☐	916 ☐	☐	☐	☐
Specify cause					
— — — — — — — — — —					
b. Without unconsciousness	917 ☐	918 ☐	☐	☐	☐
Specify cause					
— — — — — — — — — —					
7. OTHER, SPECIFY	919 ☐	920 ☐	☐	☐	☐
— — — — — — — — — —					

U. OTHER CONDITIONS

	SUSPECT	DEFINITE	(1)	(2)	(4)
U. OTHER CONDITIONS	929 ☐	930 ☐	☐	☐	☐

NONE ☐

Specify

1. _ _ _ _ _ _ _ _ _ _ _ _ _ _ _

2. _ _ _ _ _ _ _ _ _ _ _ _ _ _ _

3. _ _ _ _ _ _ _ _ _ _ _ _ _ _ _

4. _ _ _ _ _ _ _ _ _ _ _ _ _ _ _

V. PROCEDURES

NONE ☐

	SUSPECT	DEFINITE	(1)	(2)	(4)
1. BLOOD TRANSFUSIONS	941 ☐	942 ☐	☐	☐	☐
2. PARENTERAL FLUID	943 ☐	944 ☐	☐	☐	☐
3. SPINAL PUNCTURE	945 ☐	946 ☐	☐	☐	☐
4. SUBDURAL PUNCTURE	947 ☐	948 ☐	☐	☐	☐
5. VENTRICULAR PUNCTURE	949 ☐	950 ☐	☐	☐	☐
6. GENERAL ANESTHESIA	951 ☐	952 ☐	☐	☐	☐
7. SURGERY (exclude minor office surgery, specify)	953 ☐	954 ☐	☐	☐	☐
— — — — — — — — — —					
8. CHROMOSOME STUDIES	965 ☐	966 ☐	☐	☐	☐
9. E.E.G.	967 ☐	968 ☐	☐	☐	☐
10. OTHER, SPECIFY	969 ☐	970 ☐	☐	☐	☐
— — — — — — — — — —					
— — — — — — — — — —					

W. SOCIAL AND ENVIRONMENTAL CONDITIONS

NONE ☐

INFORMATION INADEQUATE ☐

	SUSPECT	DEFINITE	(1) PED-11	(2) PRIOR EXAM OR PED-29	(4) HISTORY ONLY
1. LOSS OF ONE OR BOTH PARENTS OR PARENT SURROGATE	981 ☐	982 ☐	☐	☐	☐
2. FOSTER HOME	983 ☐	984 ☐	☐	☐	☐
3. UNFAVORABLE EMOTIONAL ENVIRONMENT	985 ☐	986 ☐	☐	☐	☐
4. PROLONGED OR RECURRENT HOSPITALIZATION (totalling approximately 30 days)	987 ☐	988 ☐	☐	☐	☐
5. OTHER, SPECIFY	989 ☐	990 ☐	☐	☐	☐
— — — — — — — — — —					

FOR LOCAL USE ONLY

COLLABORATIVE RESEARCH
PERINATAL RESEARCH BRANCH, NINDB, NIH
BETHESDA 14, MD.

6-63   PAGE 8 OF 8

PED-12

326

GLOSSARY

ABORTION—A pregnancy terminating at less than twenty-weeks gestation. (Length of gestation is rounded to nearest week.)

AGE OF GRAVIDA—Years completed at last birthday at time of registration in the study.

BIRTHWEIGHT—As reported at delivery, converted from pounds and ounces to grams where necessary. For cases where delivery did not occur at the collaborating hospital, the information was obtained if possible.

CORE CASE—Case included in study because it fell in the hospital's normal sampling procedure. (A noncore case is one that is included in the study because of a special interest of the hospital.)

FIRST STUDY PREGNANCY—The first pregnancy registered in the study for a gravida. A subsequent pregnancy registered in the study for the same gravida is called a repeat pregnancy. It should be noted that the first study pregnancy was not necessarily the gravida's first pregnancy—it may have been her sixth child, but it was the first pregnancy registered in the study.

GESTATION—Gestation was calculated in days between the first day of the gravida's last menstrual period (LMP) and the date of the event (registration, delivery, etc.). Conversion to weeks was performed by dividing by seven and rounding to the nearest week.

LIVEBIRTH—A product of a conception of twenty or more weeks gestation, which at the time of complete delivery shows any sign of life (i.e., respiratory activity, heartbeat, pulsation of cord, or definite movement of voluntary muscles).

LOST-TO-STUDY CASES—Cases for which neither labor and delivery nor pediatric data were available. Includes women who refused to participate after registering, who moved and could not be located. etc.

NCPP—NINCDS Collaborative Perinatal Project.

NEONATAL DEATH—A death after birth and before 28 days.

NEONATAL PERIOD—The period from birth to 28 days.

NEUROLOGICALLY ABNORMAL AT ONE YEAR—This category in this report consists of definite abnormals only; suspects are excluded. It includes those children for whom the examiner is able to make a diagnosis of a recognized syndrome; those who he feels are definitely neurologically abnormal, but who do not fit into any specific diagnostic category; and those with conditions that may not be themselves neurological, but that are often related to central nervous system disorders (such as abnormalities of the skull, spinal anomalies, and unusual facies).

NURSERY PERIOD—The period after birth spent in the hospital nursery (usually 3–5 days).

PERINATAL DEATHS—Stillbirths plus neonatal deaths.

PLUS (+)—The plus sign on a variable line means "and over."

RACE—The race of the mother, as she reported it.

RATE—All rates are per 1000. Perinatal death rates and stillbirth rates are per 1000 births (exclusive of those terminating at less than twenty-weeks gestation).

STILLBIRTH—The product of a conception of gestation of twenty or more weeks (rounded to nearest week), which, at the time of complete delivery, shows no sign of life (i.e., respiratory activity, heartbeat, pulsation of cord, or definite movement of voluntary muscles).

SYSTEM—As used in tables, refers to cardiovascular, pulmonary, blood, etc., as shown on PED–8 (see Appendix).

INDEX

THE JOHNS HOPKINS UNIVERSITY PRESS

This book was composed in Linotype Times Roman text and foundry Times Roman display type by the Maryland Linotype Composition Co., Inc. It was printed on 70-lb. Paloma Matte paper and bound in Holliston Roxite vellum cloth by Universal Lithographers, Inc.

LIBRARY OF CONGRESS CATALOGING IN PUBLICATION DATA

Hardy, Janet B
  The first year of life.

  Includes bibliographical references and index.
  1. Infants (Newborn)—United States—Longitudinal studies. 2. Infants (Newborn)—
Diseases—United States—Longitudinal studies. 3. Infants—Diseases—United States—
Longitudinal studies. 4. Pediatric neurology. 5. Collaborative Perinatal Project. I. Drage,
Joseph S., joint author. II. Jackson, Esther C., joint author. III. National Institute of
Neurological and Communicative Disorders and Stroke. IV. Title.
[DNLM: 1. Nervous system diseases—Etiology. 2. Nervous system diseases—In infancy
and childhood. WS340.3 H269f]

RJ60.U5H37   618.9′28′0471   78-20528
ISBN 0-8018-2167-3